Dictionary of Cardiac Pacing, Defibrillation, Resynchronization, and Arrhythmias

Dictionary
of Cardiac Pacing, Defibrillation, Resynchronization, and Arrhythmias

DAVID L. **HAYES** MD • SAMUEL J. **ASIRVATHAM** MD

Second Edition

David L. Hayes, MD
Chair, Division of Cardiovascular Diseases, Mayo Clinic; Professor
of Medicine, Mayo Medical School, College of Medicine; Rochester,
Minnesota

Samuel J. Asirvatham, MD
Consultant, Division of Cardiovascular Diseases, Mayo Clinic; Associate
Professor of Medicine, Mayo Medical School, College of Medicine;
Rochester, Minnesota

cardio**text**
MINNEAPOLIS, MINNESOTA

Cover art by Mike Hoium, Slow Dog Studios
Cover and book design by Ann Delgehausen, Trio Bookworks

Library of Congress Control Number: 2007922162
ISBN-13: 978-0-9790164-0-0

Printed in the United States of America

10   09   08   07   1   2   3   4   5

To Wilma Maue-Dickson, whose wisdom and creativity spawned many lasting educational venues and tools in implantable cardiac device therapy—such as this dictionary—DLH

To Dr. Molly Thomas Sen Bhanu, who could see behind the obvious flaws—SJA

Preface

Given the aging population, continued rapid technologic advantages, and expanding indications for implantable cardiac devices, there is a constant and growing need for education about implantable devices. Because of the belief that there was a need for a source of definitions of terms related to pacemakers, implantable cardioverter-defibrillators, and arrhythmia management, a *Dictionary of Cardiac Pacing, Electrophysiology, and Arrhythmias* was published in 1993. This was an expanded version of a text published in 1986. It was written with a great deal of assistance from Marshall S. Stanton, MD, the incredible dedication and determination of Wilma Maue-Dickson, PhD, and the layout, publishing, and graphic skills and general assistance of David R. Dickson, PhD. Dr. Wilma Maue-Dickson should be credited as one of the true pioneers of education in the field of pacemakers and implantable cardioverter-defibrillators and one of the first to recognize the need for education targeted directly at allied professionals dedicated to the field. Drs. Dickson and Dickson recognized the success of the initial dictionary and, although they are no longer active in the field, agreed to allow me to proceed with a new dictionary, using the initial text and figures that were still applicable to the science.

Since the publication of the original dictionary, the field has advanced significantly. Implantable cardioverter-defibrillators and pacemakers are more sophisticated, and cardiac resynchronization was not part of our therapeutic armamentarium in 1993. This dictionary is intended to update the language of cardiac pacing, electrophysiology, and arrhythmias. Many new terms have been added, previous definitions were revised when necessary, and illustrations and tables were added to lend depth to certain concepts and definitions. The definitions are extensively cross-referenced to make it easier to find terms that have one or more synonyms and to assist readers in finding related terms and concepts. In addition, because the language is at times technical and abbreviations are used extensively, we have appended a list of accepted and commonly used abbreviations and their meanings.

A great deal of effort was made to include all relevant terms, but undoubtedly some terms were inadvertently excluded. The way in which we use the language of cardiac pacing, electrophysiology, and arrhythmia management will determine its evolution and the final, accepted definitions of its terminology.

With rare exception, we have used generic terms that can be applied to implantable cardiac rhythm devices from various manufacturers. However, there are selected trademarked terms that are important in current vocabulary, and we have selectively included such terms and credited them to the manufacturer as appropriate.

The terms for clinical trials are not all-inclusive. Of the large number of planned, ongoing, and completed clinical trials in the field, some are completed and some are not; some will make important contributions to the way we practice and some will not; and some will be recognized as manufacturer-, device-, or algorithm-specific and some will not. Our goal was to select trials, planned, ongoing, or completed, that we believed did or would potentially have an impact on the way we practice. Whenever possible, a reference is included to the description of the clinical trial.

In addition to the coauthors and contributors of the 1993 edition of *Dictionary of Cardiac Pacing, Electrophysiology, and Arrhythmias*, this text would not be possible without the hard work and dedication of my coauthor Samuel J. Asirvatham, MD; the staff of the Mayo Clinic Section of Scientific Publications, especially Jean Plote (editorial assistant), Alissa Baumgartner (proofreader), Roberta Schwartz (production editor), and LeAnn Stee (editor); the staff of Mayo Clinic Media Support Services, in particular Jim Tidwell (medical illustrator); and Mike Crouchet, Julie Sink, and the rest of the team at Cardiotext. We hope that our efforts and this text will assist persons involved in arrhythmia management as we witness the continued expansion of this discipline and the improved quality of life afforded to many patients as a result.

David L. Hayes, MD

Contents

*The symbol • indicates that a corresponding
figure or table is on an adjacent page.*

a

A. Abbreviation for *ampere*.

A (atrial). *A* is used in most pacemaker marker channels to represent a paced atrial event. See the figure *NBG code*.

A₁. In electrophysiology, the atrial response to S_1, the drive stimulus. See also *drive cycle, S_1*.

A₂. In electrophysiology, the atrial response to S_2, the first extrastimulus. See also *extrastimulus, S_2*.

A2-A3. In an assessment of sinoatrial conduction, the measured distance from an induced atrial premature depolarization (A2) to the next sinus beat (A3); represents the first return cycle.

A3-A4. In an assessment of sinoatrial conduction, the measured distance from the end of the first return cycle after an induced atrial premature depolarization (A3) to the next sinus beat (A4); represents the second return cycle.

AAD. Abbreviation for *antiarrhythmic drug*.

AAI. The NBG code for atrial-inhibited pacing. Pacing and sensing occur in the atrium, and the mode of response to sensed events is inhibited. Portions of the AAI timing cycle that must be considered include the lower rate (LR) and the

"paced" event but may at times be used for an intrinsic atrial event.

AAIR. The NBG code for atrial-inhibited rate-adaptive pacing. Pacing and sensing occur in the atrium, and the mode of response to sensed events is inhibited. The pacemaker also is capable of rate-adaptive pacing, *R*, via a sensor that monitors some physiologic or nonphysiologic parameter and adjusts the heart rate accordingly. See also *atrial-inhibited rate-adaptive pacing mode*.

AAT. The NBG code for atrial-triggered pacing. Pacing and sensing occur in the atrium, and the mode of response to sensed events is triggered. The atrial output pulse is synchronized with sensed atrial activity and, in the presence of intrinsic activity, does not contribute to atrial depolarization. See also *atrial output pulse, atrial-triggered pacing mode*.

A-A timing. A timing scheme used in pacemakers which bases all timing on atrial events, in contrast to ventricular-based timing or timing systems that incorporate a hybrid of atrial and ventricular timing.

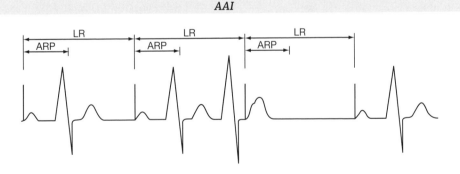

AAI

ARP, atrial refractory period; LR, lower rate.

atrial refractory period (ARP). AAI pacing also is called atrial demand pacing. See also *atrial-inhibited pacing mode*.

AA interval. The measured distance from atrial event to atrial event. *A* generally denotes a

AATR. The NBG code for atrial-triggered rate-adaptive pacing. Pacing and sensing occur in the atrium, and the mode of response to sensed events is triggered. The pacemaker also is capable of rate-adaptive pacing via a sensor that monitors some physiologic or nonphysiologic variable and adjusts the heart rate accordingly. See also *atrial-triggered rate-adaptive pacing mode*.

ABCD. See *Alternans Before Cardioverter Defibrillator*.

aberrancy. Abnormal intraventricular conduction that arises from any of several different mechanisms, such as the Ashman phenomenon, drug toxicity, electrolyte abnormalities, and acceleration-dependent or deceleration-dependent bundle branch block. Fixed bundle branch block is not considered aberrancy. See also *acceleration-dependent aberration, Ashman phenomenon, bundle branch block, deceleration-dependent aberration*.

aberration. See *aberrancy*.

ablate and pace. Terminology for atrioventricular nodal ablation and permanent pacing. Practices vary between placing the pacemaker before the ablation and placing a temporary pacemaker before the ablation and then placing the permanent pacemaker after the ablation.

ablation. The removal or destruction of tissue. Ablation can be used to eliminate the site of origin of tachycardia or to interrupt the circuit through which the arrhythmia travels. Ablation commonly is used to interrupt accessory pathways such as those found in the Wolff-Parkinson-White syndrome. Ablation techniques include cauterization, cryosurgery, diathermy, direct-current ablation, fulguration, laser ablation, microwave ablation, radiofrequency ablation, and surgical ablation.

abnormal automaticity. The formation of a tachycardia by the emergence of an ectopic rhythm at a rate faster than the normal sinus rate. The underlying mechanism is spontaneous phase 4 depolarization rather than reentry or triggered activity. Tachycardias generated by abnormal automaticity are difficult to identify by electrophysiologic testing because programmed electrical stimuli do not consistently initiate or terminate this form of tachycardia. Abnormal automaticity also is known as enhanced automaticity. See also *reentry*.

aborted shock. An instance in an implantable cardioverter-defibrillator during which the device initiates an energy charge but does not deliver a shock, often due to spontaneous termination of the tachyarrhythmia.

absolute refractory period (ARP). Physiologically, the period of time after cellular activation during which a response cannot be initiated regardless of the strength of the stimulus. The absolute refractory period typically lasts from the onset of an action potential until repolarization is approximately one-third complete. See also *relative refractory period*.

AC. Abbreviation for *alternating current*.

ACC/AHA/NASPE Guideline for Implantation of Cardiac Pacemakers and Antiarrhythmia Devices. A document endorsed by the major cardiology and heart rhythm societies which provides guidelines for when a pacemaker, implantable cardioverter-defibrillator, and cardiac resynchronization therapy are indicated. The document is updated periodically. The most recently published document is the following: Gregoratos G, Abrams J, Epstein AE, Freedman RA, Hayes DL, Hlatky MA, et al, ACC/AHA/NASPE 2002 Guideline Update for Implantation of Cardiac Pacemakers and Antiarrhythmia Devices: summary article: a report of the American College of Cardiology/American Heart Association Task Force on Practice Guidelines (ACC/AHA/NASPE Committee to Update the 1998 Pacemaker Guidelines). Circulation. 2002;106:2145-61 and Gregoratos G, Abrams J, Epstein AE, Freedman RA, Hayes DL, Hlatky MA, et al. ACC/AHA/NASPE 2002 Guideline Update for Implantation of Cardiac Pacemakers and Antiarrhythmia Devices: summary article: a report of the American College of Cardiology/American Heart Association Task Force on Practice Guidelines (ACC/AHA/NASPE Committee to Update the 1998 Pacemaker Guidelines). J Am Coll Cardiol. 2002;40:1703-19.

accelerated idioventricular rhythm. An abnormal rhythm that arises from a ventricular focus with a rate similar to and competing with the sinoatrial node. Accelerated idioventricular rhythms are thought to be largely due to abnormal automaticity, with some instances of triggered activity. The rhythm has gradual onset and termination and typically has faster than normal ventricular escape rates (30-40 beats per minute) but is slower than ventricular tachycardia. It is generally thought to be benign, because runs are usually hemodynamically well tolerated and brief.

accelerated junctional rhythm. See *nonparoxysmal junctional tachycardia*.

acceleration. A sudden and sustained increase in the rate of a cardiac rhythm and, thus, a decrease in the cardiac interval. Antitachycardia pacing used to terminate an arrhythmia may instead cause acceleration. For example, degeneration of ventricular tachycardia into ventricular fibrillation is acceleration.

acceleration-dependent aberration. Abnormal intraventricular conduction that occurs with gradual increases in heart rate, not necessarily associated with the occurrence of a premature impulse. This type of aberration is pathophysiologic and usually has a left bundle branch block configuration.

acceleration-dependent bundle branch block. Infrahisian conduction block in either the right or the left bundle branch that occurs with an increased supraventricular rate (sinus tachycardia, supraventricular tachycardia).

acceleration time. A programmable variable in rate-adaptive pacing which determines how quickly the pacing rate of an activity-sensing device will increase once an increase in the activity level is detected. See also *reaction time*.

accelerometer. A device used to measure acceleration. In some pacing systems, accelerometers have been incorporated as sensors that detect anterior-posterior motion of the patient for rate-adaptive pacing. See also *activity sensor*.

access code. In pacing, an encoded signal that allows access to the pulse generator for communication. Access is permitted only if the key entered by the person programming the device corresponds to a given identification code.

accessory pathway. An aberrant conduction pathway in which an electrical signal bypasses part or all of the normal cardiac conduction system. Conduction through accessory pathways can cause preexcitation of the ventricles. An accessory pathway, such as a Kent fiber, may provide antegrade or retrograde conduction of impulses. These accessory pathways frequently provide the anatomical basis for reentrant arrhythmias. See also *concealed bypass tract, Kent fiber, Mahaim fiber, Wolff-Parkinson-White syndrome*.

accessory pathway antegrade effective refractory period. During atrial pacing, the longest A_1 to A_2 interval at which A_2 does not conduct to the ventricle over the accessory pathway. The A_1 to A_2 interval is measured from a site as close to the accessory pathway as possible. See also *effective refractory period*.

accordion pacing. See *concertina pacing*.

Accufix/Encor leads. See *Accufix J lead*.

Accufix J lead. A specific preformed atrial J lead (Telectronics, Inc., Englewood, Colorado). The lead incorporated a "retention wire" to maintain the J shape. In some patients, the retention wire fractured, an event leading to cardiac perforation or tamponade. Another atrial lead manufactured by Telectronics, Inc., the Encor, had similar problems.

Accufix retention wires. See *Accufix J lead*.

acebutolol. A β_1-selective, β-adrenergic blocking agent with intrinsic sympathomimetic activity. Acebutolol may increase pacing and sensing thresholds. Because of its β_1-selectivity, acebutolol may tend to cause less bronchospasm than some other β-adrenergic blocking agents. Because of its intrinsic sympathomimetic activity, acebutolol may tend to cause less fatigue and bradycardia than some other β-adrenergic blocking agents. Acebutolol is metabolized by the liver but has an active metabolite that is excreted by the kidneys. For side effects, see *β-adrenergic blocking drugs*.

ACE inhibitor. Abbreviation for *angiotensin-converting enzyme inhibitor*.

acetylcholine. A neurotransmitter that stimulates muscarinic receptors and causes postganglionic efferent parasympathetic nerve transmission. Acetylcholine also is a preganglionic neurotransmitter that stimulates nicotinic receptors in both the sympathetic and the parasympathetic nervous systems.

acetylcysteine. A mucolytic agent that can be given prophylactically, in addition to hydration, to prevent the reduction in renal function sometimes induced by contrast agents in patients with heart failure. Generic name for Mucomyst.

***N*-acetylprocainamide (NAPA).** The major active metabolite of procainamide. *N*-Acetylprocainamide has class III activity and is being investigated as an antiarrhythmic drug. It prolongs refractoriness in atrial, ventricular, and accessory pathway tissue. It has efficacy in the treatment of supraventricular and ventricular arrhythmias. Unlike procainamide, NAPA does not seem to cause a lupus syndrome. The plasma half-life of NAPA is 8 hours. It is excreted by the kidneys. Side effects include gastrointestinal and central nervous system effects and proarrhythmia.

acetylstrophanthidin. A cardiac glycoside used experimentally to block the sodium-potassium pump.

acidosis. A pathologic condition caused by the accumulation of acid or loss of base in the body. Acidosis is characterized by increased hydrogen ion concentration in body tissues (decreased pH). Acidosis may alter pacing thresholds. See also *pH sensing*.

aconitine. A toxin that blocks the inward fast sodium current across cell membranes. Aconitine is used experimentally in vitro and in vivo to induce sustained arrhythmias.

acquired AV block. Atrioventricular block that is not congenital. Causes of acquired atrioventricular block are shown in the table below.

action potential is characterized by rapid depolarization followed by repolarization. During depolarization, a reversal of polarity causes the inside of the cell to become positive with respect to the extracellular fluid. During repolarization, the cell returns to its resting potential. Action potentials occur in response to intrinsic or extrinsic stimulation.

action potential duration (APD). The amount of time required for one complete action potential to occur. Action potential duration is measured from the onset of phase 0 to the return to resting membrane potential. Action potential

Acquired Atrioventricular Block: Causes

Idiopathic (senescent) block	**Collagen-vascular**	**Neuromuscular**
Coronary artery disease	·Ankylosing spondylitis	·Limb-girdle dystrophy
Calcific valvular disease	·Dermatomyositis	·Myotonic muscular
Postoperative or traumatic	·Marfan's syndrome	dystrophy
	·Polyarteritis nodosa	·Peroneal muscular atrophy,
Atrioventricular node	·Rheumatoid arthritis	Charcot-Marie-Tooth
ablation	·Scleroderma	disease
Therapeutic radiation to chest	·Systemic lupus	·Progressive external
Infectious	erythematosus	ophthalmoplegia, Kearns-
·Chagas' disease	**Infiltrative**	Sayre syndrome
·Diphtheria	·Amyloidosis	·Scapuloperoneal syndrome
·Infective endocarditis	·Hemochromatosis	**Drug effect**
·Lyme disease*	·Malignant disease	·Amiodarone
·Syphilis	(lymphomatous	·β-Blockers
·Toxoplasmosis	or solid tumor)	·Calcium blocking agents
·Tuberculosis	·Sarcoidosis	·Class IC agents:
·Viral myocarditis (e.g.,		propafenone, encainide,
Epstein-Barr, varicella)		flecainide
		·Digoxin
		·Procainamide

* Should not require permanent pacing; temporary pacing only until infection is treated.

acquired long QT syndrome. Prolongation of the QT interval which is not congenital and associated with subsequent susceptibility to ventricular arrhythmias, especially torsades de pointes. Acquired long QT syndrome most frequently is due to antiarrhythmic drugs that prolong repolarization. See also *congenital long QT syndrome, torsades de pointes*.

actin. One of several genes identified as responsible for familial dilated cardiomyopathy.

action potential. A sudden transient change in the electrical potential (voltage) across the cell membrane of muscle or nerve cell tissue. An

duration often is measured as a percentage of full recovery; for example, APD_{90} is equal to the action potential duration measured to 90% recovery of repolarization. In antiarrhythmic therapy, increasing the action potential duration, and thus refractoriness, may control arrhythmias. However, in some disease states, a long action potential may cause prolonged repolarizations and lead to arrhythmias.

activated state. One of the three states of an ion channel. According to the modulated receptor hypothesis, ion channels can exist in three states: activated (A), inactivated (I), resting (R).

In the activated state, a channel in the cell membrane is open and may conduct ions. See also *inactivated state, ion channel, modulated receptor hypothesis, resting state*.

activation front. The leading edge of depolarization propagating through tissue. See also *depolarization*.

activation mapping. A catheter mapping technique used to pinpoint the focus and circuit of a tachycardia and thus guide therapeutic intervention, such as ablation. Activation mapping uses a roving catheter in the atrium or ventricle to identify locations of the earliest signal or a progression of activation for an arrhythmia.

activation recording. Similar to activation mapping, but it also may be done for a nonmapping issue, such as a trigger for a therapy.

activation sequence. The order in which various cardiac structures are depolarized by an impulse. For example, sinus rhythm occurs in a high-to-low atrial activation sequence; that is, impulses normally spread downward from the sinus node, through the atrial myocardium, to the atrioventricular node. Similarly, impulses normally spread downward from the atrioventricular node, through the His bundle, the bundle branches, and the Purkinje fibers to the ventricular myocardium.

activation time. The amount of time required for an impulse to travel from one point to another. Activation time cannot necessarily be translated into conduction velocity because the pathway of activation is unknown and may not be linear.

active electrode. The part of a pacing lead that delivers energy to the heart from the pulse generator; usually the tip electrode of a transvenous pacing lead.

active fixation. Embedment of the distal tip of an endocardial or epicardial pacing lead directly into the myocardium by means of a special fixation device designed to ensure stable electrode placement. See also *active fixation lead*.

active fixation lead. A pacing lead with a screw, barb, prong(s), hook(s), or some other mechanical device affixed at the lead tip. During lead positioning, the device is embedded into the myocardium to ensure stable electrode placement. Active fixation leads may be particularly useful in clinical situations that necessitate atypical lead placement. See also *endocardial screw-in lead, epicardial screw-in lead*.

activities of daily living (ADL) rate. Heart rate target that a patient is expected to reach during moderate exercise, that is, with activities that would occur during the course of a normal day.

activity sensing, accelerometers in. See *accelerometer*.

activity sensing, gravitational. A device configuration in which a moving magnetic ball is surrounded by a wire coil in the pacemaker housing. Movement of the ball gives rise to an electrical signal that is interpreted into a pacing rate. Several variations of gravitational sensors have been studied as part of rate-adaptive pacing systems.

activity sensing, magnetic ball. See *activity sensing, gravitational*.

activity sensing, piezoelectric vibration sensors in. See *piezoelectric crystal*.

activity sensing, in rate-adaptive pacing. A nonmetabolic variable for rate control in pacing that has achieved wide clinical acceptance. Activity-sensing pacemakers typically react quickly to the start and end of exercise, although their performance in other areas,

---

Activity Sensors

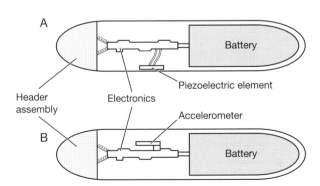

Modified from Millerhagen JO, Combs WJ. Activity sensing and accelerometer-based pacemakers. In: Ellenbogen KA, Kay GN, Wilkoff BL, editors. Clinical Cardiac Pacing and Defibrillation. 2nd ed. Philadelphia: W.B. Saunders Company; 2000. p. 249-70. Used with permission.

such as proportionality to exertion or specificity of response, continues to evolve. Activity sensors may be combined with other sensors, such as those measuring minute ventilation or QT (stimulus-T) interval.

activity sensor. A piezoelectric crystal or accelerometer used to measure the acceleration of certain muscle groups or body parts and the extent of body activity. Measured changes in sensed body motion may be used to effect a proportionate change in pacing rate. See also *accelerometer, piezoelectric crystal.* •

activity threshold. Programmable variable representing the level of activity that must be exceeded before a rate-adaptive pacing system will increase pacing rate.

acute electrical remodeling. Any change in refractoriness, conduction, or automaticity after initiation or termination of an arrhythmia or pacing sequence.

acute injury pattern. In pacing, elevation of the ST segment on the acute intracardiac electrogram. An acute injury pattern is one indication of contact between the electrode and the myocardial surface.

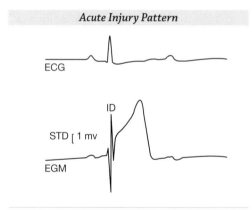

Acute Injury Pattern

acute pacing threshold. The minimal level of electrical activity required to reliably depolarize the myocardium at the time of lead placement. Acute thresholds typically are lower than chronic thresholds. The inflammatory tissue response caused by trauma at the site of electrode contact and the subsequent fibrotic tissue encapsulation around the electrode require higher pacemaker output pulses for depolarization. See also *chronic pacing threshold, pacing threshold, sensing threshold, threshold, threshold maturation.*

acute phase. Time period of the lead maturation process from implantation to the first few weeks after implantation. Stimulation thresholds can change during this phase as the lead develops mature contact with the endocardial tissue.

acute sensing threshold. The minimal intrinsic electrical signal required for consistent sensing of myocardial depolarization. See also *chronic sensing threshold, pacing threshold, sensing threshold, threshold maturation.*

acute threshold. Pacing or sensing threshold determination acquired at the time of lead implantation.

acute-to-chronic threshold change. See *threshold maturation.*

adapter. See *adaptor.*

adaptive AVI. See *rate-variable AV interval.*

adaptor. In pacing, a specialized connector that permits an electrical or mechanical connection between a lead terminal pin, its sealing mechanism, and a pacemaker header aperture of different dimensions or design. An adaptor is used to upsize or downsize the existing lead terminal pin and its sealing mechanism to enable compatibility with the pacemaker neck aperture. Defibrillation lead adaptors also permit upsizing and downsizing to different standards. Historically, adaptors have been used to adapt an inline lead configuration to a bifurcated configuration or to allow connection of a unipolar lead to a bipolar generator, or vice versa. However, few bifurcated pacing leads are still in service today.

ADC. Abbreviation for *analog-to-digital converter.*

adenosine. A naturally occurring endogenous nucleoside that slows atrioventricular nodal conduction and thus is useful as a therapeutic agent for termination of tachycardias in which the atrioventricular node is part of the circuit, such as atrioventricular nodal reentrant tachycardia or atrioventricular reentrant tachycardia involving an accessory pathway. Adenosine also can aid in the diagnosis of atrial flutter and atrial tachycardia by creating transient high-grade atrioventricular block. Adenosine decreases atrial refractoriness and increases atrioventricular nodal refractoriness. It may slightly decrease refractoriness in accessory pathways. Generally, it causes no untoward hemodynamic effects. Adenosine has a half-life of less than 10 seconds, and thus its effects are very brief. Side effects include flushing, dyspnea, and chest pain. The effects of adenosine are antagonized by theophylline and caffeine, and thus it may be ineffective in their presence.

adenosine triphosphate (ATP). Substrate for the formation of cyclic adenosine monophosphate (cAMP). Adenosine triphosphate is involved in transmitting the effects of β-adrenergic stimulation. See also *β-adrenergic receptor*.

adenylyl cyclase. The enzyme responsible for converting adenosine triphosphate to cyclic adenosine monophosphate (cAMP). Stimulation of β-adrenergic receptors results in activation of adenylyl cyclase through regulatory G proteins. See also *β-adrenergic receptor, cyclic adenosine monophosphate, G proteins*.

ADL. Abbreviation for *activities of daily living*.

generic term does not distinguish between α- and β-adrenergic stimulation.

adrenergically mediated. Occurring through or via the adrenergic nervous system.

adrenoceptor. See *adrenergic receptor*.

adrenoreceptor. See *adrenergic receptor*.

advanced heart failure. This term is not specific but is generally used to refer to New York Heart Association class III and IV heart failure.

advisory committee. In the United States, a group of independent technical experts in a specific area who review technical and clinical data presented to the U.S. Food and Drug Administration in support of action on a specific product or group of products and make recommendations on the action. This action may be

Acute Thresholds

	Atrium	Ventricle
Capture threshold*	≤ 1.5 V	≤ 1 V
Sensed P/R wave	≥ 1.5 mV	≥ 4 mV
Slew rate	≥ 0.3 V/s	≥ 0.5 V/s
Impedance†	400-1,500 ohms	400-1,500 ohms

* At 0.5-ms pulse duration.

† Dependent on electrode design; some normally functioning leads will fall outside of these impedance ranges

ADOPT-A. See *Atrial Dynamic Overdrive Pacing Trial*.

adrenaline. See *epinephrine*.

adrenergic. Pertaining to the sympathetic nervous system.

adrenergic antagonists. Agents that work to suppress sympathetic neuronal activity. See also *adrenergic receptor antagonists*.

adrenergic receptor. A type of receptor that is found on effector organs and is innervated by postganglionic adrenergic fibers of the sympathetic nervous system. Adrenergic receptors are classified as α-adrenergic and β-adrenergic receptors. Adrenergic receptors also are known as adrenoreceptors or adrenoceptors. See also *α-adrenergic receptor, β-adrenergic receptor*.

adrenergic receptor antagonists. Agents that bind to adrenergic receptors but do not activate them, including α-receptor blockers and β-receptor blockers.

adrenergic stimulation. Stimulation or excitement of the adrenergic nervous system. This

reclassification of a product, a Premarket Approval Application, or market withdrawal of a product.

AEGM. Abbreviation for *atrial electrogram*.

AEI. Abbreviation for *atrial escape interval*.

AF. Abbreviation for *atrial fibrillation*.

AF-CHF study. See *Atrial Fibrillation and Congestive Heart Failure trial*.

afferent nerves. Nerve fibers that carry impulses away from organs and back to the central nervous system. Efferent nerves, in contrast, transmit impulses from the central nervous system to end organs.

AFl. Abbreviation for *atrial flutter*.

afterdepolarization. A secondary depolarization that occurs during or just after completion of repolarization. Afterdepolarizations may reach threshold and generate a subsequent action potential, thus leading to tachycardia formation. See also *delayed afterdepolarization, early afterdepolarization, triggered activity*.

afterpolarization. A current produced in a

muscle or nerve after the conduction of an electric current through the tissue. See also *afterpotential*.

afterpotential. A small positive or negative waveform seen on an electrocardiogram or on an intracardiac electrogram after, and dependent on, the predominant electrical potential from either intrinsic or extrinsic stimulation. In pacing, an afterpotential represents the polarization at the electrode-myocardial interface after the sharp vertical or intrinsic deflection caused by the delivery of a pacemaker output stimulus. An afterpotential occurs while the pacemaker output capacitor is recharging, and it is propagated to the electrode, the lead, and the pacemaker sensing circuit. The electrical characteristics of the myocardial tissue in contact with the electrode are altered and the current is dissipated over time. Most of the effective afterpotential voltage occurs during the refractory period of the pacemaker. This timing reduces the probability that the afterpotential will be sensed by the pacemaker and cause the pacemaker to be inhibited or triggered, depending on the pacing mode. If output (voltage, current, or pulse duration) is high and the refractory period is short, the afterpotential may be sensed by the pacemaker.

AGC. Abbreviation for *automatic gain control*.

A-h. Abbreviation for *ampere-hour*.

AH interval. The amount of time that it takes for a wave of depolarization to travel from the lower right atrium to the interatrial septum to the His bundle, as measured on an intracardiac electrogram. The AH interval provides an approximation of the atrioventricular nodal conduction time. Normal adult values of the AH interval range from 55 to 130 milliseconds. See also *AV nodal conduction time*.

AICD. Abbreviation for *automatic implantable cardioverter-defibrillator*.

AID. Abbreviation for *automatic implantable defibrillator*.

air embolism. A complication that can occur when a central vein is accessed with a lead introducer sheath; may be noted as a hiss as air is taken into the sheath by negative intrathoracic pressure (e.g., deep inspiration by a snoring patient).

air entrapment. In pacing, the confinement of air in the pacemaker pocket at the time of pacemaker implantation or replacement. In a unipolar pacing system, air entrapment can cause an intermittent loss of sensing or capture. These complications are especially likely to occur after pacemaker replacement when the new pacemaker is smaller than the explanted pacemaker. Air entrapment usually can be managed by application of a pressure dressing to the pacemaker pocket. See also *dry pocket*.

ajmaline. A class IA antiarrhythmic drug that prolongs refractoriness of atrial, atrioventricular nodal, ventricular, and accessory pathway tissue. Ajmaline has efficacy in the treatment of supraventricular and ventricular arrhythmias. Currently, ajmaline is not approved in the United States.

alert interval. See *alert period*.

alert period. The portion of the atrial or ventricular timing cycle during which the pacemaker can sense intrinsic cardiac activity and respond in a preset or programmed manner. The alert period occurs after the refractory period of the pacemaker timing cycle and terminates with the next sensed or paced event. Intrinsic activity sensed during the alert period initiates an inhibited or triggered response from the pacemaker, depending on the pacing mode. The alert period also may be referred to as the alert interval. See also *atrial alert period, ventricular alert period*.

algorithm. A process or set of computational steps used to process information, that is, a set of rules that determines the characteristics of an operation or series of operations. In pacing, an algorithm may be used for automatic pacemaker functions. For example, an algorithm can be used in an antitachycardia pacemaker to process intrinsic signals for the automatic activation of a tachycardia-terminating mechanism. See also *tachycardia-terminating algorithm*.

Allen key. See *Allen wrench*.

Allen setscrew. A small screw with a hexagonal recessed socket. Allen setscrews are often used in pacing systems to secure the lead terminal pin in the pacemaker neck. See also *setscrew*.

Allen wrench. A hexagonal wrench. In pacing, an Allen wrench is used to drive Allen setscrews, which often are used to secure the lead terminal pin within the pacemaker neck aperture. The wrench may have an L-shaped shank or a straight shank. To avert damage to the lead terminal pin from the application of excessive torque to the Allen setscrew, the shank of the Allen wrench may be spring-loaded or it may be designed to yield (twist on itself) at the proper torque to prevent overtightening of the setscrew. An Allen wrench also is referred to as an Allen key.

alligator clamp. A clasping device with long, narrow, toothed, V-shaped jaws, used to make a temporary electrical connection. In pacing, an alligator clamp is used on some pacing accessories, for example, the cables and the temporary leads used for pacemaker testing before implantation. An alligator clamp also may be referred to as an alligator clip.

alligator clip. See *alligator clamp*.

alloy. A mixture of two or more metals which usually is formed when the elements are dissolved and fused together by heating. The mixture used to create alloys is designed to provide durability or other special qualities. Alloys such as cobalt-nickel and platinum-iridium are used as lead electrodes.

α-adrenergic antagonists. See *α-blocker*.

α-adrenergic receptor. A type of sympathetic nervous system receptor stimulated by norepinephrine. α-Adrenergic receptors are subdivided into α_1- and α_2-receptors. α_1-Receptors are postsynaptic. Their stimulation results in increased myocardial contractility, decreased myocardial automaticity, and increased Purkinje fiber refractoriness. α_2-Receptors are located on presynaptic nerve terminals. Their stimulation enhances the reuptake of norepinephrine from the synapse.

α-blocker. A pharmacologic agent that competitively blocks α-adrenergic receptors. A generic example is phentolamine.

α-pathway. See *slow pathway*.

alprenolol. A nonselective, β-adrenergic blocking agent with intrinsic sympathomimetic activity. For side effects, see *β-adrenergic blocking drugs*.

alternans. See *electrical alternans*.

Alternans Before Cardioverter Defibrillator (ABCD). This is a clinical trial in progress to evaluate and compare the positive predictive value of a T-wave alternans test to that of an electrophysiologic study in patients with ischemic heart disease, left ventricular dysfunction, and nonsustained tachycardia.

alternate scanning. An algorithm used in antitachycardia therapy. In alternate scanning, intervals in successive pacing trains alternately are shortened and lengthened by increasing amounts about a median that was the last successful memory value to revert a tachycardia. The process continues until the tachycardia has reverted or until the complete range of possible intervals has been covered, at which time the interval is reset to the memory value.

alternate-site pacing. Generic term used to describe implantation of pacemaker or defibrillator lead or leads in a position(s) other than the most commonly used right atrial appendage and right ventricular apical positions.

alternating current (AC). A type of electric current, sometimes used to induce ventricular fibrillation during electrophysiologic testing. Alternating-current frequency varies from country to country depending on the type of mains electricity system, but typically the frequency is 50 or 60 Hz.

alternative sites. See *alternate-site pacing*.

aluminum electrolytic capacitor. See *electrolytic capacitor*.

ambulatory electrocardiogram. A long-term (usually 24-hour) recording of two or three surface electrocardiographic leads. Ambulatory electrocardiograms are useful for assessing rhythm abnormalities, pacemaker function, heart rate variability, and ST-segment elevation. Ambulatory electrocardiography also is known as Holter monitoring.

ambulatory monitoring. See *ambulatory electrocardiogram*.

American National Standards Institute (ANSI). In the United States, the representative organization of the International Organization for Standardization (ISO).

amiloride. A potassium-sparing diuretic that has antiarrhythmic activity due to its sodium-pump blocking effect. Amiloride has a half-life of 6 to 9 hours, and it is excreted by the kidneys. Side effects include hyperkalemia and gastrointestinal distress.

4-aminopyridine (4-AP). A potassium channel blocker used experimentally to block the transient outward current (ITO) from a cell.

4-aminopyridine-sensitive potassium current. One of several ion channels responsible for sinoatrial pacemaker activity.

amiodarone. A class III antiarrhythmic drug that slows conduction through the normal atrioventricular conduction system and accessory pathways, slows sinus rate, and prolongs refractoriness in atrial, atrioventricular nodal, ventricular, and accessory pathway tissue.

Amiodarone is efficacious for the treatment of supraventricular and ventricular tachycardias, but it has potentially significant side effects. Amiodarone does not significantly affect pacing thresholds but may increase defibrillation thresholds. Amiodarone is metabolized by the liver and is excreted in the bile. Its half-life ranges from 40 to 55 days. Side effects of amiodarone include bradycardias, proarrhythmia, pulmonary fibrosis, cirrhosis, hyperthyroidism or hypothyroidism, photosensitivity, corneal microdeposits, and blue discoloration of the skin. Amiodarone currently is available only as an oral preparation in the United States, but an intravenous preparation is available elsewhere.

Amiodarone Versus Implantable Cardioverter-Defibrillator in Patients With Nonischemic Dilated Cardiomyopathy and Asymptomatic Nonsustained Ventricular Tachycardia (AMIOVIRT). This study found that mortality and quality of life were not statistically different for patients with nonischemic dilated cardiomyopathy and nonsustained ventricular tachycardia treated with amiodarone or an implantable cardioverter-defibrillator (Strickberger SA, Hummel JD, Bartlett TG, Frumin HI, Schuger CD, Beau SL, et al, AMIOVIRT Investigators. Amiodarone versus implantable cardioverter-defibrillator: randomized trial in patients with nonischemic dilated cardiomyopathy and asymptomatic nonsustained ventricular tachycardia: AMIOVIRT. J Am Coll Cardiol. 2003;41:1707-12).

AMIOVIRT. See *Amiodarone Versus Implantable Cardioverter-Defibrillator in Patients With Nonischemic Dilated Cardiomyopathy and Asymptomatic Nonsustained Ventricular Tachycardia.*

ampere (A). The international unit of measurement of electrical current. One ampere is the amount of electrical charge flowing past a specified circuit point at a rate of 1 coulomb (C) per second. One ampere of current flows in a circuit when 1 volt (V) of potential is applied across 1 ohm (Ω) of resistance. Circuit current drain and pacemaker output are expressed in microamperes and in milliamperes, respectively.

ampere-hour (A-h). A unit for the quantification of electricity and a measurement of battery capacity. One ampere-hour is the amount of electrical current flowing past a specified circuit point at a rate of 1 A per hour. One ampere-hour is equal to 3,600 C.

amplifier. An electronic device or circuit capable of magnifying an incoming electrical signal to enlarge the amplitude of the signal. The degree of magnification is known as the gain of the amplifier and is expressed either as a ratio or in decibels. In pacing, the amplifier magnifies the sensed intrinsic cardiac signal as that signal is passed through the pacemaker circuitry.

amplitude. The maximal absolute value attained by an electrical waveform, or the maximal measured value of any signal that varies periodically. In pacing, amplitude indicates magnitude of the voltage or amperage level of a pacemaker output pulse. Amplitude usually is measured in volts or in milliamperes. Typical voltage amplitude values of pacemaker output pulses are 2.5 or 5 V, although programmable options vary from 0.5 to 10 V.

amplitude modulation. The alteration and encoding of a carrier signal with an applied waveform. The alteration of the carrier signal occurs by changes in its amplitude. The amplitude of the carrier is varied in proportion to the voltage of the waveform that is applied. However, the frequency of the carrier signal stays the same. In pacing, amplitude modulation is used during programming and telemetry to encode the carrier signal transmitted between the external programmer and the implanted pacemaker. See also *carrier signal, modulation.*

AMS. Early abbreviation for *automatic mode switching.* See *mode switching.*

amyloidosis. The accumulation of a glycoprotein in body tissues. Amyloidosis may be systemic or localized within the myocardium. When there is infiltration of the cardiac conduction system with amyloid, symptomatic bradycardias that require permanent pacing may result.

analog signal. A continuous signal that varies in amplitude and direction and is an analog representation of a corresponding value. For example, an electrocardiogram or intracardiac electrogram is the visual analog of cardiac electrical activity.

analog-to-digital converter (ADC). An electronic device or circuit that changes an analog signal or electrical voltage level into discrete digital signals such as binary bits. For example, an analog-to-digital converter can be used to convert the analog signals of intracardiac electrograms into digital signals for telemetry.

analyzer. A device used to obtain physiologic or

device measurements before or during the implantation of a pacemaker or implantable cardioverter-defibrillator. See also *defibrillator systems analyzer, pacemaker systems analyzer*.

anchoring sleeve. See *suture sleeve*.

aneurysm. A sac formed by the dilatation of the wall of a vessel (artery or vein) or of the wall of a cardiac chamber. Ventricular aneurysms, particularly those of the left ventricular wall, are associated with reentrant ventricular arrhythmias.

aneurysmectomy. Excision of an aneurysm. An aneurysmectomy combined with a subendocardial resection may be used to eliminate ventricular tachycardia.

ANF. Abbreviation for *atrial natriuretic factor*.

angiotensin-converting enzyme inhibitor. A class of drugs that decrease production of angiotensin II, resulting in a decrease in arteriolar resistance and an increase in venous capacitance. As a result, these drugs are effective in the treatment of hypertension and also commonly used in the treatment of congestive heart failure.

anisotropy. Variation in conduction velocity seen as an impulse spreads through the myocardium in different directions due to differences in myocardial fiber orientation. Impulses travel more rapidly along the longitudinal axis of fibers than along the transverse axis. Anisotropy is subclassified into uniform and nonuniform anisotropic conduction.

annunciator. A dedicated visual or audio output device intended to alert a user to some condition. Some implantable cardioverter-defibrillators have an audio annunciator or beeper that signals charging for a shock or indicates elective replacement time.

anodal band. In pacing, either the contact ring on an in-line bipolar lead terminal pin or the proximal-ring electrode on an endocardial lead. See also *contact ring, proximal-ring electrode*.

anodal stimulation. In pacing, delivery of electrical current to the myocardium from the anode (positive pole). Pacing stimulation typically is done at the cathode (negative pole), but sufficient current density at the anode may result in myocardial stimulation.

anode. The positive pole of a circuit or cell, as in a battery; also, the anodal ring on a bipolar pacing lead. In an electrical system, the anode is the electrode away from which electrons move during current flow. In a unipolar endocardial pacing system, the anode usually is the pacemaker case. In a bipolar endocardial pacing system, the anode usually is the proximal-ring electrode on the lead. The anode also is referred to as the indifferent electrode. See also *anodal band, cathode*.

ANP. Abbreviation for *atrial natriuretic peptide*.

ANS. Abbreviation for *autonomic nervous system*.

ANSI. Abbreviation for the *American National Standards Institute*.

antegrade accessory pathway. An aberrant, usually muscular, conduction pathway that bypasses the normal atrioventricular nodal conduction system. This results in preexcitation of the ventricle and an abnormal early portion of the QRS complex (delta wave). See also *Mahaim fiber*.

antegrade block. Failure to conduct current in one direction, usually during stimulation of the proximal chamber. This phenomenon may be temporary or permanent.

antegrade conduction. The conduction of cardiac impulses in the normal forward direction from the atria to the ventricles via normal or accessory cardiac conduction pathways. Normal conduction occurs sequentially, as follows: from the sinus node through the atrial myocardium, the atrioventricular node, the His bundle, the left and right bundle branches, the Purkinje fibers, and the ventricular myocardium. Antegrade conduction also is referred to as anterograde conduction or atrioventricular conduction. See also *retrograde conduction*.

anterograde conduction. See *antegrade conduction*.

antiarrhythmic agent. Any drug used for the management of arrhythmias. Antiarrhythmic drugs are classified by their mechanism of action. Class I antiarrhythmic drugs block the fast sodium channel and are subdivided into three subgroups. Class IA drugs moderately depress the rise of the action potential (phase 0) and markedly prolong refractoriness. Class IB drugs decrease spontaneous depolarization, have little effect on phase 0, and shorten refractoriness. Class IC drugs markedly depress phase 0 and have little effect on refractoriness. Class II antiarrhythmic drugs are β-adrenergic receptor blockers. Class III antiarrhythmic drugs prolong action potential duration and thus refractoriness and have little effect on phase 0. Class IV antiarrhythmic drugs are calcium channel blockers. See also *depolarization phases*.

antiarrhythmic drug (AAD). See *antiarrhythmic agent*.

antiarrhythmic therapy. Treatment used for the prevention, interruption, or termination of cardiac arrhythmias. Antiarrhythmic therapies include pharmacologic agents, electrical devices

Antiarrhythmic Agents in Clinical Use

Class	Drug	Effect on conduction	Action potential duration	QRS duration	QT interval	Comments
IA	Quinidine, procainamide, disopyramide	↓	↑	↑	↑	Quinidine increases sinus rate, procainamide may be associated with lupus, disopyramide potent vagolytic and negative inotrope
IB	Lidocaine, mexiletine, phenytoin, tocainide	0	↓	0	± ↓	Lidocaine particularly effective in ischemia
IC	Flecainide, propafenone	↓↓	± ↑	↑↑	± ↑	Mostly used for atrial fibrillation
II	Propranolol, atenolol, metoprolol, carvedilol	AV node ↓ SA node ↓	0	0	0	β-Blockers
III	Amiodarone, dofetilide, sotalol, ibutilide, azimilide, NAPA	0	↑↑	0	↑↑	Azimilide blocks I_{Kr} and I_{Ks}, all others block I_{Kr} only; NAPA is a metabolite of procainamide
IV	Verapamil, diltiazem	AV node ↓ SA node ↓	0	0	0	Calcium channel blockers

Antiarrhythmics Versus Implantable Defibrillators (AVID). This study found that the implantable cardioverter-defibrillator is superior to antiarrhythmic drugs for increasing overall survival among survivors of ventricular fibrillation or sustained ventricular tachycardia causing severe symptoms (The Antiarrhythmics versus Implantable Defibrillators [AVID] Investigators. A comparison of antiarrhythmic-drug therapy with implantable defibrillators in patients resuscitated from near-fatal ventricular arrhythmias. N Engl J Med. 1997;337:1576-83).

such as pacemakers and implantable cardioverter-defibrillators, and surgical intervention.

antibiotic prophylaxis, for pacemaker, implantable cardioverter-defibrillator, or cardiac resynchronization device implantation. Administration of antibiotics before, during, or after implantation of a device. Use of and guidelines for prophylactic antibiotic administration vary. There is general agreement that intravenous antibiotics should be administered before the initial skin incision is made.

anticholinergic. Pertaining to blockage of the passage of impulses through the parasympathetic nervous system. Some antiarrhythmic drugs, such as atropine, scopolamine, and disopyramide, are anticholinergic, that is, they block the parasympathetic nervous system and thus decrease its stimulatory effects. Anticholinergic effects include sinus tachycardia, accelerated atrioventricular nodal conduction, dry mouth, blurred vision, constipation, and urinary retention. See also *cholinergic*.

anticoagulant drugs. Any agent that is used for prevention of blood clotting. It most commonly refers to intravenous or subcutaneous agents such as heparin or an oral agent such as warfarin.

antidromic. Propagation of an electrical impulse occurring opposite to the usual direction of conduction through a conductive pathway.

antidromic activation. Conduction from a distal to the proximal chamber by a conducting pathway (opposite of orthodromic).

antidromic atrioventricular reentrant tachycardia (AVRT). Reentrant tachycardia occurring antegrade over an accessory pathway and retrograde via the normal atrioventricular conduction system. Antidromic tachycardias are distinguished from orthodromic atrioventricular reentrant tachycardias by a wide QRS complex.

antidromic reciprocating tachycardia (ART). A macroreentrant rhythm in which a wave front travels from the atria down one or more accessory atrioventricular fibers to the ventricles and returns to the atria through either the ventriculoatrial conduction system (the His-Purkinje system and the atrioventricular node) or a secondary accessory pathway. Antidromic reciprocating tachycardia must be differentiated from supraventricular tachycardias with bystander conduction over an accessory pathway such as in atrial tachycardia or atrioventricular nodal reentrant tachycardia.

antidromic tachycardia. Specifically refers to a preexcited tachycardia in which the accessory pathway is critical to the circuit.

anti-inflammatory drugs, for electrode-tissue interface inflammation. Incorporating an anti-inflammatory drug in or around the electrode tip in an attempt to limit inflammation at the electrode-myocardial interface. Corticosteroids are most commonly used, but multiple anti-inflammatory drugs have been tried.

antitachycardia defibrillator. An implantable defibrillator that uses antitachycardia pacing to terminate ventricular tachycardia. See also *antitachycardia pacing*.

antitachycardia pacemaker. An implantable pacemaker that delivers programmed electrical stimuli to interrupt or terminate a tachycardia. Most antitachycardia pacemakers contain an algorithm in the pacemaker circuitry to identify tachycardias and automatically activate the preset or programmed antitachycardia pacing mechanism. In general, antitachycardia pacemakers are used only for supraventricular tachycardias. Some antitachycardia pacemakers can be activated with an external device or a magnet. See also *antitachycardia defibrillator, antitachycardia pacing, burst pacing*.

Antibiotic Recommendations (Mayo Clinic Rochester) For Implantable Device Procedure

Cefazolin 1 g intravenously if <80 kg or 2 g if ≥80 kg, within 60 minutes of start of procedure and every 8 hours for 2 doses in patients staying overnight. For pulse generator change, only the initial dose is given

If penicillin or cephalosporin-sensitive, vancomycin 20 mg/kg intravenously within 2 hours of start of procedure. If patient is staying overnight, 15 mg/kg once 12 hours later. Dose is adjusted for renal insufficiency. For pulse generator change, only the initial dose is given

For prolonged procedures, electrophysiologic or device, same prophylaxis as listed above and repeat cefazolin at 4 hours and 16 hours after start of procedure and repeat vancomycin at 12 hours

antitachycardia pacing (ATP). Pacing provided by some implantable pacemakers designed to detect and terminate tachycardias. The pacemaker circuitry contains an algorithm for identification of tachycardia. When a sensed intrinsic rhythm satisfies the criteria of the algorithm and is thereby identified as a tachycardia, the preset or programmed antitachycardia pacing mechanism is activated. See also *antitachycardia pacemaker, asynchronous antitachycardia pacing,* *autodecremental pacing, autoincremental pacing, burst pacing, critically timed stimulus, overdrive pacing, programmed electrical stimulus, scanning pacemaker, synchronous antitachycardia pacing, tachycardia-terminating algorithm, underdrive pacing.*

antitachycardia pacing algorithm. An algorithm used to control the delivery of pacing pulses to revert a tachycardia.

antitachycardia therapies. In implantable devices, programmable options designed to interrupt tachycardia or fibrillation in an attempt to restore normal sinus rhythm. Depending on the model of implantable cardioverter-defibrillator or cardiac resynchronization therapy defibrillator, therapies may include antitachycardia pacing, cardioversion, or defibrillation.

antitheft detector. See *antitheft surveillance equipment and electromagnetic interference*.

antitheft surveillance equipment and electromagnetic interference. Equipment commonly used at the exit(s) of commercial establishments to prevent theft of merchandise. It is germane to implantable devices because of potential electromagnetic interference that can occur with certain types of the antitheft equipment.

AOO. The NBG code for atrial asynchronous pacing. Pacing occurs in the atrium at a fixed rate, and there is no sensing of intrinsic cardiac activity. See also *asynchronous pacing, atrial asynchronous pacing mode*.

AOOR. Asynchronous atrial pacing mode with rate-adaptive response.

aortic bodies. Small neurovascular structures containing chemoreceptors that respond to changes in oxygen, carbon dioxide, and hydrogen ion concentration in the blood. The aortic bodies play an important role in the reflex regulation of respiration. See also *baroreceptor, carotid body, chemoreceptor*.

4-AP. Abbreviation for *4-aminopyridine*.

APC. Abbreviation for *atrial premature complex*.

APD. Abbreviation for *action potential duration, atrial premature depolarization*.

aperture. An opening. In pacing, an aperture is an opening in the pacemaker connector block into which a lead terminal pin is inserted and secured to form an electrical connection between the lead and the pacemaker circuitry.

arc welding, and electromagnetic interference (EMI). A type of welding equipment that often is mentioned as potentially causing clinically significant EMI; industrial welding, which typically operates at 500 A or more and is a likely source of EMI, should be differentiated from hobby welding, in which equipment operates at lower amperage and is much less likely to generate clinically significant EMI. See also *electromagnetic interference*.

AR interval. The amount of time between the atrial pacing stimulus and the onset of the next native ventricular event (R wave) as measured on an electrocardiogram.

ARP. Abbreviation for *absolute refractory period, atrial refractory period*.

arrest. See *cardiac arrest*.

arrhythmia. Any abnormality of cardiac rhythm. See also *bradycardia, dysrhythmia, tachycardia*.

arrhythmogenesis. The generation of arrhythmias, such as by certain antiarrhythmic drugs, ischemia, or electrolyte abnormalities. See also *proarrhythmia*.

arrhythmogenic right ventricular cardiomyopathy. See *arrhythmogenic right ventricular dysplasia*.

arrhythmogenic right ventricular dysplasia (ARVD). A pathophysiologic process that predominantly affects the right ventricle and in which myocardial cells are replaced by fibrotic and adipose tissue. Damaged areas may give rise to ventricular tachycardias.

ART. Abbreviation for *antidromic reciprocating tachycardia*.

artifact. In pacing, an extraneous signal superimposed on an electrocardiogram or an intracardiac electrogram. There are many potential sources of artifacts, including pacemaker output pulses, electromagnetic interference, myopotentials, programming transmission, and defibrillation. See also *stimulus artifact*.

ARVD. Abbreviation for *arrhythmogenic right ventricular dysplasia*.

Ashman phenomenon. A form of abnormal intraventricular conduction caused by changes in myocardial refractoriness which occur as a result of abrupt changes in cycle length. The Ashman phenomenon typically is seen as right bundle branch block that occurs after an atrial premature complex following a relatively long pause; this produces a long-short sequence. The occurrence of the Ashman phenomenon usually is physiologic, and often it explains the aberrancy of supraventricular tachycardias that begin abruptly. See also *aberrancy*.

as-shipped values. The nominal values to which a pacemaker or an implantable cardioverter-defibrillator is programmed for shipment. In most cases, as-shipped values for pacemakers are set to therapeutic levels and thus the pacemaker usually can be implanted safely without reprogramming. As-shipped values for implantable cardioverter-defibrillators may not be life-supporting. As-shipped values may be used as a reference point for programming pacemakers and implantable cardioverter-defibrillators.

asynchronous antitachycardia pacing. Antitachycardia pacing in which the pacemaker output pulses are delivered without regard to specific characteristics of the sensed tachycardia. See also *burst pacing, overdrive pacing, underdrive pacing.*

asynchronous mode. A mode of pacing without sensing and without inhibition or tracking, for example, AOO, AOOR, VOO, VOOR, DOO, DOOR. Asynchronous modes are rarely used as permanently programmed modes. Asynchronous pacing most commonly occurs with magnet placement.

asynchronous pacing. Pacing at a fixed, preset rate independent of any intrinsic cardiac activity. Because intrinsic cardiac electrical activity is not sensed during asynchronous pacing, the pacemaker output pulses may compete with the intrinsic cardiac rhythm. An asynchronous pacemaker artifact during the vulnerable period of the cardiac cycle may initiate malignant arrhythmias if the cardiac condition is acute or unstable. Asynchronous pacing usually is the magnet mode of response in pacemakers. See also *asynchronous mode, AOO, DOO, VOO.*

asynchrony. A lack of coordination between parts. From a device standpoint, this most commonly refers to lack of synchrony between the atria and ventricles and lack of synchrony between the right and left ventricles (interventricular) or intraventricular asynchrony of the left ventricle. Asynchrony and dyssynchrony are often used interchangeably when describing intraventricular lack of synchrony.

asystole. The absence of cardiac contraction; cardiac standstill.

atenolol. A β_1-selective, hydrophilic, β-adrenergic blocking agent that has no intrinsic sympathomimetic activity. Because of its β_1-selectivity, atenolol may tend to cause less bronchospasm than some other β-adrenergic blocking agents.

Because it is hydrophilic, atenolol does not pass the blood-brain barrier well and thus may have fewer central nervous system side effects than some other β-adrenergic blocking agents. For side effects, see *β-adrenergic blocking drugs.*

ATP. Abbreviation for adenosine triphosphate. Also an abbreviation for antitachycardia pacing.

atrial activation sequence. The order in which various parts of the atrial myocardium are depolarized. Analysis of the atrial activation sequence aids in distinguishing sinus rhythm from ectopic atrial foci and retrograde conduction over the atrioventricular node or accessory pathways. See also *concentric retrograde atrial activation, eccentric retrograde atrial activation.*

atrial alert period. The portion of the pacemaker timing cycle during which the atrial sensing circuit is alert. In a DDD pacemaker, the atrial sensing circuit is refractory during the atrioventricular interval and the postventricular atrial refractory period. Intrinsic atrial activity sensed during the atrial alert period will cause the pacemaker output to be inhibited or triggered in the atrial or ventricular channel of the pacemaker, depending on the pacing mode. In most pacing modes, such as AAI, DDI, and DDD, if intrinsic atrial activity is not sensed, the pacemaker releases an atrial output pulse at the end of the alert period. In other pacing modes, such as VAT and VDD, atrial activity sensed during the atrial alert period results in a triggered ventricular output pulse. In non–rate-adaptive modes, the maximal atrial alert period is equal to the minimal rate minus the sum of the atrioventricular interval and the refractory period.

atrial arrhythmias. Broad classification used to describe arrhythmias whose substrate is the atria but do not involve the atrioventricular node. Subgroups of this classification include sinus node tachycardias, atrial ectopy and tachycardia, atrial flutter, and atrial fibrillation.

atrial asynchronous pacing mode (AOO). A single-chamber pacing mode in which the atrium is paced at a preset or programmed rate independently of any intrinsic cardiac activity. In atrial asynchronous pacing, intrinsic cardiac electrical activity is not sensed; thus, competition with intrinsic rhythm may occur. An asynchronous atrial pacemaker stimulus that occurs during atrial repolarization may initiate an arrhythmia. Atrial asynchronous pacing rarely is indicated as a chronic pacing mode, but usually it is the magnet mode of response in AAI pacing. See also *AOO, asynchronous pacing.*

atrial asystole. Absence of atrial contractions.

atrial-based lower rate timing. See *atrial-based timing system.*

atrial-based pacemaker timing. See *atrial-based timing system.*

atrial-based timing system. A pacemaker timing system in which the AA interval is fixed. In contrast, in a ventricular-based system, the atrial escape interval is fixed. As long as lower rate-limit pacing is stable, there is no discernible difference between the two timing systems. In a system with atrial-based timing, a sensed R wave that occurs during the atrioventricular interval inhibits the ventricular output but does not alter the basic AA timing. Hence, the rate stays at the programmed lower rate limit during effective single-chamber atrial pacing. When a ventricular premature beat is sensed during the atrial escape interval, the timers also are reset, but it is the AA interval rather than the atrial escape interval that is reset.

depolarization or, in some cases, by normal atrioventricular conduction, as indicated by a paced atrial event followed by a QRS complex.

atrial channel. The independent circuit of a pacemaker or implantable cardioverter-defibrillator dedicated to activity in the atrium.

atrial contribution. See *atrial kick, atrial-inhibited pacing mode.*

atrial decremental pacing. Continuous atrial pacing in which the cycle length is gradually decreased, causing an increase in the pacing rate. In normal atrioventricular conduction systems, the AH interval lengthens progressively as the cycle length decreases until Wenckebach-type atrioventricular block occurs. Atrial decremental pacing can be used to analyze atrioventricular nodal and His-Purkinje function. See also *incremental pacing, ventricular decremental pacing.*

atrial defibrillator. Implantable device designed to deliver automatic or on-demand shock to terminate atrial fibrillation. Atrial-only defibrillators and combined atrial and ventricular cardioverter-defibrillators have been introduced but have not been widely accepted, largely because

Atrial-Based Timing

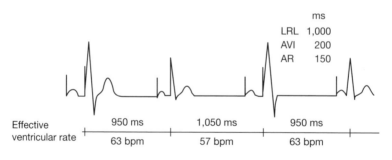

	ms
LRL	1,000
AVI	200
AR	150

AR, AR interval; LRL, lower rate limit.

atrial blanking. Interval during which the atrial channel sense amplifier is completely disabled. During the atrial blanking period, the device does not sense any electrical signals on the atrial channel.

atrial boost. See *atrial kick.*

atrial capture. The successful depolarization of the atria by a pacemaker stimulus. Atrial capture may be confirmed on an electrocardiogram or intracardiac electrogram by the presence of an atrial pacing artifact followed by atrial

of poor patient acceptance of painful shock for atrial fibrillation.

atrial demand pacing. See *atrial-inhibited pacing mode.*

atrial depolarization. The electrical process in which polarized atrial myofibrils are depolarized and produce atrial contraction. Atrial depolarization is represented by a P wave on an electrocardiographic recording.

Atrial Dynamic Overdrive Pacing Trial (ADOPT-A). This study found that overdrive atrial pacing with a specific atrial fibrillation suppression algorithm decreased the burden of symptomatic atrial fibrillation significantly in patients with sick sinus syndrome and paroxysmal atrial fibrillation (Carlson MD, Ip J, Messenger J, Beau S, Kalbfleisch S, Gervais P, et al, Atrial Dynamic Overdrive Pacing Trial [ADOPT] Investigators. A new pacemaker algorithm for the treatment of atrial fibrillation: results of the Atrial Dynamic Overdrive Pacing Trial [ADOPT]. J Am Coll Cardiol. 2003;42:627-33).

atrial dyssynchrony. Lack of synchrony between two atria or within the atria resulting in uncoordinated contraction and associated with difficulty in optimizing atrioventricular synchrony.

atrial ectopy. Spontaneous depolarization of the atria initiated by a group of myocardial cells other than the sinus node.

atrial effective refractory period. During atrial pacing, the longest S_1 to S_2 interval at which S_2 does not cause atrial depolarization. The atrial effective refractory period generally decreases at shorter drive pacing cycle lengths. See also *effective refractory period*.

atrial EGM (AEGM). See *atrial electrogram*.

atrial electrogram. An intracardiac electrogram of the atrial myocardium. See also *electrogram*.

atrial electrophysiologic remodeling. Process wherein atrial arrhythmias result in increased ease of initiation and maintenance of further atrial arrhythmia (commonly occurs in atrial fibrillation).

atrial endocardial activation. The site of origin of an atrial arrhythmia occurring on the endocardial surface rather than the epicardial surface of the atrium. Sinus rhythm has early epicardial activation, whereas most atrial tachycardias have endocardial activation.

atrial escape interval (AEI). In single-chamber atrial pacemakers that are not rate-adaptive, the maximal amount of time between a paced or sensed atrial event and the next consecutive output pulse. The atrial escape interval is equal to the programmed rate minus the atrioventricular interval. In dual-chamber pacemakers, the atrial escape interval, also referred to as the ventriculoatrial interval, is the amount of time from a ventricular paced or sensed event to the next atrial output pulse. The atrial escape interval is terminated if an intrinsic P wave or intrinsic ventricular event is sensed before the interval has been completed. The atrial escape interval is measured in milliseconds.

atrial extrastimuli. An extrinsic electrical impulse delivered in the atrium, usually delivered at a preset or programmed coupling interval.

atrial fibrillation (AF). An irregular, rapid atrial arrhythmia characterized by continuous, uncoordinated, and ineffective contractions of the atrial myocardium. The atrial rate usually is 350 to 600 beats per minute. Atrial fibrillation is thought to be due to reentry.

Atrial Fibrillation and Congestive Heart Failure (AH-CHF) trial. The primary objective of the Atrial Fibrillation and Congestive Heart Failure (AF-CHF) trial was to determine whether restoring and maintaining sinus rhythm significantly reduces cardiovascular mortality compared with a rate control strategy in patients with atrial fibrillation and congestive heart failure. It was a prospective, multicenter trial randomizing patients with New York Heart Association class II to IV congestive heart failure, left ventricular ejection fraction less than 35%, and a documented clinically significant episode of atrial fibrillation within the past 6 months to either 1) rhythm control with the use of direct-current cardioversion in combination with antiarrhythmic drugs (amiodarone or other class III agents) (and additional nonpharmacologic therapy in resistant patients) or 2) rate control with the use of β-blockers, digoxin, or pacemaker and atrioventricular node ablation if necessary. Cardiovascular mortality was the primary end point, and the intention-to-treat approach is the primary method of analysis (Rationale and design of a study assessing treatment strategies of atrial fibrillation in patients with heart failure: the Atrial Fibrillation and Congestive Heart Failure [AF-CHF] trial. Am Heart J. 2002;144:597-607).

atrial fibrillation prevention algorithm. Various pacemaker algorithms designed to alter the timing cycles in order to prevent the initiation or recurrence of atrial fibrillation. Approaches include atrial overdrive pacing, atrial rate stabilization, and specific algorithms to maintain atrial pacing after a mode-switch episode.

atrial flutter (AFl). A regular, rapid atrial arrhythmia due to macroreentry within the atrial myocardium. Atrial flutter is characterized by poorly effective contractions and an atrial rate of 250 to 350 beats per minute with variable conduction to the ventricles. On an electrocardiogram, atrial flutter typically shows a classic sawtooth pattern in the inferior leads.

atrial functional refractory period. During atrial pacing, the shortest A_1 to A_2 interval generated in response to an S_1 to S_2 interval. The atrial functional refractory period generally decreases at shorter drive pacing cycle lengths. See also *functional refractory period.*

atrial incremental pacing. See *atrial decremental pacing.*

atrial inhibited pacing. See *AAI, atrial-inhibited pacing mode.*

atrial-inhibited pacing mode (AAI). The single-chamber pacing mode in which the pacemaker inhibits its atrial output pulse in response to intrinsic atrial activity sensed during the atrial alert period. If a P wave is not sensed, the pacemaker delivers an atrial output pulse at the preset or programmed rate interval, that is, at the end of the atrial alert period. Atrial-inhibited pacing also is referred to as atrial-demand pacing. See the figure *AAI.*

atrial-inhibited rate-adaptive pacing mode (AAIR). The single-chamber pacing mode in which pacing and sensing occur in the atrium, and the mode of response to sensed atrial events is inhibited. The pacemaker also is capable of rate-adaptive pacing via a sensor that monitors some physiologic or nonphysiologic variable and adjusts the heart rate accordingly. See also *rate-adaptive pacing.*

atrial J lead. An atrial endocardial pacing lead in which the distal portion of the pacing lead is shaped like a J to facilitate appropriate secure placement of the lead in the atrium. See also *atrial lead.*

atrial kick. The normal atrial contribution to cardiac output when atrioventricular synchrony is intact. The loss of atrioventricular synchrony may decrease cardiac output by 10% to 30%. Dual-chamber pacing modes preserve the atrial kick, whereas VVI pacing does not. Atrial kick also is referred to as atrial boost or atrial contribution.

atrial lead. An epicardial or endocardial, unipolar or bipolar, active or passive fixation lead designed for use in atrial pacing or sensing. An endocardial atrial lead can be positioned in the atrial appendage, on the interatrial septum, or on the lateral wall of the atrium. On occasion, an atrial lead is positioned in the coronary sinus. Optimal endocardial atrial lead placement requires careful manipulation of the lead within the atrium to obtain the best position for sensing of the low-amplitude intrinsic atrial signal. Several different atrial lead configurations designed to ensure secure placement are available. See also *active fixation lead, atrial J lead, endocardial lead, epicardial lead, passive fixation lead, screw-in lead.*

atrial myocardium. The thin muscular walls of the upper two chambers of the heart. See also *atrium.*

atrial natriuretic factor (ANF). See *atrial natriuretic peptide (ANP).*

atrial natriuretic peptide (ANP). A naturally occurring peptide synthesized by myoendocrine cells located in the atrial myocardium. Atrial natriuretic peptide levels can be increased by atrial stretch caused by an increase of atrial pressure, volume expansion, or atrial tachycardia. In pacing, atrial natriuretic peptide levels usually are increased with any pacing mode in which loss of atrioventricular synchrony occurs. Atrial natriuretic peptide also is referred to as atrial natriuretic factor (ANF).

atrial output pulse. A pacemaker stimulus delivered to the atrial myocardium. The atrial output pulse is recorded as a vertical deflection either above or below the baseline on an electrocardiogram or an intracardiac electrogram.

atrial overdrive pacing. A method of pacing in which the pacing rate is faster than the patient's intrinsic rate or rate of the tachycardia. This method is used in certain pacemakers to prevent late coupled premature atrial complexes initiating atrial tachyarrhythmias. Its use in cardiac electrophysiology is in distinguishing automatic arrhythmias from triggered or reentrant arrhythmias. See also *overdrive suppression.*

atrial overdrive ramp. A type of antitachycardia pacing in which the cycle length decreases with each pacing stimulus. This has the advantage of terminating arrhythmias with a very small excitable gap and the disadvantage of accelerating trigger arrhythmias or inducing more rapid reentrant arrhythmias despite termination of the initial arrhythmia. See also *burst pacing, excitable gap.*

atrial oversensing. Detection of activity on the atrial sensing circuit that is something other than intrinsic atrial activity, for example, QRS, paced ventricular event, T wave, electromagnetic interference.

atrial paced event (AP). Atrial depolarization that occurs as a result of delivery of a pacing artifact in the atrium or adjacent to atrial tissue, that is, the stimulus may be delivered in the right atrium, left atrium, or coronary venous system.

atrial pacing. Pacing the atrial myocardium to control bradycardia or tachycardia. AAI or AAIR pacing is appropriate for sinus node dysfunction, but only if atrioventricular nodal function is normal. See also *AAI, AAT, AOO*.

atrial premature complex (APC). An early atrial depolarization that originates in an area of the atrial myocardium other than the sinus node. An atrial premature complex also is referred to as an atrial premature depolarization or a premature atrial complex.

atrial premature contractions. See *atrial premature complex.*

atrial premature depolarization (APD). See *atrial premature complex.*

atrial recharge pulse. See *superfast atrial recharge pulse.*

atrial refractory extension. See *postventricular atrial refractory period extension.*

atrial refractory interval. See *atrial refractory period.*

atrial refractory period (ARP). In pacing, an interval of the atrial channel timing cycle during which the atrial sensing amplifier is designed to be unresponsive to input signals. In some pacemakers, however, the sensing circuitry is alert for extraneous or noncardiac signals during a portion of the atrial refractory period. In single-chamber atrial pacing modes, the atrial refractory period occurs after a sensed or paced atrial event. In dual-chamber pacing modes, the atrial refractory period is synonymous with the postventricular atrial refractory period, that is, the atrial refractory period occurs after a sensed or paced ventricular event. The atrial refractory period is preset or programmable. A longer atrial refractory period decreases the likelihood that retrograde P waves will be sensed by the pacemaker, but this can limit upper rate responses in dual-chamber pacemakers. The atrial refractory period should not be confused with the total atrial refractory period or with the heart's intrinsic atrial refractory period. The atrial refractory period also is referred to as the atrial refractory interval (ARI). See also *total atrial refractory period.*

atrial relative refractory period. During atrial pacing, the longest S_1 to S_2 interval at which the S_2 to A_2 interval exceeds the S_1 to A_1 interval. See also *relative refractory period.*

atrial resynchronization. A pacing stimulation technique in which near simultaneous right and left atrial excitation is targeted. This can often be achieved with bifocal pacing in the right atrium, biatrial pacing, or pacing in the posterior (coronary sinus) or superior (Bachmann's bundle) interatrial site.

atrial sensed event (AS). An event that is recognized on the atrial sensing circuit as an intrinsic cardiac event arising from the atrium. Events that are extrinsic to the atrium, for example, QRS, paced ventricular event, T wave, electromagnetic interference, that are sensed on the atrial sensing circuit could mistakenly be recognized as an atrial sensed event.

atrial sensing. Ability of the pacemaker or implantable cardioverter-defibrillator to recognize and respond to electrical activity that is recognized on the atrial sensing circuit.

atrial standstill. An unusual situation in which there is atrial asystole and failure of either a junctional or a ventricular focus to activate the atrium retrogradely. See also *asystole, atrial asystole.*

atrial stimulation. Delivery of a pacemaker output pulse in the atrium or tissue adjacent to the atrium which results in depolarization of atrial tissue.

atrial stimulus. A pacemaker output pulse delivered in the atrium or tissue adjacent to the atrium, for example, delivered in the right or left atrium or coronary venous system.

atrial-synchronized pacing. See *P-wave synchronous pacing.*

atrial-synchronized ventricular-inhibited pacing mode (VDD). The pacing mode in which pacing occurs only in the ventricle, sensing occurs in both the atrium and the ventricle, and there is a dual mode of response, that is, ventricular pacing is triggered in response to sensed ventricular events.

atrial synchronous (P-tracking) pacing. Pacing in which sensing occurs in the atrium, and pacing occurs in the ventricle with a tracked mode of response. Intrinsic atrial activity is sensed, a programmable PV interval is initiated, and the ventricle is paced at the end of the PV interval. P-wave synchronous pacing maintains atrioventricular synchrony. Pacing modes capable of P-wave synchronous pacing include VDD, VDDR, DDD, and DDDR. See also *P-wave synchronous pacing, VDD*.

atrial systole. Contraction of the atria which may be initiated by an intrinsic or paced activity.

atrial tachycardia. An arrhythmia that arises from the atrium at a rate of 100 to 250 beats per minute. Atrial tachycardias may be due to abnormal automaticity, triggered activity, or reentry. Digitalis toxicity should be suspected in the setting of paroxysmal atrial tachycardia with atrioventricular block.

as myopotentials and electromagnetic interference. See also *AV block, triggered pacing*.

atrial-triggered rate-adaptive pacing mode (AATR). The single-chamber pacing mode in which pacing and sensing occur in the atrium, and the mode of response to sensed atrial events is triggered. The pacemaker also is capable of rate-adaptive pacing via a sensor that monitors some physiologic or nonphysiologic variable and adjusts the heart rate accordingly. See also *rate-adaptive pacing*.

atriofascicular fibers. Fibers that form a type of accessory pathway connecting the right atrium with the right bundle branch. These fibers exhibit atrioventricular nodal-like properties and participate in tachycardias. Although

Atrial Tachycardia

Spontaneous onset of atrial tachycardia. The first two complexes show sinus rhythm, and the last three show atrial tachycardia. Note change in atrial activation sequence and also change in atrial electrogram morphology from the mapping catheter, which is located at the site of tachycardia origin (RFDIST, radiofrequency ablation catheter—distal). The third complex shows fusion in the atrial electrogram recorded from the site of origin as tachycardia begins. RFPROX, radiofrequency ablation catheter—proximal.

atrial tracking. See *tracking*.

atrial tracking preference. Feature in some cardiac resynchronization therapy devices with defibrillation-cardioversion capabilities in which the postventricular atrial refractory period shortens at high rates to maintain atrial tracking and more hemodynamic pacing.

atrial-triggered pacing mode (AAT). The single-chamber pacing mode in which an atrial output pulse is delivered synchronously with each sensed P wave. Atrial-triggered pacing is used to avoid inhibition of an atrial output pulse in response to something other than a P wave sensed by the atrial sensing circuit, such

sometimes called Mahaim fibers, atriofascicular fibers are not the exact anatomical structures described by Mahaim. See also *Mahaim fiber*.

atriohisian fibers. Fibers that form a type of accessory pathway connecting the atrium with the His bundle, thus bypassing the atrioventricular node. These fibers are associated with a short PR interval and no prolongation of the PR or AH intervals of atrial premature complexes. Although these fibers have been described anatomically, their participation in tachycardias is controversial. Atrio-hisian fibers commonly are referred to as James fibers. See also *Lown-Ganong-Levine syndrome*.

atrioventricular. Pertaining to the atria and ventricles of the heart; commonly abbreviated AV. See also *antegrade conduction, AV node.*

atrioventicular accessory pathway. An aberrant, usually muscular, conduction pathway connecting atrium to ventricle and bypassing the atrioventricular node. These pathways cause preexcitation of a portion of the ventricle and may form one limb of reentrant arrhythmia also involving the atrioventricular node. Some atrioventricular accessory pathways exhibit atrioventricular nodal-type property (Mahaim fibers).

atrioventricular block. See *AV block.*

atrioventricular conduction. See *antegrade conduction.*

atrioventricular conduction axis. See *AV conduction axis.*

atrioventricular conduction system effective refractory period. See *AV conduction system effective refractory period.*

atrioventricular conduction system functional refractory period. See *AV conduction system functional refractory period.*

atrioventricular conduction system relative refractory period. See *AV conduction system relative refractory period.*

atrioventricular conduction time. See *AV conduction time.*

atrioventricular delay. See *AV interval.*

atrioventricular delay hysteresis. See *rate-variable AV interval.*

atrioventricular dissociation. See *AV dissociation.*

atrioventricular fibers. Fibers that form the most common type of accessory pathway that crosses the atrioventricular groove and connects the atria with the ventricles. Atrioventricular fibers participate in tachycardias and, when they conduct in the antegrade direction, may cause a delta wave on the surface electrocardiogram. Atrioventricular fibers also are referred to as Kent fibers. See also *accessory pathway, Kent fiber, Wolff-Parkinson-White syndrome.*

atrioventricular groove. A groove on the external surface of the heart, separating the atria from the ventricles. Portions of the atrioventricular groove are occupied by the major arteries and veins of the heart.

atrioventricular interval. See *AV interval.*

atrioventricular interval, differential. See *differential AV interval.*

atrioventricular interval, hysteresis. See *AV interval, hysteresis.*

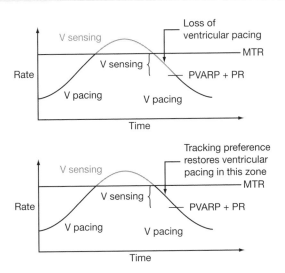

Atrial Tracking Preference

From Guidant Corporation [homepage on the Internet]. Natick (MA): Boston Scientific Corporation; c2006 [updated 2004 Jun; cited 2007 Jan 19]. CONTAK RENEWAL (trademark) TR: Cardiac Resynchronization Therapy Pacemaker. Available from: http://www.guidant.com/products/ProductTemplates/CRM/Contak_Renewal_TR.shtml. Used with permission.

atrioventricular interval optimization. See *AV interval optimization.*

atrioventricular interval, programming. Setting criteria for variations of atrioventricular timing. Many options exist including differential atrioventricular delay, positive atrioventricular hysteresis, negative atrioventricular hysteresis, and rate-adaptive atrioventricular interval.

atrioventricular interval, rate-adaptive. See *AV interval, rate-adaptive.*

are being paced or that the pacemaker has the capability to pace both chambers.

atrioventricular reentrant tachycardia (AVRT). See *AV reentrant tachycardia.*

atrioventricular sequential asynchronous (DOO) pacing. See *dual-chamber asynchronous pacing mode.*

atrioventricular sequential pacemaker (DVI) mode. See *AV sequential ventricular-inhibited pacing mode.*

atrioventricular synchrony. See *AV synchrony.*

Atypical AV Nodal Reentry

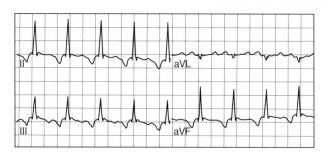

atrioventricular junction. Tissue capable of conducting electrical impulses from the atria to the ventricles. The atrioventricular junction is comprised of the atrioventricular node and the His bundle.

atrioventricular junction, ablation of. See *AV junction, ablation of.*

atrioventricular nodal bypass tract. See *AV nodal bypass tract.*

atrioventricular nodal conduction time. See *AV nodal conduction time.*

atrioventricular nodal disease. See *AV nodal disease.*

atrioventricular nodal effective refractory period. See *AV nodal effective refractory period.*

atrioventricular nodal functional refractory period. See *AV nodal functional refractory period.*

atrioventricular nodal reentrant tachycardia (AVNRT). See *AV nodal reentrant tachycardia.*

atrioventricular nodal reentry. See *AV nodal reentrant tachycardia.*

atrioventricular nodal relative refractory period. See *AV nodal relative refractory period.*

atrioventricular node. See *AV node.*

atrioventricular (AV) pacing. Generic term implying either that both atrium and ventricle

atrioverter. See *atrial defibrillator.*

atrium. One of the upper two chambers of the heart. Blood from the right and left atria passes into the respective right and left ventricles. In atrial pacing, the pacing lead is placed in contact with the right atrial endocardium or myocardium, and successful stimulation causes depolarization of both atria. The two atria together form one functional syncytium that is separate from the ventricular syncytium. The atrial and ventricular syncytia are connected both anatomically and physiologically by the atrioventricular conduction axis. Because of this connection, in patients with normal atrioventricular conduction, atrial pacing alone causes sequential contraction of the atria and the ventricles and closely mimics normal nonpaced cardiac contractions. See also *AV conduction axis, ventricle, ventricular myocardium.*

atropine. An anticholinergic drug that, by blocking the muscarinic receptors, increases the sinus rate and enhances atrioventricular nodal conduction. Atropine is used to treat sinus bradycardia, sinus arrest, or sinus node block. In electrophysiologic studies, atropine can be used to assess sinus node disorders and suspected hypervagotonia. Atropine has no significant effect on pacing thresholds.

Attain system. Trademark used for a system of guiding catheters, sheaths, and over-the-wire pacing leads to enable left ventricular stimulation (Medtronic, Inc., Minneapolis, Minnesota).

atypical atrial flutter. All macroreentrant tachycardias involving the atrium which are not dependent on the cavotricuspid isthmus. Common types are lower loop reentry, mitral isthmus flutter, and scar-related flutters.

atypical atrioventricular nodal reentry. See *atypical AV nodal reentry.*

atypical AV nodal reentry. A type of atrioventricular node reentrant tachycardia that utilizes the slow pathway of the atrioventricular node for retrograde conduction. The earliest site of atrial activation in this arrhythmia is in the region of the coronary sinus ostium, a feature that distinguishes this arrhythmia from typical atrioventricular node reentry, in which the earliest site is just behind the tendon of Todaro. Both long RP and short RP tachycardias can be the result of this arrhythmia circuit.

atypical AVNRT. See *atypical AV nodal reentry.*

audio transducer. A device that converts electrical impulses into sound. In pacing, audio transducers are used in some pulse generators to provide an audible tone, such as a beep, to confirm that specific programming functions have been completed successfully.

auto-adjusting sensitivity threshold. A programmable variable in implantable cardioverter-defibrillators for ventricular sensing in which the sensitivity threshold decreases over the duration of the cardiac cycle while maintaining a fixed signal gain.

AutoCapture. A trademark used for a pacemaker algorithm that assesses threshold and adjusts pacing output values accordingly. Designed to accommodate a patient's dynamic threshold changes without having to program a generous safety margin, thereby reducing the amount of energy the device uses. The interval at which the autocapture threshold is assessed varies by programming option selected and by manufacturer.

autodecrement. The automatic progressive shortening of the interval between paced impulses in a pacing burst or of the coupling interval of an extrastimulus that follows a drive train. Autodecremental delivery of programmed electrical stimuli sometimes is used in electrophysiologic testing and in antitachycardia pacemakers.

autodecremental pacing. A type of pacing used in electrophysiologic studies and in some antitachycardia pacemakers to terminate a tachycardia. When used in programmed electrical stimulation, the coupling interval of the extrastimulus is progressively reduced on each successive pacing drive, that is, the pacing rate is increased gradually as each successive cycle length is decreased by a small preset or programmable amount. In antitachycardia pacemakers and defibrillators, the cycle length of the pacing burst is progressively shortened and thus the pacing rate is increased gradually on each successive delivery.

autoincrement. The automatic progressive lengthening of the interval between paced impulses in a pacing burst or of the coupling interval of an extrastimulus that follows a drive train. Autoincremental delivery of programmed electrical stimuli is sometimes used in electrophysiologic testing and in antitachycardia pacemakers.

autoincremental pacing. A type of pacing used in electrophysiologic studies and in some antitachycardia pacemakers to terminate tachycardias. When used in programmed electrical

AutoCapture

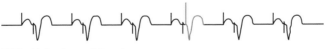

ECG with backup safety pulse

From St. Jude Medical [homepage on the Internet]. St. Paul (MN): St. Jude Medical, Inc.; c2007 [cited 2007 Jan 19]. Auto-Capture Pacing Systems. Available from: http://www.sjm.com/devices/device.aspx?name=AutoCapture%26%23153%3b+Pacing+Systems&location=us&type=1. Used with permission.

stimulation, the initial pacing rate is faster than the rate of the tachycardia, and the coupling interval of the extrastimulus is progressively lengthened on each successive pacing drive. Thus, the paced rate is decelerated gradually as each successive cycle length is increased by a small preset or programmable amount. In antitachycardia pacemakers and defibrillators, the cycle length of the pacing burst is increased progressively and thus the pacing rate is decreased gradually on each successive delivery.

automatic atrial tachycardia. A paroxysmal supraventricular tachycardia whose mechanism is enhanced automaticity of a group of atrial cells. Automatic atrial tachycardias may be chronic or transient. In electrophysiologic testing, an automatic atrial tachycardia may be suspected as the mechanism for the arrhythmia if an atrial premature beat does not predictably initiate or terminate the tachycardia. At their onset, these arrhythmias also generally demonstrate warm-up (a gradual acceleration of rate).

automatic capture verification. Monitoring every beat for the presence of an evoked response (the signal resulting from the electrical activation of the myocardium by a pacemaker stimulus).

automatic cardioverter-defibrillator analyzer. A noninvasive testing device that reveals the functional status, including power supply, of older models of the automatic implantable cardioverter-defibrillator. A magnet within the analyzer triggers the release of charge from the device into a capacitor. When the capacitor is fully charged, it unloads to a special test resistor. A progressive increase in the amount of time it takes for the capacitor to fully charge, normally 10 seconds or less, indicates battery depletion. The automatic cardioverter-defibrillator analyzer is not used with current models of implantable cardioverter-defibrillators.

automatic gain control (AGC). A feedback mechanism in which the gain of an amplifier can be adjusted automatically according to the sensed magnitude of the input or output signal in order to sense both small and large inputs without undersensing or oversensing. This allows the internal cardioverter-defibrillator to maintain adequate sensing during polymorphic ventricular tachycardia and during ventricular fibrillation (i.e., rhythms that may have marked variations in signal amplitude).

The input amplitude usually can be measured within the atrial refractory period, which determines the response time of the system.

automatic implantable cardioverter-defibrillator (AICD). A device designed to automatically detect an arrhythmia and deliver an electrical shock to terminate ventricular tachycardia or ventricular fibrillation. See also *implantable cardioverter-defibrillator*.

automatic implantable defibrillator (AID). A device designed to automatically detect ventricular tachycardias and deliver an electrical shock to defibrillate the heart. This was the earlier version of the automatic implantable cardioverter-defibrillator (AICD). See also *implantable cardioverter-defibrillator*.

automatic mode switching. See *mode switching*.

automatic output regulation. Automatic adjustment of a pacemaker's output (voltage amplitude or pulse duration) to result in the pacing output being set just above the measured threshold, ensuring the lowest energy level required for capture and thus optimizing device longevity.

automatic refractory period regulation. Automatic regulation of the refractory period, a potentially desirable feature for rate-adaptive pacemakers. As sensor-driven increases in pacing rate occur, unless the refractory period is shortened proportionally to the cycle length, the sensing channel will be refractory for an inappropriate duration of the total cycle length.

automatic rhythm. The rhythm generated by enhanced phase 4 depolarization in cells firing at a rate faster than the sinus node. In electrophysiologic studies, an automatic rhythm may be suspected when the application of programmed electrical stimuli does not predictably initiate or terminate a tachycardia. See also *depolarization*.

automatic sensitivity adjustment. In pacing, a feedback mechanism in which the reference level to the sensing system comparator is adjusted automatically in keeping with the measured amplitude of the input signal in order to avoid undersensing and oversensing. The input amplitude usually can be measured within the atrial refractory period, which determines the response time of the system. In the corresponding figure at the (*), a QRS is sensed, and sensitivity is lowered to prevent T-wave oversensing. The sensitivity progressively increases over the cardiac cycle to permit sensing of small-amplitude fibrillation wavelets, should they occur. Some defibrillators dynamically adjust the gain while maintaining a fixed sensitivity, with a similar effect on sensing cardiac events over time.

automatic stimulation threshold search. Measuring pacing thresholds on a regular basis to determine the output energy level requirement.

old generically could refer to a pacing or sensing threshold that was automatically determined.

autothreshold test. In pacing, an automatic sequential decrease in output (voltage, current, or pulse duration) for a specific number of cycles, the purpose of which is to determine the pacing threshold. The mechanism by which such a noninvasive test may be activated varies.

Automatic Sensitivity Adjustment

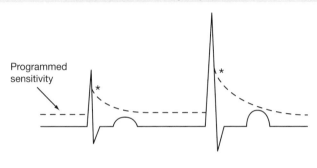

Programmed sensitivity

From Hayes DL, Lloyd MA, Friedman PA. Cardiac pacing and defibrillation: a clinical approach. Armonk: Futura Publishing Company, Inc; 2000. p. 347-451. Copyrighted and used with permission of Mayo Foundation for Medical Education and Research.

automaticity. See *intrinsic automaticity*.

autonomic disorder. A clinical abnormality of the neural network that innervates the heart, blood vessels, glands, smooth muscle, and viscera. The autonomic nervous system is subdivided into the sympathetic and parasympathetic nervous systems and controls many functions that are predominantly involuntary. There are many potential clinical manifestations of autonomic disorder which may result from overactivity or imbalance of either the sympathetic or the parasympathetic nervous system. Cardiac manifestations include tachyarrhythmias and bradyarrhythmias. See also *inappropriate sinus tachycardia, neurocardiogenic syncope, postural orthostatic tachycardia syndrome*.

autonomic nervous system (ANS). Anatomically and physiologically, the neural network that innervates the heart, blood vessels, glands, smooth muscle, and viscera. The autonomic nervous system is subdivided into the sympathetic and parasympathetic nervous systems and controls many functions that are predominantly involuntary. See also *parasympathetic nervous system, sympathetic nervous system*.

autothreshold. Automatic determination by the pulse generator of some threshold. Autothresh-

AV. Abbreviation for *atrioventricular*.

AV block. A delay or interruption of conduction along the normal conduction pathway from the atria to the ventricles. Atrioventricular block is classified as first-degree, second-degree (type I and type II), and third-degree (complete) block. See also *first-degree AV block, second-degree AV block, third-degree AV block*. •

AV conduction. See *antegrade conduction*.

AV conduction axis. The normal pathway that provides a connection between the atrial myocardium and the ventricular myocardium for the conduction of intrinsic electrical impulses. The atrioventricular axis consists of compact atrioventricular node, the transitional zone, and the His bundle. See also *AV node, His bundle, transition zone*.

AV conduction system effective refractory period. During atrial pacing, for a given drive cycle (S_1 to S_1), the longest A_1 to A_2 interval at which A_2 does not cause a ventricular depolarization. See also *effective refractory period*.

AV conduction system functional refractory period. During atrial pacing, for a given drive cycle (S_1 to S_1), the shortest V_1 to V_2 interval generated in response to an S_1 to S_2 interval. See also *functional refractory period*.

AV conduction system relative refractory period. During atrial pacing, for a given drive (S_1 to S_2), the longest A_1 to A_2 interval at which the A_2 to V_2 interval exceeds the A_1 to V_1 interval.

a portion of the total atrial refractory period. It is also referred to as the AV delay and is measured in milliseconds. See also *crosstalk sensing window*.

AV Block (High-Grade)

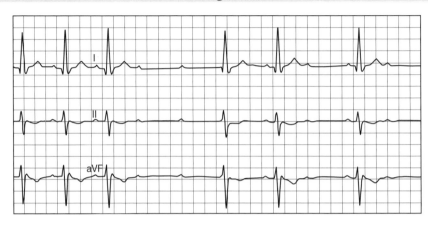

AV conduction time. The amount of time required for an impulse to propagate from the atria to the ventricles.

AV crosstalk. See *crosstalk*.

AVD. Abbreviation for *AV delay*.

AV delay (AVD). See *AV interval*.

AV dissociation. Independent rates and rhythms of the atria and ventricles. Atrioventricular dissociation occurs due to three general causes: 1) slowing of the sinus node rate to a degree such that a subsidiary pacemaker takes over but does not conduct back to the atria; 2) acceleration of a lower focus without retrograde conduction to the atria, such as in ventricular tachycardia; and 3) complete interruption of atrioventricular conduction, such as in third-degree atrioventricular block. Atrioventricular dissociation is not, in itself, a rhythm diagnosis.

AVI. Abbreviation for *AV interval*.

AVID. See *Antiarrhythmics Versus Implantable Defibrillators*.

AV interval (AVI). In a dual-chamber pacemaker timing cycle, the period between the initiation of the paced or sensed atrial event and the delivery of a consecutive ventricular output pulse. Depending on the preset or programmed pacing mode, the atrioventricular interval may be truncated if an intrinsic QRS complex is sensed before the interval has been completed. The atrioventricular interval is a programmable function in dual-chamber pacing systems and is

AV interval, differential. See *differential AV interval*.

AV interval hysteresis. A confusing term used synonymously with differential atrioventricular interval. See *differential AV interval, rate-variable AV interval*.

AV interval latency. An early term used to describe the differential atrioventricular interval. See also *differential AV interval*.

AV interval optimization. Determining the atrioventricular delay value that provides best (optimal) hemodynamic response. An optimized atrioventricular interval is one that allows complete filling of the ventricles and causes ventricular contraction to occur immediately after ventricular filling. It also may be defined as the shortest possible atrioventricular delay that allows complete ventricular filling. This delay thereby optimizes stroke volume and minimizes presystolic mitral regurgitation.

AV interval, rate-adaptive. Capability of some pacemakers to shorten the atrioventricular interval as the atrial rate increases, either by an increase in sinus rate or by a sensor-driven increase in paced rate. It is intended to mimic the normal physiologic decrease in the PR interval as the atrial rate increases.

AV junction, ablation of. See *AVN ablation*.

AVN. Abbreviation for *AV node*.

AVN ablation. Removal or destruction of the atrioventricular junction in order to control rapid ventricular response in atrial fibrillation; typically used when medications fail to manage ventricular response and resulting iatrogenic complete heart block requires permanent pacemaker implantation.

AV nodal blockade. Pharmacologic or nonpharmacologic intervention aimed at slowing ventricular rates during supraventricular arrhythmias. A commonly used strategy to control symptoms in patients with atrial fibrillation. It is contraindicated in patients with atrial fibrillation and antegradely conducting accessory pathways.

AV nodal bypass tract. An auxiliary rapid-conduction pathway through or around the atrioventricular node. Atrioventricular nodal bypass tracts reduce the total atrioventricular conduction time. The AH interval in a conduction system with atrioventricular nodal bypass tracts typically is 60 milliseconds or less and is prolonged minimally with atrial premature extrastimuli. See also *atriohisian fibers.*

AV nodal conduction time. The time that it takes for an impulse to traverse the atrioventricular node. This period is measured as the AH interval on an intracardiac electrogram. Variations from the normal adult atrioventricular nodal conduction time of 55 to 130 milliseconds may indicate conduction system disease in the atrioventricular node, or they may be the result of changes in autonomic tone. Changes in overall atrioventricular conduction time most commonly are due to changes in atrioventricular nodal conduction time. See also *AH interval.*

AV nodal disease. Any pathophysiologic process that affects the specialized atrioventricular nodal tissue and alters electrical conduction through the specialized conduction system.

AV nodal effective refractory period. In antegrade conduction, for a given cycle (A_1 to A_1), the longest A_1 to A_2 interval at which the response to A_2 does not propagate to the His bundle; in retrograde conduction, for a given cycle (H_1 to H_1), the longest H_1 to H_2 interval at which the response to H_2 does not propagate to the atrium. The atrioventricular nodal effective refractory period generally increases with shorter drive pacing cycle lengths. See also *effective refractory period.*

AV nodal functional refractory period. In antegrade conduction, the shortest H_1 to H_2 interval in response to an A_1 to A_2 interval; in retrograde conduction, the shortest A_1 to A_2 interval generated in response to an H_1 to H_2 interval. The atrioventricular nodal functional refractory period generally decreases with shorter drive pacing cycle lengths. See also *functional refractory period.*

AV nodal reentrant tachycardia (AVNRT). A supraventricular arrhythmia involving dual atrioventricular nodal pathways: a fast pathway and a slow pathway. The fast pathway has

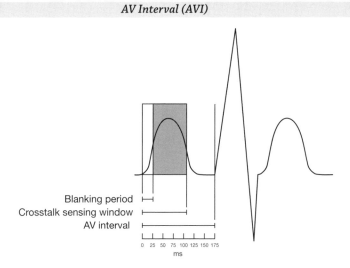

AV Interval (AVI)

Blanking period
Crosstalk sensing window
AV interval

0 25 50 75 100 125 150 175
ms

Modified from Hayes DL, Levine PA. Pacemaker timing cycles. In: Ellenbogen KA, editor. Cardiac pacing. Boston: Blackwell Scientific Publications; 1992. p. 263-308. Used with permission.

rapid conduction but a relatively long refractory period. The slow pathway has slow conduction but a short refractory period. Typical atrioventricular nodal reentrant tachycardia involves an impulse that travels to the His bundle via the fast pathway. In a less common form of atrioventricular nodal reentry, atypical atrioventricular nodal reentrant tachycardia, the direction of the circuit is reversed. In the corresponding figure, there is initiation of atrioventricular nodal reentrant tachycardia by a single atrial extrastimulus (S_2), following an atrial drive (S_1). Antegrade conduction occurs down the slow pathway (long AH), and retrograde conduction occurs up the fast pathway (short HA). HA, 90 milliseconds; VA, 50 milliseconds.

node, which transmits electrical signals from the atria to the ventricles, is capable of serving as the pacemaker of the heart. The node conducts impulses relatively slowly and accounts for the greatest delay in the transmission of impulses from the atria to the ventricles.

AVNRT. Abbreviation for *AV nodal reentrant tachycardia.*

AV/PV hysteresis. Programmable feature that automatically alters the duration of the atrioventricular interval on the basis of the presence or absence of intrinsic ventricular activity after the atrial event. See also *negative AV interval hysteresis, positive AV interval hysteresis.*

AV reentrant tachycardia (AVRT). An arrhythmia involving an accessory pathway. In orthodromic reciprocating tachycardia, impulses

AV Nodal Reentrant Tachycardia

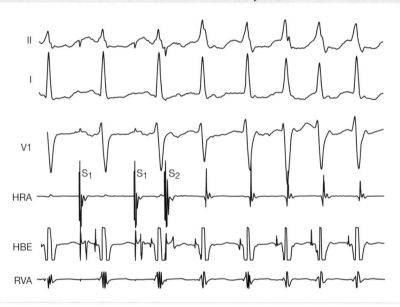

AV nodal relative refractory period. In antegrade conduction, the longest A_1 to A_2 interval at which the A_2 to H_2 interval exceeds the A_1 to H_1 interval; in retrograde conduction, the longest H_1 to H_2 interval at which the H_2 to A_2 interval exceeds the H_1 to A_1. The atrioventricular nodal relative refractory period generally increases with shorter drive pacing cycle lengths. See also *relative refractory period.*

AV node. A small concentration of specialized conductive tissue at the base of the atrial septum. If the sinus node fails, the atrioventricular

travel from the atria to the ventricles over the normal atrioventricular conduction system and return to the atria via the accessory pathway. In antidromic reciprocating tachycardia, impulses travel to the ventricles over the accessory pathway and return to the atria via the normal atrioventricular conduction system or via a second accessory pathway. See also *antidromic reciprocating tachycardia, orthodromic reciprocating tachycardia.*

AVRT. Abbreviation for *AV reentrant tachycardia.*

AV sequential dual-chamber inhibited pacing mode (DDI). A type of atrioventricular sequential pacing in which pacing occurs in both the atrium and the ventricle, sensing occurs in both chambers, and the mode of response to sensed events is inhibited. Sensed atrial activity inhibits the atrial output pulse but does not result in triggered ventricular pacing or "tracking." In DDI pacing, the timing cycle of each channel typically is controlled by the ventricular channel of the pacemaker to maintain a constant RV or VV interval. See also *AV sequential pacing*.

AV sequential pacing. Atrial pacing followed by a paced or sensed ventricular event. This pacing was used initially to describe the DVI pacing mode. However, this pacing also may occur with DDD and DDI pacing and the rate-adaptive counterparts of each (DVIR, DDDR, DDIR). See also *AV sequential ventricular-inhibited pacing mode (DVI), dual-chamber asynchronous pacing mode (DOO)*.

AV sequential ventricular-inhibited pacing mode (DVI). A type of atrioventricular sequential pacing in which pacing occurs in both the atrium and ventricle, sensing occurs only in the ventricle, and the mode of response to sensed events is inhibited. The DVI mode may demonstrate two types of response: committed and noncommitted. In committed DVI pacing, there is no sensing in the ventricle during the atrioventricular interval, whereas in noncommitted DVI pacing, there is ventricular sensing during the atrioventricular interval. See also *AV sequential pacing, committed DVI pacing, noncommitted DVI pacing*.

AV synchrony. Physiologically, the sequence of atrial depolarization by an appropriate PR interval and ventricular depolarization. In pacing, the PR interval is the preset or programmed atrioventricular interval. Maintenance of atrioventricular synchrony enhances cardiac output. Loss of atrioventricular synchrony may reduce cardiac output by 10% to 30%.

AV universal pacing. An early descriptive term used for DDD pacing. DDD pacing is not truly "universal" because it is not capable of restoring a physiologic conduction system in all patients.

a waves. Portion of a recording, such as a mitral flow velocity curve or pulmonary capillary wedge pressure tracing, that represents atrial contraction.

axillary vein. Large venous structure, representing a continuation of the basilic vein, that terminates beneath the clavicle at the outer border of the first rib.

axillary vein, thrombosis of. Occurrence of thrombus (asymptomatic or symptomatic) in the axillary vein. Axillary venous thrombosis may be due to many causes, but relative to device therapy it may occur as a result of the presence of one or more intravascular leads.

axillary venous approach in implantation. A transvenous approach for lead placement. The axillary vein is, by definition, extrathoracic. Therefore, the axillary puncture technique that is properly performed should not place the patient at risk for pneumothorax.

axillary puncture. See *axillary venous approach in implantation*.

azimilide. An antiarrhythmic agent with potassium channel blocking property, primarily with atrial effects. A potential treatment option for patients with atrial fibrillation.

azygos vein lead implantation. Use of the azygos vein typically draining the posterior mediastinum into the superior vena cava. Leads placed in this site may be used for cardiac defibrillation.

b

Bachmann's bundle. A branch of the anterior internodal pathway. Bachmann's bundle traverses the interatrial septum and may aid in synchronizing the atria. See also *intra-atrial block*.

background potassium current. A potassium current that rectifies with membrane depolarization.

backup mode. A pacing mode that is automatically activated in some pacemakers when the pacing system is subjected to electromagnetic interference such as defibrillation or electrocautery, or when pacemaker component malfunction occurs. See also *backup pacing*.

backup pacing. An independent secondary pacing system that provides protection in the event of pacemaker component malfunction or exposure of the pacemaker to electromagnetic interference such as defibrillation or electrocautery. The backup system is driven by an independent pacing circuit that usually functions in an asynchronous mode with a high output. Backup pacing also is used to describe a VVI pacing system programmed to a relatively slow ventricular pacing rate for a patient with rare episodes of symptomatic bradycardia.

backup safety pulse. High-output pulse delivered to ensure capture after a failed capture attempt when output is lowered as part of an automatic capture or automatic threshold determination.

Bainbridge reflex. An automatically mediated reflex in which afferent nerves located in the right atrium can sense increased atrial pressure and stimulate the cardiovascular regulatory center to increase heart rate. See also *cardiovascular regulatory center, Marey's reflex, sympathetic nervous system*.

balloon-flotation lead. A temporary, endocardial passive fixation pacing lead with a distal-tip balloon that facilitates transvenous insertion and proper placement of the lead in the appropriate heart chamber. Balloon-flotation temporary pacing catheters can be placed with or without fluoroscopic guidance. See also *temporary lead*.

balloon venoplasty. Percutaneous procedure in which a balloon-tipped catheter is inserted into a stenosed vein and the vein is dilated with inflation of balloon. In procedures related to implantation of a permanent pacemaker, implantable cardioverter-defibrillator, or cardiac resynchronization device, venoplasty is sometimes performed to allow passage of the permanent transvenous lead.

ball-tip electrode. An endocardial lead-tip electrode configuration designed to provide a relatively small stimulation surface area to maximize electrical field strength. The ball-tip electrode is a small metal ball that protrudes from the distal end of some passive fixation leads. See also *electrical field strength*.

band-pass filter. A component of an electronic circuit that is designed to process a selected band of frequencies and to attenuate all others. In pacing, a band-pass filter modifies incoming signal characteristics by passing selected frequencies in the range of atrial or ventricular depolarizations. The appropriate frequency range selected for depolarization signals varies among pacemaker manufacturers and pacemaker models. Frequency is measured in hertz (Hz), and typical ranges for intracardiac signals are 20 to 40 Hz for P waves, 18 to 50 Hz for R waves, 0 to 10 Hz for T waves, and 7 to 25 Hz for premature ventricular contractions. •

baroceptor. See *baroreceptor*.

baroreceptor. One of many sensory nerve endings that are stimulated by changes in pressure and are found primarily in the walls of blood vessels. Baroreceptors also are called pressoreceptors. See also *aortic bodies, carotid body, chemoreceptor*.

baroreflex. One of a number of autonomic reflexes, such as slowing of the heart rate in response to an increase in blood pressure. Baroreflex sensitivity is a marker of vagal tone. Diminished baroreflex sensitivity seems to be associated with an increased risk of sudden cardiac death after myocardial infarction. See also *Bainbridge reflex, Marey's reflex*.

barotrauma in direct-current ablation. Direct-current energy used to ablate arrhythmogenic substrate that so often is associated with pressure-related collateral trauma.

basal mechanical dyssynchrony. Dyssynchronous movement of the basal segments of the left ventricle, usually comparing the septal and lateral segments.

Setting the Pace in Rhythm Management: Global Leadership in Medical Technology. Available from: http://www.medscape.com/infosite/sjm/sjm-settingpace).

basic interval. A specific timing interval that refers to the most basic or fundamental portion of the timing cycle. For example, in a VVI pacemaker the basic interval is "V to V", in an AAI

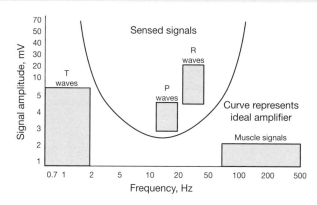

Band-Pass Filter

Modified from Kay GN. Basic aspects of cardiac pacing. In: Ellenbogen KA, editor. Cardiac pacing. Boston: Blackwell Scientific Publications; 1992. p. 32-119. Used with permission.

baseline. A zero-voltage horizontal reference line on graphic representations such as oscilloscopic tracings. The baseline is used in electrocardiogram and intracardiac electrogram analysis to interpret the amplitude of waveforms such as intrinsic cardiac depolarizations.

baseline electrophysiologic study. The initial electrophysiologic study, performed in the drug-free state. The baseline electrophysiologic study also is known as the control electrophysiologic study.

base rate. Generally used to refer to programmed lower rate.

base rate behavior. Function of the pacemaker at the programmed lower (base) rate. Slight variations in the programmed lower rate may occur as a result of specific ventricular-based timing systems.

Base Rest Rate Elevation for Apnea Therapy (BREATHE). This multicenter study evaluated the effects of high heart rate pacing for treating sleep apnea (closed to enrollment) (Medscape [homepage on the Internet]; St. Jude Medical. New York: Medscape [cited 2006 Dec 25].

pacemaker the basic interval is "A to A", and in a dual-chamber pacemaker the basic rate defines the programmed lower rate limit.

basic pacing rate interval. See *base rate*.

basic sinus cycle length. The length of time between one complete cardiac cycle and the next consecutive cardiac cycle of the intrinsic sinus rhythm, that is, the cycle length of the intrinsic sinus rhythm.

basket catheter. Method of electrical mapping with multiple electrodes placed collinearly in a basketlike fashion. This configuration allows mapping with only a few beats of arrhythmia.

batch programming. The capability to program more than one programmable variable simultaneously, as do all contemporary programmers.

battery. One or more power source cells that produce electrical energy. A battery consists of a negative pole (cathode), a positive pole (anode), and an electrolyte through which electrically charged particles are transported. The chemical interaction between the anode and cathode causes current flow through an external circuit. In most modern pacemaker batteries, the anode is lithium and the cathode usually is cupric sulfide or lithium iodide. Such batteries often are referred to as lithium batteries. See also *lithium-cupric sulfide, lithium iodide, silver-vanadium cell chemistry, zinc-mercuric oxide*.

battery capacity. The capability of a battery to store a charge and the quantity of electric current that a battery can deliver under specified conditions. Battery capacity is expressed in ampere-hours, or sometimes in joules. Battery capacity varies as a function of battery chemistry, size, and design. See also *battery status, deliverable battery capacity, maximum available battery capacity, theoretical battery capacity*.

battery current drain. See *current drain*.

battery depletion. A decrease in the deliverable capacity of a battery, that is, the remaining deliverable charge and its associated voltage when the battery is nearly depleted. In pacing, battery depletion is significant when the energy delivered decreases to a level that may impair pacemaker function. See also *battery status, elective replacement indicator, end of life*.

battery impedance. Opposition to the current flow within a battery. Battery impedance varies depending on battery chemistry. In some chemistries, the battery impedance increases over the life of the battery and limits the available battery voltage and current. Battery impedance also is known as cell impedance.

battery life. The projected longevity of a battery. Battery life is affected by many variables, including programmed output values, impedance, and percentage pacing.

battery longevity. See *battery life*.

battery status. A relative measurement of battery voltage. In pacing, battery status is nominally determined by application of a magnet to the pacemaker and measurement of the magnet rate or pulse duration. When specific rate or pulse duration changes established by the manufacturer are observed, the pacemaker should be replaced. In some pacemakers and implantable cardioverter-defibrillators, battery status may be included in the information transmitted from the device during real-time telemetry. See also *battery capacity, battery depletion, end of life*.

baud. A measurement of communication speed. A baud is a specific amount of digital data transmitted over a given time. One baud is equal to the number of code elements (pulses and spaces) transmitted per second. In pacing, baud may be used as a measurement of the amount of information transmitted during programming or telemetry.

Bayes' theorem. Theorem that elucidates the importance of the likelihood of disease in a given population in understanding the utility of a given test.

Bazett's formula. Formula attempting to normalize QT interval over varying heart rates: corrected QTc interval is equal to $QT/\sqrt{R-R}$.

BBB. Abbreviation for *bundle branch block*.

BBR. Abbreviation for *bundle branch reentry*.

BCL. Abbreviation for *burst cycle length*.

beats per minute (bpm). A unit of measure of the heart rate expressed as the number of cardiac contractions in 60-seconds. The number of beats per minute is equal to 60,000 divided by the cycle length in milliseconds. See also *pulses per minute*.

beat-to-beat gain adjustment. Changes in sensitivity gain on a beat-by-beat basis to maximize sensing of low-amplitude signals that occur randomly.

beat-to-beat heart rate variability. Method of analyzing heart rate variability as a marker of autonomic tone.

beeper. An audio annunciator used in some implantable cardioverter-defibrillators to signal charging or other conditions. See also *annunciator*.

beepergram. An older term that was specific to one of the earlier implantable cardioverter-defibrillators that had an audio output mode that represented sensed events.

beginning of life (BOL). In pacing, the predicted voltage and charge capacity of a pacemaker battery at the time of implantation. The battery capacity at the beginning of life is the deliverable portion of battery capacity. The longevity prediction for a battery at the beginning of life is calculated from the average battery self-discharge losses, pacing rates, and pacing modes, which together determine the current drain. In some pacemakers, a magnet placed over the pacemaker causes asynchronous pacing at a preset rate at the beginning of life. A decrease in rate is apparent as the battery status changes. See also *elective replacement indicator, end of life*.

BELIEVE. See *Bi vs Left Ventricular Pacing: an International Pilot Evaluation on Heart Failure Patients With Ventricular Arrhythmias*.

benign vasovagal syncope. See *neurocardiogenic syncope*.

BEST-ICD. See *Beta-Blocker Strategy Plus Implantable Cardioverter-Defibrillator*.

β-adrenergic blocking drugs. Class II antiarrhythmic drugs that block β-adrenergic receptors. β-Blockers may be $β_1$-selective and may have intrinsic sympathomimetic activity. Aside from blunting sympathetic activity, these drugs generally increase atrioventricular nodal refractoriness. They have little other direct electrophysiologic effect at therapeutic concentrations. β-Blockers decrease heart rate, reduce the force of cardiac contractions, and lower blood pressure. They are used to treat angina, hypertension, and arrhythmias. Side effects of β-adrenergic blocking drugs include bradycardias, congestive heart failure, exacerbation of asthma, depression, nightmares, fatigue, impotence, blunted response to hypoglycemia in diabetics, and Raynaud's phenomenon. See also *antiarrhythmic agent*.

was a multicenter, prospective, randomized trial to evaluate the usefulness of an electrophysiologic study-guided/implantable cardioverter-defibrillator strategy in patients at high risk of sudden death early after myocardial infarction. The BEST-ICD trial found that despite optimal therapy, mortality remains significant in high-risk patients after myocardial infarction. Although there was a trend in favor of electrophysiologic study-guided/implantable cardioverter-defibrillator, the data were insufficient to show a survival benefit of this strategy early after myocardial infarction (Raviele A, Bongiorni MG, Brignole M, Cappato R, Capucci A, Gaita F, et al, BEST + ICD Trial Investigators. Early EPS/ICD strategy in survivors of acute myocardial infarction with severe left ventricular dysfunction on optimal beta-blocker treatment: the BEta-blocker STrategy plus ICD trial. Europace. 2005;7:327-37).

Bezold-Jarisch reflex. A normal reflex caused by activation of myocardial mechanoreceptors

β-Adrenergic Blocking Drugs

Intrinsic sympatho-mimetic activity	Agent		
	Cardioselective	Noncardioselective	With α-blocking activity
Yes	Acebutolol	Alprenolol	Bucindolol
		Carteolol	Labetalol
		Oxprenolol	
		Penbutolol	
		Pindolol	
No	Atenolol	Nadolol	
	Betaxolol	Propranolol	
	Esmolol	Sotalol	
	Metoprolol	Timolol	

β-adrenergic receptor. A sympathetic nervous system cellular receptor that may be stimulated by norepinephrine or epinephrine. β-Adrenergic receptors are subdivided into $β_1$ and $β_2$ subtypes. Stimulation of $β_1$ receptors leads to increased sinus rate, increased conduction velocity, and shortening of refractoriness in the atrioventricular node, His-Purkinje tissue, and accessory pathways. $β_1$-stimulation also causes increased automaticity in His-Purkinje tissue. One of the effects of $β_2$-receptor stimulation is relaxation of smooth muscle, which leads to vasodilatation.

β-blockade. See *β-adrenergic blocking drugs*.

β-blocker. See *β-adrenergic blocking drugs*.

Beta-Blocker Strategy Plus Implantable Cardioverter-Defibrillator (BEST-ICD). This

that transmit vagal afferent impulses via C fibers. This causes withdrawal of efferent sympathetic activity to peripheral blood vessels, which leads to hypotension, and an increase in efferent vagal output, which leads to bradycardia. The Bezold-Jarisch reflex is thought to be a major cause of vasodepressor syncope.

biatrial linear ablation. Method of ablating in both atria with ablation lines anchored at electrically inert sites, scars, or other ablation lines. Method of ablation to treat atypical atrial flutters or atrial fibrillation.

biatrial pacing. Nonspecific term to signify pacing the atria in two sites. It is most commonly used to designate pacing the right atrium from two simultaneous sites. However, it could also refer to pacing right and left atria or multisite epicardial pacing.

Biatrial Pacing

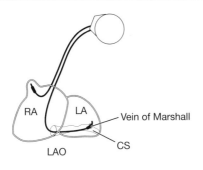

CS, coronary sinus; LA, left atrium;
LAO, left anterior oblique; RA, right atrium.

bidirectional programming. A pacemaker-programmer interaction in which commands are transmitted from the programmer to the pacemaker and information is transmitted from the pacemaker to the programmer, as in telemetry.

bidirectional shock. A defibrillation shock configuration in which two phases, typically of the same polarity, are delivered in quick succession via two different path or lead pathways. See also *sequential shock.*

bidirectional telemetry. The transmission of encoded signals between two electronic units. Most pacing systems use radiofrequency signals to telemeter information from the pulse generator back to the programmer to confirm correct transmission of programming. See also *bidirectional programming, telemetry.*

bidirectional ventricular tachycardia. A form of ventricular tachycardia with a right bundle branch block morphology and with the axis shifting on every other complex from a left anterior fascicular block pattern to a left posterior fascicular block pattern. Bidirectional ventricular tachycardia usually is associated with digitalis toxicity.

bidisomide. An investigational antiarrhythmic drug that is said to have class IA and class IB antiarrhythmic effects. Side effects include possible increase of liver enzyme values and, as with other drugs that prolong repolarization, lengthening of the QT interval.

bidomain model. Mathematical model of cardiac

tissue conduction that takes into account cardiac anisotropic properties. See also *anisotropy.*

bifascicular block. A delay or interruption in conduction through two of the three divisions of the bundle branches, such as right bundle branch block with left anterior fascicular block.

bifocal pacing. Pacing from two sites or foci.

bifurcated bipolar lead. An older type of bipolar pacing lead in which the proximal end of the lead is divided into two branches. One of the lead terminal pins completes the circuit between the pacemaker and the distal-tip negative electrode (cathode); this pin is marked with a white band or the word *distal.* The other lead terminal pin completes the circuit between the pacemaker and the proximal-ring positive electrode (anode). The bifurcated bipolar lead terminal pins were inserted into two separate pacemaker header apertures to ensure alignment between the lead terminal pin electrodes and the pacemaker circuitry. See also *bipolar lead, coaxial lead.* See the figure *Bipolar leads.*

bigeminy. Coupling of an atrial, junctional, or ventricular premature complex to every beat of the dominant rhythm such that every other beat is premature, for example, coupling of a QRS complex and a premature ventricular contraction. In pacing, bigeminy may occur with the coupling of a paced beat and an intrinsic cardiac depolarization.

bin. In relation to device therapy, this refers to a single rate "spread" within a rate histogram, such as 60 to 69 beats per minute. In the figure shown, each bin is represented by a bar of the graph and indicates the percentage of beats that occurred within each rate spread of 10 beats per minute. •

binary code. A communication code based on the binary number system, which uses only the digits 0 and 1. The binary code is used in all digital computers to represent, store, and process information. In pulse generators, binary codes can be the basis for communication from an external noninvasive programmer to an implanted pacemaker. The codes are transmitted via pulsed magnetic fields or pulsed radiofrequency signals. The use of binary codes allow more information to be transferred in a relatively small number of pulses than would be possible with a pulse count code.

binary counter. A device used to record or count

binary codes. Binary counters in pulse generator circuitry are used to count sequential events such as timing circuit cycles and tachycardia beats. See also *binary code*.

binding potential. Electrical potential at which optimal chemical binding occurs. Changes in binding potential are used to indicate alteration in transmitter levels in response to electrical stimulation.

biphasic. Description of energy delivery or measured current that has both a positive and a negative component. Either component may occur first, and each component may have a different amplitude or duration of energy delivery.

biphasic waveform. A waveform configuration in which signal polarity reverses such that it has consecutive positive and negative components. In pacing, biphasic output signals are used for

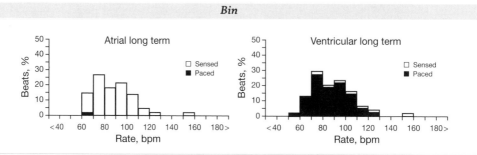

Bin

biocompatible material. A material that, when used in biologic systems, is not subject to rejection, induces little or no inflammation in tissue, and is noncarcinogenic. Biocompatible materials such as titanium, platinum-iridium, silicone elastomer, and polyurethane are used in pacing systems. See also *platinum-iridium, polyurethane, silicone elastomer, titanium*.

biodegradation. The breakdown in structure or reduction in chemical composition of materials used in biologic systems. Biodegradation can be a desirable feature in materials such as absorbable sutures, or an undesirable feature in materials such as lead insulation.

biofeedback. The use of output information from a biologic system as input back into the system to control its function(s). Biofeedback is the underlying principle in closed-loop pacing systems that, for example, monitor heart rate, respiratory rate, or other physiologic variables and then use the acquired information to automatically adjust pacing variables such as heart rate. See also *closed-loop control system*.

biogalvanic batteries. Battery system in which the anode and cathode act as fuel and are consumed in the electrolytic process, with implanted tissue serving as electrolytes and at times depolarizer.

BIOPACE. See *Biventricular Pacing for Atrioventricular Block to Prevent Cardiac Desynchronization*.

equal charge and discharge throughout the tissue to allow faster recovery of the pacemaker sensing circuit. The improved recovery time provides capability for improved noise sensing and for shorter refractory periods. In defibrillation, the biphasic waveform typically is asymmetric, with a ratio such as 60:40. In an implantable cardioverter-defibrillator with a one-capacitor circuit, the leading edge of phase 2 is equal to the trailing edge of phase 1; however, this is not true in a two-capacitor circuit. Biphasic shock waveforms frequently reduce the energy required for defibrillation compared with monophasic waveforms. The biphasic configuration may become the standard for defibrillation.

biplane coronary venography. Obtaining angiographic images of the coronary venous system by simultaneously imaging in two planes.

biplane Simpson's equation. Equation that allows volume calculations when two-dimensional axes measurements are known.

bipolar electrode system. An electrical system with two poles. In a bipolar pacing system, the two electrodes (anode and cathode) are external to the pacemaker case and are located in proximity to each other on the distal portion of the pacing lead. Bipolar pacing systems are less susceptible to myopotential inhibition and electromagnetic interference than unipolar systems. See also *bipolar lead, electrode configuration, unipolar electrode system*.

Bipolar Electrode System

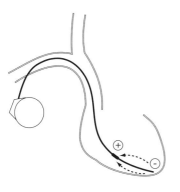

bipolar lead. A lead with two electrical poles. The stimulating cathode typically is located at the distal tip of the endocardial lead. The anode is a metal ring encircling the lead several millimeters proximal to the lead tip. Both electrodes must be placed in the chamber of the heart that is to be paced or sensed. Current bipolar pacing leads have an in-line design and older bipolar leads were bifurcated. See also *bifurcated bipolar lead, bipolar electrode system, in-line bipolar lead, unipolar electrode system, unipolar lead.*

be simultaneous, or there may be offset with either left or right ventricular stimulation first followed by stimulation in the other ventricle.

Biventricular Pacing for Atrioventricular Block to Prevent Cardiac Desynchronization (BIOPACE). This is a trial to evaluate whether patients with a standard pacing indication will benefit from biventricular pacing for the prevention of left ventricular remodeling. Patients must have an indication for pacing but no specific left ventricular ejection fraction or QRS duration. End points include patient survival time, 6-minute hall walk, and quality-of-life (Funck RC, Blanc J-J, Mueller H-H, Schade-Brittinger C, Bailleul C, Maisch B, BioPace Study Group. Biventricular stimulation to prevent cardiac desynchronization: rationale, design, and endpoints of the 'Biventricular Pacing for Atrioventricular Block to Prevent Cardiac Desynchronization [BioPace]' study. Europace. 2006;8:629-35).

biventricular sensing. Sensing in both the right and the left ventricle.

biventricular trigger. When an event is sensed by the right ventricular lead, either a conducted beat or a premature ventricular contraction,

Bipolar Leads

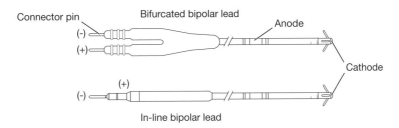

Connector pin — Bifurcated bipolar lead — Anode — Cathode — In-line bipolar lead

bipolar-to-bipolar adapter. A connector that allows two bipolar leads to be connected.

bipolar-to-bipolar Y adapter. An adaptor that allows two bipolar leads to be adapted into a single bipolar lead.

bit. In computer systems, an acronym for *binary digit*. A bit is the smallest unit of information that can be recognized by a computer, and it can have only two possible values: the digits 0 or 1. Bits make up the binary code used in noninvasive pacemaker programming and telemetry. See also *binary code.*

biventricular pacing. Stimulation of both the right and the left ventricle. Stimulation may

both ventricles are paced immediately after the event in an effort to promote synchronization. This is a "triggered" mechanism, like that of VVT pacing mode. This has also been termed "ventricular sense response."

Biventricular Versus Left Univentricular Pacing With Implantable Cardioverter-Defibrillator Back-Up in Heart Failure Patients (B-LEFT-HF). This is a prospective, randomized, double-blind parallel study that compares optimized biventricular pacing to only left ventricular pacing (Leclercq C, Ansalone G, Gadler F, Boriani G, Perez-Castellano N, Grubb N, et al, B-LEFT HF Investigators. Biventricular vs. left univentricular pacing in heart failure: rationale, design, and endpoints of the B-LEFT HF study. Europace. 2006;8:76-80).

Biventricular Versus Right Ventricular Pacing in Heart Failure Patients With Atrioventricular Block (BLOCK-HF). This trial includes patients in New York Heart Association class I, II, or III heart failure with advanced atrioventricular block and left ventricular ejection fraction of 45% or less who are not currently indicated for cardiac resynchronization therapy. The objective is to assess whether biventricular pacing limits the clinical progression of heart failure when compared with atrial synchronous right ventricular pacing. The primary end point is a composite of mortality, morbidity, and cardiac function (ClinicalTrials.gov [homepage on the Internet]. Bethesda: U.S. Department of Health and Human Services National Institutes of Health [updated 2006 Oct 16; cited 2006 Dec 25]. Biventricular Versus Right Ventricular Pacing in Heart Failure Patients With Atrioventricular Block [BLOCK HF]. Available from: http://www.clinicaltrials.gov/ct/show/NCT00267098).

Bi vs Left Ventricular Pacing: an International Pilot Evaluation on Heart Failure Patients With Ventricular Arrhythmias (BELIEVE). This was a randomized pilot study of biventricular and left ventricular pacing which included patients with an ejection fraction less than 35%, left ventricular end-diastolic dimension more than 55 mm, and QRS more than 130 milliseconds. The primary end points were echo indices (left ventricular ejection fraction, left atrial and left ventricular dimensions, interventricular mechanical delay, and Doppler measurements) and freedom from device complications (Gasparini M, Bocchiardo M, Lunati M, Ravazzi PA, Santini M, Zardini M, et al, BELIEVE Investigators. Comparison of 1-year effects of left ventricular and biventricular pacing in patients with heart failure who have ventricular arrhythmias and left bundle-branch block: the Bi vs Left Ventricular Pacing: an International Pilot Evaluation on Heart Failure Patients with Ventricular Arrhythmias [BELIEVE] multicenter prospective randomized pilot study. Am Heart J. 2006;152:155.e1-7).

blanking. See *blanking period*.

blanking period. The temporary disabling of pacemaker sensing amplifiers after the delivery of an output pulse. The blanking period prevents inappropriate sensing of residual energy from the pacemaker output pulse and, in dual-chamber pacemakers, prevents sensing of pacemaker output pulses or intrinsic events in the chamber other than that in which the event occurred. For example, in dual-chamber pacing, blanking prevents sensing in the ventricle of an output pulse delivered to the atrium. The duration of the blanking period is usually programmable. See also *crosstalk, ventricular blanking period*.

B-LEFT-HF. See *Biventricular Versus Left Univentricular Pacing With Implantable Cardioverter-Defibrillator Back-Up in Heart Failure Patients*.

blended sensor. A rate-adaptive sensor that combines more than one, normally two, sensor technologies. Examples include 1) accelerometer and minute ventilation and 2) accelerometer and stimulus-T (QT) interval sensor.

blind subclavian puncture. See *subclavian puncture*.

BLOCK-HF. See *Biventricular Versus Right Ventricular Pacing in Heart Failure Patients With Atrioventricular Block*.

block response. An upper rate response in some dual-chamber pacemakers that occurs when the rate of intrinsic atrial activity exceeds the maximal tracking rate of the pacemaker. The interval between consecutive P waves is shorter than the total atrial refractory period. As a consequence, some of the P waves fall into the total atrial refractory period and are not sensed. Ventricular pulses occur only after sensed P waves, and a blocked response results. The apparent degree of block, such as 4:3, 3:2, 2:1, depends on the maximal tracking rate of the ventricular channel and the intrinsic atrial rate. The maximal tracking rate interval of the blocked response is equal to the total atrial refractory period. See also *maximum tracking rate, maximum tracking rate interval, pseudo-Wenckebach response, total atrial refractory period, 2:1 block response, upper rate response, variable block response*.

blood temperature sensors. Rate-adaptive sensor used clinically in the past which achieved rate-adaptive pacing by adjusting heart rate based on changes of temperature measurements made via a temperature sensor incorporated in the pacing lead.

BNP. Abbreviation for *B-type natriuretic peptide*.

body motion sensing. The use of a piezoelectric

crystal or accelerometer to measure the acceleration of certain muscle groups or body parts and the extent of body activity. In pacing, sensed body motion may be used to produce a proportionate change in pacing rate. See also *accelerometer, piezoelectric crystal*.

body surface mapping. An investigational technique using more than 100 electrodes on the skin to analyze changes in electrical potential throughout the cardiac cycle.

BOL. Abbreviation for *beginning of life* of a pulse generator battery.

Boltzmann's constant. Physical constant that relates the energy of a molecule to its absolute temperature. Important in current/potential calculations with semiconductors.

Boltzmann's relations. See *Boltzmann's constant*.

boot. In pacing, a silicone rubber cover that may be placed over the pacemaker case at the time of implantation to prevent local muscle stimulation around the pacemaker pocket or to minimize myopotential inhibition. A boot is rarely required with contemporary pulse generators.

Borrelia burgdorferi. The organism responsible for Lyme disease, which may cause atrioventricular block.

BPEG. Abbreviation for *British Pacing and Electrophysiology Group*.

BPG. See *BPEG*.

bpm. Beats per minute.

bradyarrhythmia. See *bradycardia*.

bradyasystolic arrest. Bradycardia as a result of asystole.

bradycardia. A slow heart rate, that is, a heart rate that has declined to a level physiologically inappropriate for the patient's age, condition, or activity level. Although bradycardia is traditionally defined as a rate less than 60 beats per minute, an absolute value may not be appropriate for an individual patient.

bradycardia pacing. Cardiac stimulation for the purpose of treating a clinically significant bradycardia.

bradycardia-tachycardia syndrome. A syndrome affecting the electrical conduction system of the heart, specifically, the sinus node and sometimes the atrioventricular node. Atrial tachycardias, most often atrial fibrillation, often are associated with sinus bradycardia or sinus arrest when they terminate. Bradycardia-tachycardia syndrome also is known as sick sinus syndrome and tachycardia-bradycardia syndrome. See also *sinus node dysfunction*.

brady-tachy syndrome. See *bradycardia-tachycardia syndrome*.

braided conductor. A pacing lead in which the conductor is composed partially or completely of multiple wires that are woven around a central conductor wire. See also *drawn-brazed strand*.

breakthrough site. The first site of ventricular endocardial activation. This is usually in the left ventricle either at the interventricular septum or in the anterior region.

BREATHE. See *Base Rest Rate Elevation for Apnea Therapy*.

bretylium. A class III antiarrhythmic drug that prolongs atrial and ventricular refractoriness without exerting any significant effect on atrioventricular nodal or accessory pathway tissue. Bretylium increases myocardial contractility and increases heart rate slightly. It is used predominantly to control refractory ventricular tachycardia or ventricular fibrillation. Bretylium depletes norepinephrine stores in sympathetic nerve terminals and may cause orthostatic hypotension. It also may initiate or accelerate ventricular arrhythmias.

British Pacing and Electrophysiology Group (BPEG). A specialty society of British physicians with an interest in pacing and electrophysiology; this group contributed to the NBG pacemaker code for antibradycardia, rate-adaptive, and antitachycardia devices. See also *NBG code*.

broad complex tachycardia. See *wide complex tachycardia*.

Brownlee code. A detailed system of letters developed to describe the actual operating modes of a pacemaker. The Brownlee code was intended to complement the original code of pacing nomenclature established by the Intersociety Commission of Heart Disease Resources (ICHD). It provided information on atrial and ventricular functions individually. The numerator indicated the functions of the atrial pacing channel, and the denominator indicated the functions of the ventricular pacing channel. The code was easy to visualize but difficult to verbalize in discussions on pacing modes and pacemaker function. See also *ICHD code, NBG code*.

Brugada syndrome. Inherited disorder associated with sudden death and syncope, often during sleep. Particularly common in Southeast Asian males and associated with a mutation in the *SCN5A* gene that codes for the cardiac sodium channel.

branch reentrant ventricular tachycardia is reported to be the mechanism for about one-third of the monomorphic sustained ventricular tachycardias occurring in patients with dilated

Brugada Syndrome

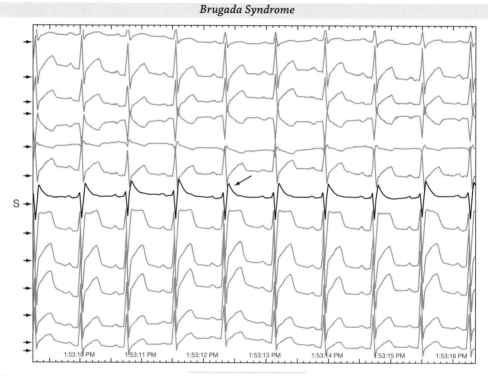

Electrocardiogram from a patient with Brugada syndrome, showing the characteristic abnormal ST segment in the chest leads, particularly V_1 and V_2.

B-type natriuretic peptide (BNP). A polypeptide (32–amino-acid sequence) secreted by the ventricular myocardium in response to excessive myocyte stretch. The levels of B-type natriuretic peptide are increased in patients with left ventricular dysfunction.

buddy wire. Second or third wire placed via a sheath into a cardiac vein or artery to enhance support for the primary wire or pacing lead.

bundle branch block (BBB). A delay or interruption of conduction through the right or left bundle branch which results in characteristic patterns of wide QRS complexes on an electrocardiogram. Bundle branch block may be physiologic or pathophysiologic.

bundle branch reentrant tachycardia. A form of ventricular tachycardia in which there is a succession of bundle branch reentrant complexes. His bundle deflections can be recorded preceding each ventricular depolarization. Bundle

cardiomyopathy. This form of ventricular tachycardia is cured easily by ablation of the right bundle branch. See also *bundle branch reentry*.

bundle branch reentry (BBR). A ventricular extrasystole that occurs when a spontaneous or stimulated premature ventricular complex blocks in the retrograde direction within the ipsilateral bundle branch, conducts across the interventricular septum, enters the contralateral bundle branch in the retrograde direction, and conducts back to the His bundle. The impulse then travels antegradely down the previously blocked ipsilateral bundle branch and activates the ventricles. The bundle branch reentrant complex typically has the same morphology as the initiating beat. A His bundle deflection can be recorded before the bundle branch reentrant complex.

bundle of His. See *His bundle*.
bundle of Kent. See *Kent fiber*.

burst cycle length (BCL). The specific cycle length at which burst pacing is performed.

burst duration. The duration during which a rapid sequence of pacing pulses is delivered by a pacemaker or defibrillator. See also *burst pacing, burst stimulation*.

burst pacing. The delivery of a train of pacing pulses by a pacemaker or defibrillator. Burst pacing may be delivered asynchronously or synchronously at a fixed, decreasing, or increasing cycle length. Antitachycardia pacemakers typically use burst pacing for treatment of supraventricular tachycardia, whereas antitachycardia defibrillators use burst pacing to terminate ventricular tachycardia. In some cases, burst pacing may disorganize or accelerate an arrhythmia instead of terminating it. Accordingly, antitachycardia pacemakers should not be used to treat ventricular tachycardia without an implanted cardioverter-defibrillator as a backup. In electrophysiologic testing, burst pacing may be used to induce tachycardias or to evaluate the effectiveness of pacing therapy. See also *burst stimulation*.

burst rate. The rate of the pacing train delivered by an antitachycardia pacemaker or defibrillator during an attempt to terminate a sensed tachycardia. See also *burst pacing, burst stimulation*.

burst scanning mechanism. In antitachycardia pacing, the automatic progressive shortening of the coupling intervals of the first impulse of each pacing burst delivered in a series of attempts to terminate a tachycardia. See also *autodecremental pacing, autoincremental pacing, burst pacing, coupling interval, scanning pacemaker, termination window*.

burst stimulation. The delivery of a rapid pacing train. In electrophysiologic testing, the use of burst stimulation is one method of arrhythmia induction. In antitachycardia pacing and defibrillation, burst stimulation is used to attempt to terminate an arrhythmia.

bypass tract. Abnormal connections other than the atrioventricular node capable of conducting current between atria and ventricles.

bypass tract-mediated macroreentrant tachycardia. Tachycardia circuits requiring atrial tissue, ventricular tissue, and an accessory bypass tract.

bypass tract-mediated supraventricular tachyarrhythmia. See *bypass tract-mediated macroreentrant tachycardia*.

Byrd dilator sheath. A type of sheath used for extraction of permanent transvenous pacing or defibrillation leads (Cook Medical, Inc., Bloomington, Indiana). Its product description is "A pair of long and moderately flexible cannulae, one fitting coaxially inside the other and capable of moving freely. The sheath set is advanced over the lead to break up fibrous adhesions. It also aids in 'countertraction' by stabilizing the heart wall when the lead tip is pulled out of the endocardial scar mass."

Byrd extraction technique. A technique used for extraction of chronically implanted pacing leads. The technique involves intravascular countertraction using a stylet locked inside the lead to reinforce the lead. Telescoping sheaths are advanced over the lead to free it from vascular scar tissue and to provide countertraction at the myocardium. See also *Cook Lead Extraction device*.

Byrd Workstation. Trademark for a set of equipment sometimes used for extraction techniques approached via the femoral vein (Cook Medical, Inc., Bloomington, Indiana). The company product description is "A 16 Fr sheath containing a coaxial 12 Fr inner sheath pre-loaded with a Dotter Helical Loop Basket and a Tip Deflecting Wire Guide." The pre-loaded cannula passes through the outer cannula to carry these two instruments, via the femoral vein, into the right atrium.

C. Abbreviation for *capacitor, carbon,* and *coulomb.*

CABG Patch trial. See *Coronary Artery Bypass Graft trial.*

cable properties. A passive property of cardiac cells whereby current flows more readily through the intracellular fluid and across the intercalated disks into adjacent cells than through the intracellular fluid and across the cell membrane into the extracellular fluid. Cardiac cells behave like an electrical cable that conducts electricity.

Cabrera's sign. Notching of more than 0.05 second in the ascending part of the S wave, usually in leads V_3 and V_4, signifying myocardial infarction despite the presence of left bundle branch block. Because right ventricular pacing results in left bundle branch block, this finding may be helpful in evaluating patients who have pacemakers.

CACAF. See *Catheter Ablation for Cure of Atrial Fibrillation.*

cadmium-nickel batteries. See *nickel-cadmium.*

CAEP. Abbreviation for *chronotropic assessment exercise protocol.*

calcium channel blockers. Any of a class of drugs that block the flow of calcium and thus may affect smooth muscle contraction of the heart. Some calcium blockers may slow conduction at the sinus node or the atrioventricular node.

calcium channels. Sarcolemmal passageways that allow calcium ions to flow across a cell membrane. Cardiac cells have two types of calcium channels: L and T. More is known about L-type calcium channels than about T-type calcium channels. L-type calcium channels are responsible for the slow inward current during phase 0; they maintain an inward current flow during phase 2, the plateau phase; they are blocked by verapamil, diltiazem, and the dihydropyridines (e.g., nifedipine); and they are stimulated by β-adrenergic agonists. T-type calcium channels may participate in the gradual spontaneous depolarization during phase 4 in cells possessing automaticity, and they are not affected by dihydropyridines or by β-adrenergic agonists.

calcium chloride. A calcium-containing compound that may reverse the effects of calcium channel blocking drugs. Calcium chloride increases muscle contractility, automaticity, and conduction of electrical impulses through the myocardium. It may cause hypotension, cardiac slowing, and hypercalcemia with bradycardia, arrhythmias, syncope, or cardiac arrest. Calcium chloride temporarily reverses the electrophysiologic effects of hyperkalemia. It may be dangerous in the setting of digitalis toxicity. Calcium chloride does not affect pacing thresholds directly, but it may allow capture that has been lost due to hyperkalemia.

calcium current. See I_{Ca-L}, I_{Ca-T}.

calcium pumps. Referring to one of several ionic pumps responsible for the diastolic clearance of cytosolic calcium. See also *calcium-sodium channels.*

calcium-sodium channels. Exchange pump that clears cytosolic calcium in exchange for sodium in a 3:2 ratio.

calibration waveform. In pacing, a square waveform that may be transmitted from some pacemakers via telemetered intracardiac electrograms. Calibration waveforms provide a reference from which the deflections of the intracardiac electrogram can be measured appropriately. See also *electrogram.*

CAMIAT. See *Canadian Amiodarone Myocardial Infarction Arrhythmia Trial.*

cAMP. Abbreviation for *cyclic adenosine monophosphate.*

can. The metal casing of the pulse generator. Usually made from titanium.

Canadian AF-CHF study. See *Atrial Fibrillation and Congestive Heart Failure trial.*

Canadian Amiodarone Myocardial Infarction Arrhythmia Trial (CAMIAT). A randomized, double-blind, placebo-controlled trial designed to assess the effect of amiodarone on the risk of resuscitated ventricular fibrillation or arrhythmic death among survivors of myocardial infarction with frequent or repetitive ventricular premature contractions (≥10 per hour or ≥1 run of ventricular tachycardia). Amiodarone reduces the incidence of ventricular fibrillation or arrhythmic death among survivors of acute myocardial infarction with frequent or repetitive ventricular premature contractions (Cairns JA, Connolly SJ, Roberts R, Gent M. Canadian Amiodarone Myocardial Infarction Arrhythmia Trial Investigators. Randomised trial of outcome after myocardial infarction in patients with frequent or repetitive ventricular premature depolarisations: CAMIAT. Lancet. 1997;349:675-82. Erratum in: Lancet. 1997;349:1776).

Canadian Implantable Defibrillator Study (CIDS). Patients with resuscitated ventricular fibrillation or ventricular tachycardia or with unmonitored syncope were randomized to receive an implantable cardioverter-defibrillator or amiodarone. The primary outcome measure was all-cause mortality, and the secondary outcome was arrhythmic death. A relative risk reduction of 20% occurred in all-cause mortality and a reduction of 33% occurred in arrhythmic mortality with implantable cardioverter-defibrillators compared with amiodarone; this reduction did not reach statistical significance (Connolly SJ, Gent M, Roberts RS, Dorian P, Green MS, Klein GJ, et al, CIDS Co-Investigators. Canadian Implantable Defibrillator Study [CIDS]: study design and organization. Am J Cardiol. 1993;72:103F-8F; Connolly SJ, Gent M, Roberts RS, Dorian P, Roy D, Sheldon RS, et al. Canadian implantable defibrillator study [CIDS]: a randomized trial of the implantable cardioverter defibrillator against amiodarone. Circulation. 2000;101:1297-302).

Canadian Trial of Atrial Fibrillation (CTAF). A prospective, multicenter trial to assess the effectiveness of low doses of amiodarone compared with sotalol or propafenone for preventing recurrent atrial fibrillation. The primary end point was the duration to a first recurrence of atrial fibrillation. Investigators concluded that amiodarone is more effective than sotalol or propafenone for the prevention of recurrences of atrial fibrillation. (Roy D, Talajic M, Dorian P, Connolly S, Eisenberg MJ, Green M, et al, Canadian Trial of Atrial Fibrillation Investigators. Amiodarone to prevent recurrence of atrial fibrillation. N Engl J Med. 2000;342:913-20).

Canadian Trial of Physiologic Pacing (CTOPP). Patients without chronic atrial fibrillation who were scheduled for a first implantation of a pacemaker to treat symptomatic bradycardia were eligible for enrollment and were randomized to receive either a ventricular pacemaker or a physiologic pacemaker. They were followed for an average of 3 years. The primary outcome was stroke or death due to cardiovascular causes. Secondary outcomes were death from any cause, atrial fibrillation, and hospitalization for heart failure. The trial concluded that physiologic pacing provides little benefit over ventricular pacing for the prevention of stroke or death due to cardiovascular causes. (Connolly SJ, Kerr CR, Gent M, Roberts RS, Yusuf S, Gillis AM, et al, Canadian Trial of Physiologic Pacing Investigators. Effects of physiologic pacing versus ventricular pacing on the risk of stroke and death due to cardiovascular causes. N Engl J Med. 2000;342:1385-91).

Candesartan in Heart Failure: Assessment of Reduction in Mortality and Morbidity (CHARM). This study examined the effect of candesartan (n=1,013) compared with placebo (n=1,015) in 2,028 patients with heart failure who were intolerant to angiotensin-converting enzyme inhibitors but were receiving other standard therapy for heart failure. The trial found that the use of candesartan resulted in a 23% (P<.001) relative risk reduction in cardiovascular death or heart failure hospitalization. The findings were independent of background therapy or ejection fraction (Frenk J, Sepulveda J, Gomez-Dantes O, Knaul F. Evidence-based health policy: three generations of reform in Mexico. Lancet. 2003;362:1667-71).

cannon _a_ waves. See _cannon waves_.

cannon waves. Large waves in the jugular venous pulse that occur when the right atrium contracts against a closed tricuspid valve. Cannon waves indicate a lack of atrioventricular synchrony or tricuspid stenosis. Cannon waves also are referred to as cannon _a_ waves and venous Corrigan waves.

capacitance. The property of a circuit element that allows it to store an electrical charge.

capacitive voltage doubler. A capacitor charge pump circuit that produces an output voltage that is twice the input voltage.

capacitor (C). An electronic circuit component that temporarily stores an electrical charge and blocks the flow of direct current or regulates the flow of alternating current. In pacemakers, capacitors receive energy from the power source (battery), store the energy until it is needed for a pacemaker output pulse, and then release the energy to the output circuit. In implantable cardioverter-defibrillators, large electrolytic capacitors are used to gather and store energy for defibrillation shocks.

capacitor maintenance. See *capacitor*.

captopril. A short-acting angiotensin-converting enzyme-inhibitor that blocks the formation of angiotensin in the kidneys, resulting in vasodilatation; used in the treatment of hypertension and congestive heart failure.

capture. In pacing, the depolarization and contradiction of the atria or ventricles in response to an electrical stimulus emitted by a pacemaker. One-to-one capture occurs when each electrical stimulus causes a corresponding depolarization and cardiac contraction. Loss of capture occurs when the voltage or current at the electrode-myocardial interface decreases below threshold. See also *stimulation threshold*.

capture threshold. See *pacing threshold*.

capture verification. The process of determining effective capture of a given cardiac chamber at a given output. Capture verification has been incorporated in several pacemakers.

carbon (C). A nonmetallic, corrosion-resistant, chemical element. In pacing, carbon may be used as an electrode material or, in thin filaments, as a lead conductor material.

cardiac action potential. See *action potential*.

cardiac activation sequence. See *activation sequence*.

cardiac arrest. A marked decrease in, or absence of, cardiac output due to ventricular tachycardia, ventricular fibrillation, or asystole. Cardiac arrest leads to death if not treated rapidly.

Cardiac Arrest Study Hamburg (CASH) trial. Randomized trial designed to compare the incidence of recurrence of cardiac arrest, sudden cardiac death, cardiac mortality, and total mortality in patients treated with antiarrhythmic drugs or an implantable cardioverter-defibrillator. The primary end point was total mortality. Device therapy was associated with a 23% (nonsignificant) reduction of all-cause mortality rates compared with treatment with amiodarone or metoprolol. The benefit of device therapy was more evident during the first 5 years after the index event (Kuck KH, Cappato R, Siebels J, Ruppel R. Randomized comparison of antiarrhythmic drug therapy with implantable defibrillators in patients resuscitated from cardiac arrest: the Cardiac Arrest Study Hamburg [CASH]. Circulation. 2000;102:748-54).

Cardiac Arrhythmia Suppression Trial (CAST). A multicenter trial that investigated the effect of treating asymptomatic complex ventricular ectopy after myocardial infarction. This study showed higher mortality rates in patients treated with encainide, flecainide, or moricizine than in patients given a placebo (Ruskin JN. The cardiac arrhythmia suppression trial [CAST]. N Engl J Med. 1989;321:386-8). See also *encainide, flecainide, moricizine*.

Cardiac Arrhythmia Suppression Trial II (CAST II). A randomized, double-blind, placebo-controlled study to determine whether the suppression of asymptomatic or mildly symptomatic arrhythmias after myocardial infarction, by moricizine, reduces the mortality rate. Patients were randomized to receive moricizine or placebo. The trial was stopped early because the first 2-week treatment period with moricizine was associated with excess mortality and morbidity (The Cardiac Arrhythmia Suppression Trial II Investigators. Effect of the antiarrhythmic agent moricizine on survival after myocardial infarction. N Engl J Med. 1992;327:227-33; Greene HL, Roden DM, Katz RJ, Woosley RL, Salerno DM, Henthorn RW. The Cardiac Arrhythmia Suppression Trial: first CAST ... then CAST-II. J Am Coll Cardiol. 1992;19:894-8; Brooks MM, Gorkin L, Schron EB, Wiklund I, Campion J, Ledingham RB. Moricizine and quality of life in the Cardiac Arrhythmia Suppression Trial II [CAST II]. Control Clin Trials. 1994;15:437-49).

Cardiac Compass. Registered trademark used for a graphic display of 14 months of a patient's clinical progress, including the total amount of atrial and ventricular pacing (Medtronic, Inc., Minneapolis, Minnesota). The intent of the information is to assist caregivers in managing device and drug therapy while monitoring disease progression. •

cardiac conduction system. The specialized conduction system of the heart, consisting of the sinus node, atrioventricular node, His bundle, bundle branches, and Purkinje network.

Cardiac Compass

Cardiac Compass Report

| Device: EnRhythm P1501DR | Serial Number:PNP123456Q | Date of Visit: 4-Jan-2005 15:15:11 |
| Patient: | ID: | Physician: |

From Medtronic, Inc [homepage on the Internet]. Minneapolis: Medtronic, Inc; c2006 [cited 2006 Nov 24]. Cardiac Compass Trends. Available from: http://www.medtronic.com/physician/brady/enrhythm/cardiaccompass.html. Used with permission.

cardiac contractility modulation. The application of non-excitatory electrical currents to the myocardium during the refractory period for the purpose of improving cardiac contractility.

cardiac dyssynchrony. The absence of synchronous left ventricular systolic contraction. Left bundle branch block is used as a clinical marker of dyssynchrony, although dyssynchrony can be present when the QRS is narrow. There are multiple echocardiographic and Doppler definitions of dyssynchrony. (Before the development of cardiac resynchronization therapy, the term *asynchrony* was more commonly accepted. *Asynchrony* and *dyssynchrony* currently are used synonymously.)

cardiac glycosides. A group of cardioactive drugs that block the sodium-potassium pump and thus increase cardiac contractility. Digoxin, the most commonly used of these drugs, slows sinus nodal automaticity, decreases atrial refractoriness, and increases atrioventricular nodal refractoriness and conduction time. Cardiac glycosides include digoxin, digitoxin, acetylstrophanthidin, and ouabain.

cardiac loop recorder. See *event recorder.*

cardiac mapping. An invasive electrophysiologic procedure used to identify accessory pathways in Wolff-Parkinson-White syndrome and other dysrhythmias, to identify atrial activation, to delineate the course of atrioventricular conduction, and to locate the origin of tachycardias. Cardiac mapping involves the placement of numerous electrodes on different sections of the myocardium, the delivery of electrical stimuli through these electrodes, and subsequent analysis of conducted stimuli. The electrodes may be passed into the heart via a vein or an artery. If a thoracotomy is used to expose the heart during arrhythmia surgery, cardiac mapping can be done epicardially and endocardially. See also *endocardial catheter mapping, endocardial surface mapping, epicardial ventricular mapping.*

cardiac output (CO). The amount of blood pumped by either ventricle during a specific amount of time; a measurement of the heart's performance. Cardiac output is calculated as the product of heart rate and stroke volume (CO = HR × SV). Typical values at rest range from 5 to 8 L/min. A hemodynamic goal of physiologic pacing is to achieve maximal cardiac output. See also *heart rate, stroke volume.*

cardiac repolarization. See *repolarization.*

Cardiac Resynchronization-Heart Failure (CARE-HF) trial. A randomized, controlled trial comparing cardiac resynchronization and optimal medical therapy with optimal medical therapy only. The patients receiving cardiac resynchronization had a 37% reduction in combined all-cause mortality (death) or unplanned cardiovascular hospitalization (primary end point), a 36% reduction in all-cause mortality (secondary end point), reduced hospitalizations for heart failure, and improved symptoms of heart failure and quality of life (Cleland JG, Daubert JC, Erdmann E, Freemantle N, Gras D, Kappenberger L, et al, Cardiac Resynchronization-Heart Failure [CARE-HF] Study Investigators. The effect of cardiac resynchronization on morbidity and mortality in heart failure. N Engl

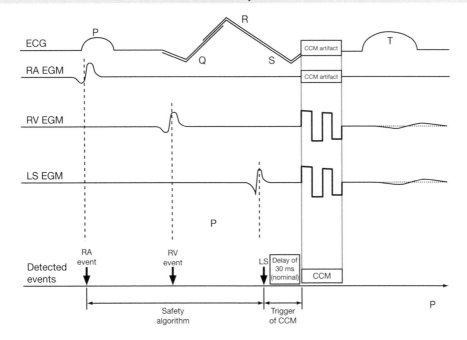

Cardiac Contractility Modulation

From Pappone C, Augello G, Rosanio S, Vicedomini G, Santinelli V, Romano M, et al. First human chronic experience with cardiac contractility modulation by nonexcitatory electrical currents for treating systolic heart failure: mid-term safety and efficacy results from a multicenter study. J Cardiovasc Electrophysiol. 2004;15:418-27. Used with permission.

J Med. 2005 Apr 14;352:1539-49. Epub 2005 Mar 7).

cardiac resynchronization therapy (CRT). Term applied to reestablishing synchrony between left ventricular free wall and ventricular septal contraction in an attempt to improve left ventricular efficiency and subsequently improve functional class. This may be biventricular pacing in some patients and left ventricular pacing only in others.

Cardiomyopathy Trial (CAT). Trial that randomized patients with recent onset of dilated cardiomyopathy (9 months) and a left ventricular ejection fraction of 30% or less to therapy with an implantable cardioverter-defibrillator or to a control group. The primary end point of the trial was all-cause mortality at 1 year of follow-up. The trial was terminated after the inclusion of 104 patients because the all-cause mortality rate at 1 year did not reach the ex-

Cardiac Resynchronization Therapy

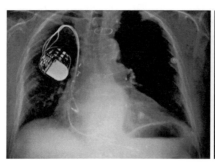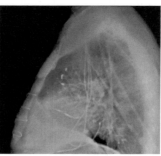

From Hayes DL, Lloyd MA. Radiography of implantable arrhythmia management devices. In: Kusumoto FM, Goldschlager NF, editors. Cardiac pacing for the clinician. Philadelphia: Lippincott Williams & Wilkins; 2001. p. 353-76. Used with permission.

cardiac standstill. See *asystole*.

cardiac tamponade. A compromise in cardiac filling and cardiac output by fluid in the pericardial cavity. Cardiac tamponade may be associated with dyspnea, dizziness, syncope, sweating, and shock. It is a potential complication after pacemaker implantation and during electrophysiologic testing if a lead perforates the myocardium. A decrease in systolic blood pressure of more than 10 mm Hg on inspiration (pulsus paradoxus) occurs with hemodynamically significant pericardial effusions (cardiac tamponade). See also *perforation*.

cardioinhibitor reflex. Relative bradycardia that results from increased parasympathetic tone and decreased sympathetic tone. It is often characterized by a vasodepressor response.

cardiomyopathy. A disease or disorder of the myocardium. Although there are many causes of a cardiomyopathic process, the most common is ischemia (i.e., ischemic cardiomyopathy) or an idiopathic dilated type. Many infiltrative diseases also may result in a cardiomyopathic state.

pected 30% in the control group. The trial did not provide evidence in favor of prophylactic implantation of a cardioverter-defibrillator in patients with dilated cardiomyopathy of recent onset and impaired left ventricular ejection fraction (Bansch D, Antz M, Boczor S, Volkmer M, Tebbenjohanns J, Seidl K, et al. Primary prevention of sudden cardiac death in idiopathic dilated cardiomyopathy: the Cardiomyopathy Trial [CAT]. Circulation. 2002;105:1453-8).

cardiopulmonary resuscitation (CPR). An emergency life-support procedure used during cardiac arrest to establish effective circulation and respiration and to prevent irreversible cerebral damage resulting from anoxia. It consists of artificial respiration and manual external cardiac massage.

cardiovascular regulatory center. An area of the medulla (lower part of the brainstem) that is the primary extrinsic center for control of heart rate. Impulses from the cardiovascular regulatory center reach the heart via sympathetic and parasympathetic pathways. Sympathetic stimuli, which travel to the heart via the cardiac plexus, cause acceleration of the heart rate and increased force of myocardial contractions. Parasympathetic stimuli, transmitted to the heart primarily through the vagus nerve and cardiac plexus, have an inhibitory effect on the heart and cause both decreased heart rate and lowered blood pressure. The cardiovascular regulatory center also receives stimuli from higher centers of the brain. Emotional stimuli such as fear, anger, and excitement can be transmitted via the hypothalamus to the cardiovascular regulatory center and activate sympathetic stimuli to the heart. See also *parasympathetic nervous system, sympathetic nervous system.*

cardioversion. The delivery of an electrical shock to the heart to synchronize the action potentials of all myocardial cells and terminate arrhythmias. Traditionally, external cardioversion is accomplished by the delivery of electrical energy via two paddles placed on the patient's thorax. The shock usually is synchronized with an R wave and delivered in a typical range of energy from 50 to 400 J. Biphasic energy delivery increases the success rate for cardioversion and is now the standard mode for cardioversion. Cardioversion also can be accomplished internally by means of endocardial or epicardial leads. The procedure is not always successful and, in some cases, may accelerate tachycardia. In implantable cardioverter-defibrillators, there is no longer a clear distinction between cardioversion and defibrillation. From the standpoint of energy levels delivered to convert an arrhythmia, energy levels of 1 to 5 J may be used for internal cardioversion and energy levels more than this, for defibrillation.

However, ventricular fibrillation sometimes converts at less than 5 J, especially with biphasic waveforms. Another distinction between cardioversion and defibrillation pertains to R-wave synchronization. If the energy delivered is R-wave synchronized, it may be called cardioversion, whereas if it is not R-wave synchronized, it may be referred to as defibrillation. Another distinction pertains to the type of arrhythmia converted. Conversion of ventricular tachycardia often is referred to as cardioversion, whereas conversion of ventricular fibrillation often is referred to as defibrillation. See also *implantable cardioverter-defibrillator.*

cardioverter-defibrillator. See *implantable cardioverter-defibrillator.*

CARE-HF. See *Cardiac Resynchronization-Heart Failure trial.*

carotid body. A small neurovascular structure containing chemoreceptors that respond to changes in oxygen saturation of the blood and play an important role in reflex regulation of respiration. The carotid body is located at the bifurcation of the carotid arteries. See also *aortic bodies, baroreceptor, chemoreceptor.*

carotid sinus hypersensitivity. Overreaction of the carotid sinus reflex, causing one of three responses: cardioinhibitory (bradycardia or asystole), vasodepressor (hypotension), or mixed cardioinhibitory and vasodepressor. See also *carotid sinus massage.*

carotid sinus massage (CSM). Manual compression of the carotid sinus, typically for up to 5 seconds, that causes reflex vagal nervous outflow. Carotid sinus massage may be used diagnostically, with electrocardiography, to determine

Cardioversion

Apex-anterior   Apex-posterior   Lateral view

whether symptomatic syncope and paroxysmal dizziness are due to a hypersensitive carotid sinus. An asymptomatic pause of up to 3 seconds is physiologic. Carotid sinus massage also is used to terminate paroxysmal supraventricular tachycardia and to evaluate atrioventricular nodal conduction disorders. Carotid sinus massage is not an innocuous procedure; it can produce cardiac standstill and can aggravate the degree of atrial block. It should not be performed in the presence of carotid artery atherosclerosis or simultaneously on both sides of the neck. See also *carotid sinus syndrome*.

carotid sinus syncope. See *carotid sinus hypersensitivity*.

carotid sinus syndrome. Hypersensitivity of the carotid sinus manifested by syncope and paroxysmal dizziness due to cardioinhibitory (sinus pause or arrest) or vasodepressor (hypotensive) effects. Carotid sinus syndrome is diagnosed from the response to carotid sinus massage. See also *carotid sinus massage*.

carrier signal. A waveform that serves as a medium for the transmission of information. The carrier signal may be a continuous or pulsed magnetic field, an electromagnetic field of a specific radiofrequency, an ultrasonic signal, or a light beam. The amplitude or frequency of the carrier signal is altered by encoding or by modulation with another signal, according to the information to be conveyed. In pacing, a carrier signal is emitted, for example, from the external programmer to the implanted pacemaker during programming or telemetry. Information transmitted from the pacemaker to the programmer is encoded onto the carrier signal by modulation. See also *modulation, programming, telemetry*.

CARTO system. Trademark used for an electroanatomic mapping system in which catheter position in three dimensions is cataloged with its corresponding measured contact electrogram. This system aids ablation for automatic tachycardias and helps delineate relevant reentrant circuit and scars.

carvedilol. An α- and β-adrenergic blocker used specifically for the reduction of symptoms of heart failure.

Carvedilol Or Metoprolol European Trial (COMET). In this study, patients with New York Heart Association class III or IV heart failure were randomized to receive carvedilol or metoprolol. Primary end points were all-cause mortality and the composite of all-cause mortality or all-cause hospitalization. The study found that treatment with carvedilol resulted in a decrease in the primary end point of all-cause mortality but not in the composite end point of all-cause mortality or all-cause hospitalization (Poole-Wilson PA, Swedberg K, Cleland JG, Di Lenarda A, Hanrath P, Komajda M, et al, Carvedilol Or Metoprolol European Trial Investigators. Comparison of carvedilol and metoprolol on clinical outcomes in patients with chronic heart failure in the Carvedilol Or Metoprolol European Trial [COMET]: randomised controlled trial. Lancet. 2003;362:7-13).

CASH trial. See *Cardiac Arrest Study Hamburg*.

CAST. See *Cardiac Arrhythmia Suppression Trial*.

CAST II. See *Cardiac Arrhythmia Suppression Trial II*.

CAT. See *Cardiomyopathy Trial*.

catecholamine. One of a group of similar chemicals with sympathomimetic activity. Endogenously produced catecholamines include epinephrine, norepinephrine, and dopamine.

catechol-dependent triggered activity. Arrhythmias caused by triggered automaticity specifically brought on by catecholamines. See *outflow tract ventricular tachycardia*.

catechol *O*-methyltransferase. The enzyme that metabolizes norepinephrine into normetanephrine and epinephrine into metanephrine.

catheter. A tubular device designed to be passed into a vessel, an orifice, a duct, or a body cavity. Electrode catheters are used to record intracardiac electrical activity and to deliver current to pace the heart. Other cardiac catheters are used to measure cardiac output, record pressures, inject radiopaque fluids to visualize the cardiovasculature, or draw blood samples from various locations within the heart and circulatory system. Pacing leads also are referred to as catheters.

catheter ablation. The technique of delivering energy through a catheter to destroy tissue. Catheter ablation is used to terminate arrhythmias by eradicating the site of origin or critical parts of the arrhythmogenic circuit. The ventricular response to atrial arrhythmias can be controlled by atrioventricular nodal ablation.

Catheter Ablation for Cure of Atrial Fibrillation (CACAF). The Catheter Ablation for Cure of Atrial Fibrillation study is the first multicenter, controlled, randomized study that has shown the higher efficacy of a single session of catheter ablation in combination with antiarrhythmic therapy compared with antiarrhythmic therapy alone for preventing the recurrence of atrial arrhythmias in patients with paroxysmal or persistent atrial fibrillation (Medscape [homepage on the Internet]. New York: Medscape; c2005 [cited 2006 Dec 7]. CACAF: Catheter Ablation for the Cure of Atrial Fibrillation Study. Available from: http://www.medscape.com/viewarticle/501551).

catheter mapping. See *endocardial catheter mapping*.

catheter maze procedure. Ablation procedure for atrial fibrillation in which ablative lines are placed mimicking the surgical maze procedure (endocardial maze procedure).

cathodal pin. In pacing, the negative pole of a bipolar lead. The cathodal pin is the metal lead terminal pin that provides contact between the pacemaker circuitry and the distal-tip electrode of the lead. See also *bipolar lead, coaxial lead, in-line connector, lead terminal pin*.

cathode. The negative pole or electrode, as in a battery. In an electrical system, the cathode is the electrode toward which electrons move during current flow. In both unipolar and bipolar endocardial pacing systems, the cathode usually is located at the distal tip of the pacing lead. See also *anode*.

cation. Positively charged ion attracted to the cathode.

cauterization. The destruction of tissue by thermal, electrical, or chemical means. See also *ablation*.

caval region. Specifically refers to the atrial tissue located between the tricuspid anulus and the inferior vena cava. More generally applies to the atrium near to and within the vena cava.

cavoatrial junction. Refers to the ostial region of the vena cava where they empty into the right atrium. Sometimes an arrhythmogenic site targeted for circumferential ablation.

cavotricuspid isthmus. Atrial tissue between the inferior vena cava and tricuspid valve, often containing the slow zone for typical atrial flutter.

CED. Abbreviation for *Coverage with Evidence Determination*.

cell. Synonym for *battery*.

cell impedance. See *battery impedance*.

Centers for Medicare and Medicaid Services (CMS). Formerly Healthcare Finance Administration (HCFA), this government agency regulates all Medicare and Medicaid services. It is part of the U.S. Department of Health and Human Services. It establishes which services are billable to Medicare and Medicaid and the level of reimbursement (U.S. Department of Health & Human Services: Centers for Medicare & Medicaid Services [homepage on the Internet]. Baltimore: Centers for Medicare & Medicaid Services [cited 2006 Nov 27]. Available from: http://www.cms.hhs.gov/).

central venous access. Access to a central vein; the subclavian, axillary, and femoral veins are all central veins that are often accessed percutaneously; the cephalic vein often is accessed by cutdown. Central venous access is used for lead placement during implantation of a pacemaker, cardioverter-defibrillator, or cardiac resynchronization pulse generator.

central venous oxygen saturation. Venous oxygen saturation measured within a central venous structure such as the vena cava or right heart chambers. Central venous oxygen saturation is a physiologic variable used to adjust heart rate in some rate-adaptive pacemakers. There is an inverse correlation between oxygen saturation and heart rate.

central venous temperature. The temperature measured within a central venous structure such as the vena cava or right heart chambers. Central venous temperature is a physiologic variable used to adjust heart rate in some rate-adaptive pacemakers. There is a direct but variable correlation between temperature and heart rate.

cephalic vein approach. Use of cephalic vein for lead placement; generally accomplished by cutdown technique.

ceramic substrate. A type of printed circuit board composed of ceramic layers with embedded metal interconnections, sometimes including integrated circuitry. A ceramic substrate allows a higher density of components within a given space.

cesium (Cs). A chemical element that blocks the delayed rectifier current (I_K). Cesium is used experimentally to induce early afterdepolarizations.

C fibers. Unmyelinated vagal afferent fibers that

are located predominantly on the inferior wall of the ventricle. See also *Bezold-Jarisch reflex*.

cGMP. Abbreviation for *cyclic guanine monophosphate*.

Chagas' disease. A form of trypanosomiasis that occurs in humans. The organism responsible for the disease is *Trypanosoma cruzi (Schizotrypanum cruzi)*, transmitted to humans by the bite of bloodsucking insects. The disease may involve the conduction system and result in symptomatic bradycardias that respond to pacemaker therapy. Chagas' disease is the most common cause of atrioventricular block in South America and is a common cause of congestive heart failure due to chagasic cardiomyopathy.

CHAMP. See *Congestive Heart Failure Atrial Arrhythmia Monitoring and Pacing study*.

channel. In cellar electrophysiology, a passageway that allows ions to flow through cell membranes. Channels may be selective, allowing only a particular ion to pass through, or nonselective, allowing several different ions to pass through. In pacing, an independent electronic circuit dedicated to a specific heart chamber and designed to distinguish between atrial and ventricular pacemaker variables or events. Conventionally, in dual-chamber pacemakers, channel 1 controls atrial sensing, and channel 2 controls ventricular sensing or pacing.

channelopathies. Disorders of ion channel structure or function. These disorders may be acquired or congenital and often result in arrhythmias.

chaos. A mathematic description of events that occur in an aperiodic (nonrepeating) but not truly random fashion. Chaos may explain some complex rhythms such as fibrillation. Chaos also is known as nonlinear dynamics.

chaotic meander. Multiple reentrant excitation waves and daughter wavelets occurring in the three-dimensional myocardium. Occurs in complex arrhythmias, including atrial fibrillation, ventricular fibrillation, and some forms of polymorphic ventricular tachycardia.

chaperone. A protein that is needed for assembly or folding of another protein.

charge (Q). The quantity of electrons accumulated on the surface of a substance through which electricity flows. In pacing, charge is used to describe the actual amount of electricity delivered to the myocardium during an atrial or ventricular output pulse. Charge may be used to quantify the output pulse in either constant-current or constant-voltage pacing systems. Charge is the product of the pulse duration in milliseconds and pacemaker output current in milliamperes. With respect to pacing systems, charge usually is expressed in microcoulombs. See also *coulomb*.

charge content. The integral of current over time, or the product of the average current and the amount of time during which current is delivered. In pacing, charge content is the product of the average current and pulse duration. Charge content provides an effective method for quantifying the electrical requirement for stimulation of the heart. Charge content usually is expressed in microcoulombs. See also *charge, coulomb*.

charge density. The charge per unit area on a surface or per unit volume in a space. In batteries, charge density is the charge stored in the battery per volume or weight. In pacing, charge density refers to the amount of charge delivered to the myocardium at the electrode-myocardial interface per unit surface area. When a stimulus of the same amplitude is delivered, an electrode with a large surface area has a lower charge density than an electrode with a small surface area.

charge dump. A function of the pacemaker circuitry that allows any residual charge on the output capacitor and at the electrode-myocardial tissue to be dissipated quickly. Charge dump maximized the pacing lead system sensing capability by reducing the recovery time of the sense amplifier. On an electrocardiogram, charge dump is evident as the exponentially decreasing waveform immediately after the deflection caused by the pacemaker output pulse.

charge pump. The use of arrays of capacitors to increase voltage in a circuit.

charge time. The amount of time required for a capacitor to charge in an implantable cardioverter-defibrillator. Charge times are dependent on battery status and integrity of the dielectric. See also *capacitor*.

CHARM. See *Candesartan in Heart Failure: Assessment of Reduction in Mortality and Morbidity*.

CHB. Abbreviation for *complete heart block*.

chemical ablation. The use of chemicals to destroy tissue. Ethanol has been used clinically to ablate the atrioventricular node and ventricular tachycardia foci via injection into the coronary artery that feeds the region to be destroyed.

chemical sensing. In pacing, the use of sensors to measure variables such as oxygen saturation and pH. Chemical sensors are incorporated into an endocardial lead, and measured changes in biologic variables are used to control pacing rate. See also *closed-loop control system, oxygen saturation sensing, pH sensing*.

chemoceptor. See *chemoreceptor*.

chemoreceptor. A receptor sense organ that is sensitive to chemical changes in the bloodstream, such as oxygen saturation, and reflexly causes a change in respiration and blood pressure. Chemoreceptors are also referred to as chemoceptors. See also *aortic bodies, baroreceptor, carotid body*.

chest wall stimulation (CWS). The delivery of electrical pulses to the external chest wall. Chest wall stimulation has been used to underdrive or overdrive an implanted pacemaker to assess the sensing function of the pacemaker, to assess the refractory periods, to perform therapeutic or diagnostic tests, and to control heart rate. Skin electrodes are connected to an external device capable of overdrive pacing or to an external pacemaker. One of the electrodes usually is placed over the heart and the other usually is placed over the pulse generator. The implanted pacemaker interprets the external pulses as spontaneous intracardiac signals and produces a triggered (AAT, VTT, DDT) or inhibited (AAI, VVI, DDD) mode of response, depending on the preset or programmed pacemaker mode. See also *external overdrive*.

CHF-STAT. See *Congestive Heart Failure Survival Trial of Antiarrhythmic Therapy*.

chip. An integrated microcircuit or integration of many microcircuits on a small silicon wafer. Chips perform many functions. In pacing circuitry, they allow an increase in pacemaker functions such as multiprogrammability, patient data storage, and telemetry. Chips also have made it possible to reduce pacemaker size.

chloride current. See I_{Cl}.

cholinergic. Activated, stimulated, or transmitted by acetylcholine. A cholinergic response is caused by the stimulation of parasympathetic nerves, which secrete acetylcholine.

cholinergic receptor. A receptor that is innervated by cholinergic nerve fibers and responds to acetylcholine secreted by these nerve fibers. See also *cholinergic*.

chordae tendineae. The small, tendinous fibers connecting each cusp of the mitral and tricuspid valves to the papillary muscles. In pacing, endocardial passive fixation leads may become entangled and lodged in the chordae tendineae of the tricuspid valve.

chronaxie. The pulse duration of an electrical stimulus that has a strength twice that of the minimum stimulus required to excite tissue. Chronaxie may be useful in the selection of an effective pacemaker output (voltage, current, or pulse duration). It is identified on a strength-duration curve as the value that is twice rheobase. Chronaxie is influenced by electrode size, electrode material, and mode of stimulation. See also *rheobase, strength-duration curve*.

chronic pacing threshold. In pacing, the minimum pacemaker output stimulus required to depolarize the myocardium after early physiologic response to pacemaker and lead implantation has subsided. Chronic thresholds

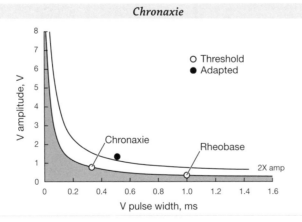

Chronaxie

usually are reached within 2 to 6 weeks after pacemaker implantation. See also *acute pacing threshold, chronic sensing threshold, threshold maturation.*

chronic sensing threshold. In pacing, the minimum intrinsic electrical signal required to consistently sense myocardial depolarization by a pulse generator after early physiologic responses to pacemaker and lead implantation have subsided. Chronic threshold usually is reached by 2 to 6 weeks after pacemaker implantation. See also *acute sensing threshold, chronic pacing threshold, threshold maturation.*

chronic threshold. See *chronic pacing threshold, chronic sensing threshold, threshold maturation.*

chronotropic. Descriptive of any process or substance that affects time or rate. The term *chronotropic* commonly is used in reference to the change in the rate of contraction of the heart in response to specific physiologic stimuli, such as exercise or pharmacologic treatment.

chronotropic assessment exercise protocol (CAEP). A treadmill exercise protocol originally developed for the assessment of chronotropic competence. It is based on 2-minute stages of exercise. See also *exercise capacity.*

chronotropy. Heart rate measurement during physiologic activities.

CIDS. See *Canadian Implantable Defibrillator Study.*

circadian events. Events or functions that occur on a 24-hour period, that is, within the span of a full day, as in a circadian rhythm.

circuit. A pathway or group of pathways made up of electronic components and capable of carrying electrical currents. In pacing, the circuit usually is composed of resistors, capacitors, transistors, semiconductors, and the power source. Pacemaker output circuits control the voltage, current, amplitude, pulse duration, and timing of output stimuli. Pacemaker sensing circuits amplify spontaneous intrinsic cardiac signals, filter out noise, and differentiate between ventricular and atrial signals. In rate-adaptive pacemakers, specially designed circuitry monitors physiologic or nonphysiologic variables and uses this information to control heart rate. Pacemaker circuits also control functions such as programming, telemetry, and analog-to-digital conversion. In electrophysiology, the arrhythmogenic substrate for reentrant arrhythmias.

Circuit (Simplified) of a Pacemaker

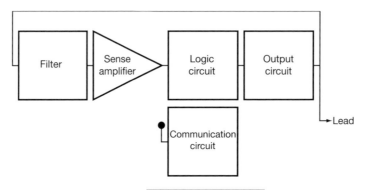

From Kenny T. *The Nuts and Bolts of Cardiac Pacing.* Malden (MA): Blackwell Futura; 2005. p. 35-42. *Copyrighted and used with permission of St. Jude Medical Inc.*

chronotropic competence. The ability to increase heart rate appropriately in response to physiologic needs.

chronotropic incompetence. Inability to increase intrinsic heart rate appropriately in response to physiologic need.

chronotropic response. Heart rate response to physiologic activities.

circuit redundancy. The duplication of critical circuit components or functions to permit continued pacing therapy in the event of component failure.

circuitry. The functional assembly of electronic elements that compose a circuit, or the assembly plan for such a circuit. In pacing, the circuitry is the portion of the pacemaker that processes the continuous power from the battery to provide pacemaker functions such as output pulses, sensing, data storage, and telemetry. The circuitry contains either discrete components or integrated and hybrid circuits enclosed in a hermetically sealed metal case. See also *discrete component, hybrid circuit, integrated circuit.*

circular multi-electrode catheter. Close or widely spaced bipoles placed in a circular configuration, typically used to aid electrical isolation

of the pulmonary and other veins. Circumferential catheters also may be used in the aortic and pulmonary arterial root. See also *Lasso catheter.*

circumferential ostial radiofrequency ablation. Common ablation procedure for atrial fibrillation in which radiofrequency energy is delivered at or near the ostium of the pulmonary vein. This technique also can be used for the vena cava, coronary sinus, and branches and in the great arteries.

Chronotropic Assessment Exercise Protocols

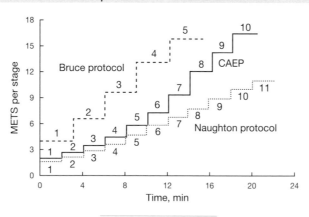

METS, metabolic equivalents.

From Hayes DL, Lloyd MA, Friedman PA. Cardiac pacing and defibrillation: a clinical approach. Armonk: Futura Publishing Company, Inc; 2000. p. 325-46. Copyrighted and used with permission of Mayo Foundation for Medical Education and Research.

Chronotropic Assessment Exercise Protocols

Stage	m/hour	Grade, %	Time, min	Cumulative time, min	Metabolic equivalents
Warm-up	1.0	0	...	...	1.5
1	1.0	2	2.0	2.0	2.0
2	1.5	3	2.0	4.0	2.8
3	2.0	4	2.0	6.0	3.6
4	2.5	5	2.0	8.0	4.6
5	3.0	6	2.0	10.0	5.8
6	3.5	8	2.0	12.0	7.5
7	4.0	10	2.0	14.0	9.6
8	5.0	10	2.0	16.0	12.1
9	6.0	10	2.0	18.0	14.3
10	7.0	10	2.0	20.0	16.5
11	7.0	15	2.0	22.0	19.0

From Hayes DL, Lloyd MA, Friedman PA. Cardiac pacing and defibrillation: a clinical approach. Armonk: Futura Publishing Company, Inc; 2000. p. 325-46. Copyrighted and used with permission of Mayo Foundation for Medical Education and Research.

circus movement tachycardia. The sustained, repetitive propagation of a wave of depolarization, most commonly involving the normal atrioventricular conduction system as one of the limbs of the tachycardia circuit. The pathways through which the circus movement travels may involve the atria, the atrioventricular node, the His bundle, the bundle branches, the ventricles, or accessory pathways. Circus movement thus is the mechanism of some reentrant tachycardias. See also *reentry.*

class I antiarrhythmic drugs. Class of drugs that include the sodium channel blockers. Class I drugs are divided into three groups depending on the effect that the drug has on the duration of the action potential. Class IA drugs increase the action potential duration, class IB drugs decrease the action potential duration, and class IC drugs do not affect the action potential duration.

class I indication. Condition for which there is evidence or general agreement that a given procedure or treatment is useful and effective.

class I recall. See *recall.*

class II antiarrhythmic drugs. Class of drugs composed of β-blockers. Drugs in this class differ in their β-receptor selectivity and pharmacokinetic properties, but all slow conduction and decrease automaticity.

class II indication. Condition for which there is conflicting evidence or a divergence of opinion about the usefulness or efficacy of a procedure or treatment.

class IIA indication. A class II indication for which the weight of evidence or opinion is in favor of usefulness or efficacy.

class IIB indication. A class II indication for which usefulness or efficacy is less well established by evidence or opinion.

class II recall. See *recall.*

class III antiarrhythmic drugs. Class of drugs that prolong repolarization. This may occur as a result of potassium channel blockade. Class III drugs include amiodarone, ibutilide, and dofetilide.

class III indication. Condition for which there is evidence or general agreement that the procedure or treatment is not useful or effective and in some cases may be harmful.

class III recall. See *recall.*

class IV antiarrhythmic drugs. Calcium channel blockers.

clavicular crush. Mechanical compression of a transvenous lead, usually one that has been implanted via subclavian puncture. Although originally the damage was believed to occur because of compression of the lead between the clavicle and the first rib, anatomic studies have shown that the damage actually may occur by compression from the subclavius muscle.

closed-loop control system. Automatic modification of an adjustable variable (such as pacing rate) that is under the control of a variable (such as minute ventilation) that is itself affected by the adjustable variable. Feedback from the output of the system to the input of the system affects the operation of the system. A closed-loop control system with negative feedback can be self-regulating, requiring no adjustments to maintain its stability. In pacing, closed-loop control requires the use of sensors located within the heart or circulatory system. The control systems are designed within the pacemaker circuitry to continuously monitor and process information collected by the sensors. See also *open-loop control system, sensor.*

closed-loop sensor. Sensors designed to monitor physiologic variables located in the heart or circulatory system. A closed-loop sensor allows adjusting of the pacing rate automatically, when appropriate, in response to changes in the monitored variables. See also *closed-loop control system, sensor.*

Closed-Loop Sensor

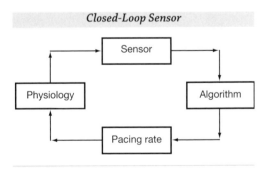

CMOS. Abbreviation for *complementary metal-oxide semiconductor.*

CMRR. Abbreviation for *common-mode rejection ratio.*

CMS. Abbreviation for *Centers for Medicare and Medicaid Services.*

CMS National ICD Registry. See *ICD Registry.*

CO. Abbreviation for *cardiac output.*

coaxial connector. See *in-line connector.*

coaxial lead. In pacing, a bipolar lead in which one helically wound conductor is placed concentrically inside of, and insulated from, a second outer helically wound conductor. Coaxial leads also are referred to as in-line bipolar leads.

Coaxial Lead

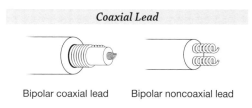

Bipolar coaxial lead   Bipolar noncoaxial lead

combipolar sensing. A trademark used for an atrial sensing method developed by St. Jude Medical (St. Paul, Minnesota) in which bipolar sensing is achieved with a dedicated unipolar lead (or the unipolar tip configuration of a bipolar lead). Atrial sensing occurs between the atrial tip electrode and the ventricular tip electrode. Ventricular sensing is standard unipolar sensing and is accomplished from the tip of the lead to the pulse generator can.

COMET. See *Carvedilol Or Metoprolol European Trial*.

commanded shock. An implantable cardioverter-defibrillator shock that is specifically initiated via the programmer. Also referred to as a "programmer-controlled" or "programmer-commanded" shock.

committed AV sequential pacing. See *committed DVI pacing*.

committed DVI pacing. A type of atrioventricular sequential pacing in which ventricular sensing does not occur during the preset or programmed atrioventricular interval. A ventricular output pulse follows each atrial output pulse after the completion of the atrioventricular interval. A committed DVI pacing system can compete with spontaneous atrial activity, thereby disrupting atrioventricular synchrony, and can potentially induce atrial fibrillation or other atrial rhythm disturbances. Theoretically, if the committed ventricular output pulse occurs during repolarization after an intrinsic ventricular event, ventricular rhythm disturbances could be induced. See also *AV sequential ventricular-inhibited pacing mode (DVI), noncommitted DVI pacing*.

committed implantable cardioverter-defibrillator. Device in which a shock is delivered automatically without reconfirmation once arrhythmia detection criteria are met and the capacitors are fully charged. In a committed system, even if the arrhythmia terminates before the capacitor is fully charged, the shock is still delivered.

committed pacing. A type of atrioventricular sequential pacing in which an atrial output pulse always is followed by a ventricular output pulse after the preset or programmed atrioventricular interval. The ventricular output pulse occurs regardless of intrinsic ventricular activity. See also *committed DVI pacing*.

committed shocks. In some implantable cardioverter-defibrillators, shocks that automatically are delivered, without reconfirmation, once an arrhythmia is detected and the capacitors have completely charged. In a committed system, shocks are delivered even if the arrhythmia self-terminates before the completion of capacitor charging. Committed shock delivery is a programmable feature in some implantable cardioverter-defibrillators. See also *noncommitted shocks*.

common atrial flutter. Atrial flutter that involves the cavotricuspid isthmus.

common atrioventricular bundle. See *His bundle*.

common-mode rejection. A function of some bipolar pacing systems whereby intrinsic cardiac events can be distinguished from extraneous noise, and extraneous noise can be rejected. A differential amplifier amplifies the difference between two electrical input signal levels applied to the two input terminals. The measured difference between the signals typically represents the intrinsic cardiac event. A common-mode signal (a signal level common to both input terminals) is characteristic of noise and is rejected. Differential amplifiers with common-mode rejection are incorporated into the sensing circuit of some bipolar pacing systems to distinguish intrinsic cardiac events and extraneous noise. See also *differential amplifier, differential bipolar sensing, differential input, sensing circuit*.

common-mode rejection ratio (CMRR). A quantity that serves as a figure of merit for a differential amplifier. The common-mode rejection ratio of the differential amplifier is the ratio of the amplified differential signal to the amplified common-mode signal, which can be as high as 1,000,000:1 in modern amplifiers. See also *common-mode rejection*.

common ventricular channel. A cardiac resynchronization device in which the right and left ventricular pacing and sensing channels are "in common."

COMPANION. See *Comparison of Medical, Pacing, and Defibrillation Therapies in Heart Failure.*

comparator circuit. An electronic circuit, typically with a single binary output, that measures one input signal level against a reference level. The output is active, or high, when the input is of a greater magnitude than the reference level. The output of a comparator in a pacemaker or implantable cardioverter-defibrillator consists of sensed events. The reference level may be fixed, programmable, or variable. In pacemakers, the reference level typically is a programmable constant. In automatic sensitivity tracking in implantable cardioverter-defibrillators, the reference level is variable.

Comparison of Medical, Pacing, and Defibrillation Therapies in Heart Failure (COMPANION). This was a multicenter, prospective, randomized, controlled clinical trial that assessed optimal pharmacologic therapy alone or with cardiac resynchronization using either a pacemaker or a combination of pacemaker-defibrillator in patients with a dilated cardiomyopathy, intraventricular conduction delay, New York Heart Association class III or IV heart failure, and no indication for a device. The primary end point was a combination of all-cause mortality and all-cause hospitalization. Secondary end points included various measures of cardiovascular morbidity. The trial was terminated prematurely after randomization of 1,520 patients at the recommendation of an independent data and safety monitoring board. The primary composite end point of all-cause death or any hospitalization was decreased by approximately 20% with use of either device therapy compared with pharmacologic therapy alone. Further, a "pacing only" resynchronization device reduced the risk of death from any cause (secondary end point) by 24% (*P*=.059) and a resynchronization device with defibrillation reduced the risk by 36% (*P*=.003) (Carson P, Anand I, O'Connor C, Jaski B, Steinberg J, Lwin A, et al. Mode of death in advanced heart failure: the Comparison of Medical, Pacing, and Defibrillation Therapies in Heart Failure [COMPANION] trial. J Am Coll Cardiol. 2005;46:2329-34).

Comparison of Metoprolol and Sotalol in Preventing Ventricular Tachyarrhythmias After the Implantation of a Cardioverter-Defibrillator. The study was designed to evaluate the efficacy of *dl*-sotalol versus metoprolol for the prevention of ventricular tachyarrhythmias (ventricular tachycardia or ventricular fibrillation) in patients receiving an implantable cardioverter-defibrillator. For patients who received implantable cardioverter-defibrillators for life-threatening ventricular tachycardia or ventricular fibrillation, treatment with metoprolol was associated with a reduction in recurrent ventricular tachyarrhythmia compared with treatment with sotalol (Seidl K, Hauer B, Schwick NG, Zahn R, Senges J. Comparison of metoprolol and sotalol in preventing ventricular tachyarrhythmias after the implantation of a cardioverter/defibrillator. Am J Cardiol. 1998;82:744-8).

compensatory pause. The occurrence of a pause after a premature complex. In the instance of a fully compensatory pause, the PP interval bracketing the premature complex equals twice the baseline PP interval because the sinus node is not reset, but the sinus node impulse cannot conduct to the ventricular myocardium because the atrioventricular node is refractory. With a noncompensatory pause, the PP interval enclosing the premature complex is less than twice the baseline PP interval because the sinus node is reset. Compensatory pauses usually, but not necessarily, are full after premature ventricular complexes and are noncompensatory after atrial premature complexes.

competition. In pacing, the asynchronous delivery of a pacemaker output pulse at the same time as, or immediately after, spontaneous intrinsic activity. Competition may be caused in either the atrium or the ventricle by certain pacing modes (e.g., AOO, DOO, VOO, and DVI), by magnet application, or by loss of pacemaker sensing. If a competitive pacemaker output pulse falls within the vulnerable period of the intrinsic repolarization, an arrhythmia may result. See also *asynchronous pacing.*

complementary metal-oxide semiconductor (CMOS). A technology used for integrated circuitry. Complementary metal-oxide semiconductor technology is characterized by low-power consumption and thus is suitable for use in electronic systems that have a limited battery capacity. In pacing, complementary metal-oxide semiconductor is the standard integrated circuitry technology and is used to provide the logic function in several different circuits.

complete AV block. See *third-degree AV block.*

complete heart block (CHB). See *third-degree AV block.*

concealed atrioventricular bypass tract. Refers to an atrioventricular bypass tract that conducts current only from the ventricle to the atrium and thus does not manifest as preexcitation on the 12-lead electrocardiogram.

concealed atrioventricular conduction. Electrical conduction between the ventricle to the atrium via a bypass tract responsible for orthodromic reentrant tachycardia.

to demonstrate any of the four classic criteria of entrainment because the pacing site is within the zone of slow conduction of the circuit and thus fusion never occurs. Pacing during the tachycardia yields no change in surface electrocardiographic morphologic features, and when pacing is discontinued the first post-pacing complex occurs at the pacing cycle length before the rhythm resumes the tachycardia cycle length on the following beat. Concealed entrainment is one phenomenon sought when searching for a site to ablate reentrant ventricular tachycardia. See also *entrainment.*

concentric retrograde atrial activation. The pattern of retrograde activation of the atria whereby activation occurs first in the region

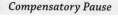

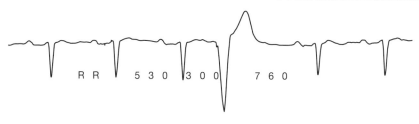

RR intervals are shown in milliseconds.

concealed bypass tract. An accessory pathway that conducts in the retrograde direction only; thus, no delta wave is present on the surface electrocardiogram under any conditions. Concealed bypass tracts may be on either the left or the right side of the heart, either on the free wall or septum, and are capable of sustaining orthodromic reciprocating tachycardia. See also *accessory pathway.*

concealed conduction. An incompletely penetrating depolarization that reaches myocardial cells before complete repolarization of the cells has occurred. The impulse prolongs repolarization and thereby affects the formation or conduction of subsequent impulses. Concealed conduction occurs most commonly in the atrioventricular node, but it may take place anywhere in the atrioventricular conduction system or in accessory pathways. Electrocardiographic recordings of concealed conduction may mimic heart block.

concealed entrainment. The process of entraining a reentrant tachycardia without being able

of the atrioventricular node, as seen on the His-bundle lead, and then spreads outward to activate the remainder of the atria. At times, normal earliest atrial activation may occur at the coronary sinus os just before (less than 30 milliseconds before) activity recorded on the His-bundle lead. Concentric retrograde atrial activation is consistent with, but not diagnostic of, conduction over the normal ventriculoatrial conduction system. See also *eccentric retrograde atrial activation.*

concertina pacing. A type of antitachycardia pacing in which the cycle length within a train of impulses alternately decreases and increases. Concertina pacing also is known as accordion pacing.

concordant alternans. Fluctuation by more than 25% of the R, T, or U wave occurring in the same axis (opposite is discordant alternans, in which inversion of the axis occurs during alternans).

conditional ventricular tracking limit. A programmable function in some older DDDR pacemakers that reduces the ventricular tracking limit as a function of the motion sensor output. This feature usually is activated in order to prevent high-rate ventricular pacing in the presence of conditions such as atrial tachycardias or atrial myopotential sensing. During exercise, the ventricular pacing rate due to atrial sensing is limited solely by the programmed upper rate limit. However, during rest, the ventricular pacing rate due to atrial sensing is further limited by the conditional ventricular tracking limit.

conducted atrial fibrillation response. Ventricular response rates during atrial fibrillation. May occur via the atrioventricular node or an accessory pathway.

conduction. The transmission of sound, heat, or an electrical charge by the passage of energy from one particle to another. Cardiac conduction is the active propagation of a wave of depolarization through the myocardium. See also *cardiac conduction system*.

conduction block. Inability of an impulse to continue to travel along the path that it was following. Conduction block may be due to functional reasons such as refractory tissue or anatomic reasons such as fibrotic tissue. Conduction block often is the initiating event in a reentrant arrhythmia.

conduction velocity. The speed at which a wave of depolarization propagates through the myo-cardial tissue. Conduction velocity is dependent on numerous physiologic factors, including electrolyte composition, fiber size and orientation, resting membrane potential, the rate at which the action potential rises, action potential amplitude, and cellular threshold level.

conductor. A material that has a low resistance to the flow of electrical current. In pacing, the conductor is the internal core of a pacemaker lead that conducts current to the electrode-myocardial interface. The conductor also transmits sensed intracardiac signals from the electrode-myocardial interface to the pacemaker. Conductors usually are made of alloys that are resistant to corrosion and have low resistivities, for example, alloys of cobalt-nickel or platinum-iridium. Titanium, also used as a conductor, is not an alloy.

conductor fracture. In pacing, the cracking or breaking of the pacemaker lead conductor, caused by excessive flexing, stress, or physical damage such as scalpel cuts, suture ligation, or compression of the lead between the clavicle and first rib. Conductor fracture causes an increase in impedance and a decrease of current flow to the electrode(s), which, in turn, affects pacemaker function. Failure of an atrial or ventricular lead to pace or sense appropriately may indicate conductor fracture. The most common

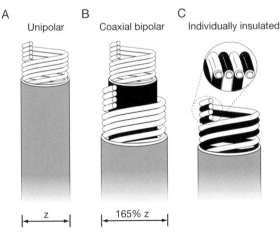

Conductors

A Unipolar   B Coaxial bipolar   C Individually insulated

|← z →| |← 165% z →|

A, Multifilar unipolar lead design. B, Coaxial bipolar lead design.
C, Individually insulated strands of wire, which allow for multiple conductive pathways in a single coil.

Modified from Callaghan F, Christensen M. Current and future lead technology. In: Singer I, Kupersmith J, editors. Clinical manual of electrophysiology. Baltimore: Williams & Wilkins; 1993. p. 211-21. Used with permission.

site of endocardial conductor fracture is near the proximal end of the lead where it enters the vein. However, fracture also may occur immediately distal to the pacemaker connector or at the point of lead curvature within the heart near the distal end of the lead. Conductor fracture also is referred to as lead fracture.

confirmation. The process or act of testing the continuing presence of tachycardias after their detection but before the delivery of shock therapy by an implantable cardioverter-defibrillator. Confirmation is used to reduce the probability of inappropriate shock delivery in cases of spontaneous reversion. Confirmation is programmable in some implantable cardioverter-defibrillators. See also *committed shocks*.

congenital complete heart block. Atrioventricular block present at birth. Congenital heart block may be structural (i.e., failure of the atrioventricular conduction system to connect) or autoimmune, a cause that may result from transplacental passage of maternal antibodies, which in turn affect the atrioventricular conduction tissues.

congenital long QT syndrome. A disorder of ventricular repolarization that predisposes to lethal ventricular arrhythmias, especially torsades de pointes. Two forms of congenital long QT syndrome that have been described are Jervell and Lange-Nielsen syndrome, an autosomal recessive form that is associated with congenital deafness, and Romano-Ward syndrome, an autosomal dominant form that is not associated with congenital deafness. See also *acquired long QT syndrome, torsades de pointes*.

Congestive Heart Failure Atrial Arrhythmia Monitoring and Pacing (CHAMP) study. This study is intended to characterize atrial arrhythmias in patients with indications for cardiac resynchronization therapy and to monitor changes in atrial arrhythmias while the therapy is provided. The primary outcome is the burden of atrial fibrillation at 6 months. The study is a diagnostic, nonrandomized, open-label, uncontrolled, single-group assignment, efficacy study. The study has completed enrollment (ClinicalTrials.gov [homepage on the Internet]. Bethesda: U.S. Department of Health and Human Services National Institutes of Health [updated 2006 Jan 4; cited 2006 Dec 7] Study to Characterize Atrial Fibrillation in CHF Patients Indicated for CRT.

Available from: http://www.clinicaltrials.gov/ct/show/NCT00156728).

Congestive Heart Failure Survival Trial of Antiarrhythmic Therapy (CHF-STAT). This was a multicenter, double-blind, placebo-controlled study that assessed the long-term effects of amiodarone on morbidity and mortality in patients with congestive heart failure and atrial fibrillation. The trial concluded that in patients with congestive heart failure, amiodarone had significant potential to spontaneously convert atrial fibrillation to sinus rhythm. Patients who had conversion had a lower mortality rate than those who did not. The drug prevented the development of new-onset atrial fibrillation and significantly reduced the ventricular rate in those with persistent atrial fibrillation (Deedwania PC, Singh BN, Ellenbogen K, Fisher S, Fletcher R, Singh SN, The Department of Veterans Affairs CHF-STAT Investigators. Spontaneous conversion and maintenance of sinus rhythm by amiodarone in patients with heart failure and atrial fibrillation: observations from the Veterans Affairs Congestive Heart Failure Survival Trial of Antiarrhythmic Therapy [CHF-STAT]. Circulation. 1998;98:2574-9).

connector. See *lead connector*.

connector block. In pacing, the portion of the pacemaker header into which the lead connector is inserted. The connector block completes the conduction pathway from the pacemaker circuitry to the electrode(s) on the lead(s) for the delivery of pacemaker output pulses and for the sensing of intrinsic activity. See also *lead connector, lead terminal pin, pacemaker header*.

connector pin. The terminal pin, or "male" plug, on the lead which is inserted into the connector block and then secured into place. •

connexin. A subunit of a connexon. Six connexins make up a connexon. See also *connexon*.

connexon. In cellular electrophysiology, a single channel within a gap junction. Each gap junction contains tens to thousands of connexons. Connexons of one cell line up with those of the adjacent cell and permit efficient cell-to-cell communication.

conscious sedation. The use of medication to minimally depress the level of consciousness in a patient while allowing the patient to continually and independently maintain a patent airway and respond appropriately to verbal commands or gentle stimulation.

consecutive interval counting. Implanted defibrillator sensing methods in which each consecutive beat-to-beat interval is counted to diagnose tachycardia. Frequently used for ventricular tachycardia and not ventricular fibrillation.

constant-current device. A device that maintains a steady current output over a wide range of impedance values by altering the output voltage as needed to maintain a constant-current value.

constant-current source. An electrical system in which the current remains constant regardless of the impedances within the system. The output voltage level in a constant current system is dependent on the external impedance. If the external impedance is high, the constant current system eventually becomes voltage-limited. In pacing, a constant current system maintains the current level during the delivery of a pacemaker output pulse to the myocardium regardless of the impedance either within the lead or at the electrode-myocardial interface or both. See also *constant-voltage source*.

constant-voltage device. A device that maintains a steady voltage output over a wide range of impedance values by altering the output current as needed to maintain a constant-voltage value.

constant-voltage source. An electrical system in which the voltage remains constant regardless of the impedances within the system. The deliverable current of a constant-voltage system is dependent on the external impedance. In pacing, a constant voltage system maintains the voltage level in the lead and across the electrode-myocardial interface during the delivery of a pacemaker output pulse to the myocardium. See also *constant-current source*.

contact ring. In pacing, the ground or positive pole on a bipolar lead. The contact ring is a metal band around the lead terminal pin that provides contact between the pacemaker circuitry and the proximal-ring electrode at the distal portion of the lead. The contact ring also is referred to as the anodal band. See also *coaxial lead, in-line connector, lead terminal pin*.

CONTAK-CD trial. A randomized, controlled, double-blind study comparing active cardiac resynchronization therapy with no pacing. For the primary end point, a composite of mortality, hospitalizations for heart failure, and episodes

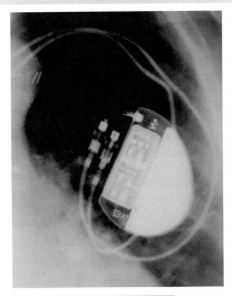

Connector Pin

Courtesy of John D. Symanski, MD, Sanger Clinic, Charlotte, North Carolina. Used with permission.

of ventricular tachycardia or ventricular fibrillation, the study found an insignificant trend favoring the resynchronization group. However, peak oxygen consumption, 6-minute hall walk distance, quality of life, and New York Heart Association class were significantly improved in the active pacing group compared with the inactive control subjects, particularly in the subgroup of patients in New York Heart Association class II or III (Lozano I, Bocchiardo M, Achtelik M, Gaita F, Trappe HJ, Daoud E, et al, VENTAK CHF/CONTAK CD Investigators Study Group. Impact of biventricular pacing on mortality in a randomized crossover study of patients with heart failure and ventricular arrhythmias. Pacing Clin Electrophysiol. 2000;23[11 Pt 2]:1711-2).

continuous diastolic activity. Fractionated electrical potentials recorded throughout electrical diastole, possibly arising in the zone of slow conduction in ventricular tachycardia.

contrast electrophysiologic study. See *baseline electrophysiologic study*.

contrast staining. During angiography (e.g., venography, arteriography, transseptal puncture), persistent staining with contrast of the tissue. Often signifies inadvertent intramyocardial injection, perforation, or dissection.

contrast venography. Injection of contrast material into a venous structure or vein to provide radiographic visualization. In pacing, contrast venography can be used to facilitate the subclavian puncture technique. Contrast material is injected via a peripheral intravenous line on the same side as the subclavian puncture. Subclavian puncture can then be directed fluoroscopically.

control electrophysiologic study. See *baseline electrophysiologic study*.

Cook Extraction Registry. A registry, no longer active, of patients undergoing lead extraction which was originally established by a company that manufactured extraction equipment.

Cook Lead Extraction device. A system used for extraction of chronically implanted pacing leads (Cook Medical, Inc., Bloomington, Indiana). The technique uses intravascular counteraction techniques with a stylet locked inside the lead to reinforce the lead, and telescoping sheaths are advanced over the lead to free it from vascular scar tissue and provide counteraction at the endocardial surface. See also *Byrd extraction technique*.

Cook locking stylet. A specialized stylet that is introduced into the lumen of a lead at its proximal end (after the electrical connector has been removed) and locks into position at the lead's distal end (Cook Medical, Inc., Bloomington, Indiana). This allows for the delivery of tractional forces. The locking mechanism at the stylet's distal end is activated to engage the coils of the lead.

cooled tipped catheter. Either closed or open saline irrigation used to cool the catheter tip during radiofrequency ablation. This technique allows greater energy delivery without catheter-related coagulum formation.

Cordis Corporation. A medical device company and a pioneer in innovative devices and products for interventional vascular medicine and electrophysiology. At one time, Cordis (Miami Lakes, Florida) was a major manufacturer of implantable devices.

Coronary Artery Bypass Graft trial (CABG Patch trial). The Coronary Artery Bypass Graft trial randomized patients with a reduced left ventricular ejection fraction and an abnormal signal-averaged electrocardiogram undergoing elective coronary artery bypass grafting to receive an implantable cardioverter-defibrillator prophylactically or not to receive one. The trial found no evidence of improved survival among patients in whom the device was placed (Bigger JT Jr, Coronary Artery Bypass Graft [CABG] Patch Trial Investigators. Prophylactic use of implanted cardiac defibrillators in patients at high risk for ventricular arrhythmias after coronary-artery bypass graft surgery. N Engl J Med. 1997;337:1569-75).

coronary sinus. The largest vein in the heart. The coronary sinus wraps around the left atrioventricular groove and empties into the low right atrium. The coronary sinus is of great importance in electrophysiologic studies of supraventricular arrhythmias because electrode catheters can be inserted into it to allow pacing and recording from the left atrium. •

coronary sinus cannulation. Engaging the coronary sinus with a lead or catheter and subsequently placing the lead or catheter within the coronary vein(s).

coronary sinus electrode. A catheter passed into the coronary sinus to pace or defibrillate the heart or to record from the left atrium.

coronary sinus lead. In pacing, an endocardial lead designed for placement in the coronary sinus. Placing the lead in the proximal portion of the coronary sinus usually results in ventricular pacing, whereas positioning the lead in the distal portion of the coronary sinus usually results in atrial pacing. A coronary sinus lead position may be difficult to determine on a posterior chest radiograph, but on a lateral chest radiograph the lead is directed posteriorly. Coronary sinus leads used for defibrillation have a large electrode surface area and no fixation device.

coronary sinus ostium. The opening or mouth of the coronary sinus.

coronary sinus pacing. Stimulation of cardiac structures via a lead placed in the coronary veins. See the figure *Coronary sinus and coronary veins*.

coronary sulcus. Atrioventricular groove separating the left atrium and left ventricle through which the coronary sinus traverses.

coronary venography. Diagnostic imaging of the coronary venous system obtained by injecting contrast agents. Coronary venography often is performed during implantation of a cardiac resynchronization device. Coronary venography allows the implanter to assess coronary venous anatomy and to determine optimal routes and sites for lead placement. •

corrected QT interval. See *QTc interval*.

Coronary Venography

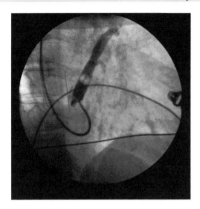 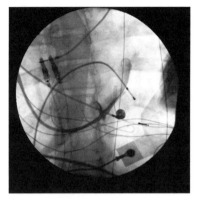

From Asirvatham SJ. Biventricular device implantation. In: Hayes DL, Wang PJ, Sackner-Bernstein J, Asirvatham SJ, editors. Resynchronization and defibrillation for heart failure: a practical approach. Oxford (UK): Blackwell Publishing; 2004. p. 99-137. Copyrighted and used with permission of Mayo Foundation for Medical Education and Research.

corrected sinus node recovery time (CSNRT). The standardized value of the sinus node recovery time derived by subtracting the basic sinus cycle length from the sinus node recovery time. Corrected sinus node recovery time is used in electrophysiologic testing. Normal values are less than 550 milliseconds. See also *sinus node recovery time.*

corridor operation. A surgical procedure for atrial fibrillation that creates an electrically isolated pathway for impulses to travel from the sinus node to the atrioventricular node while the atria remain in chronic fibrillation.

coulomb (C). The unit of measurement of an electrical charge; a quantification of electrons. One coulomb is equal to the amount of electrical charge transported by one ampere of current for 1 second through a cross-section of a conductor. In pacing, charge usually is expressed in microcoulombs. See also *charge.*

counters. In implantable devices, counters usually refer to a mechanism by which the device tracks numbers of events (i.e., atrial sensed, atrial paced, ventricular sensed, ventricular paced).

coupled electrical stimulus. A programmed electrical stimulus that is delivered at some preset or programmable interval after an intrinsic or paced complex. See also *programmed electrical stimulus.*

coupled extra stimulus. Ventricular or atrial extra stimulus placed after a predetermined coupling interval following typically 8 beats of pacing from the same chamber.

coupling. The relationship between paired beats. See also *coupling interval.*

coupling interval. The time between paired beats. During spontaneous intrinsic rhythm, the coupling interval is the amount of time between a normal beat and a subsequent premature contraction within the same chamber. In pacing and in electrophysiologic testing, the coupling interval either is the time between the

Counters

Initial Interrogation Report

Pacing, % of total		Event counters	
AS-VS	< 0.1%	PVC singles	20,618
AS-VP	37.0%	PVC runs	1,435
AP-VS	< 0.1%	PAC runs	275
AP-VP	63.0%		

AP, atrial paced; AS, atrial sensed; VP, ventricular paced; VS, ventricular sensed.

Coronary Sinus and Coronary Veins

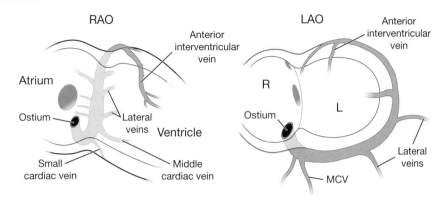

CS, coronary sinus; L, left; LAO, left anterior oblique;
MCV, middle cardiac vein; R, right; RAO, right anterior oblique.

Modified from Asirvatham SJ. Biventricular device implantation. In: Hayes DL, Wang PJ, Sackner-Bernstein J, Asirvatham SJ, editors. Resynchronization and defibrillation for heart failure: a practical approach. Oxford (UK): Blackwell Publishing; 2004. p. 99-137. Copyrighted and used with permission of Mayo Foundation for Medical Education and Research.

Coronary Venous Anatomy

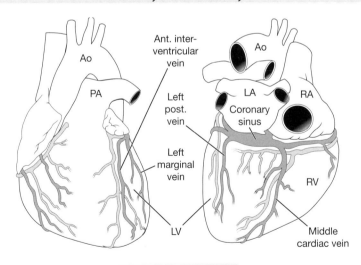

Ant, anterior; Ao, aorta; LA, left atrium; LV, left ventricle;
PA, pulmonary artery; post, posterior; RA, right atrium; RV, right ventricle.

Modified from Hayes DL, Lloyd MA, Friedman PA. Cardiac pacing and defibrillation: a clinical approach. Armonk: Futura Publishing Company, Inc; 2000. p. 159-200. Copyrighted and used with permission of Mayo Foundation for Medical Education and Research.

delivery of two consecutive programmed electrical stimuli or the time between a spontaneous intrinsic event and an electrical stimulus.

Coverage with Evidence Determination (CED). A new method used by the Centers for Medicaid and Medicare Services to determine how newly approved therapies perform in patient populations outside the confines of a randomized clinical trial. The initial example of this was the mandated formation of the ICD Registry to track patients who receive primary prevention therapy with an implantable cardioverter-defibrillator.

CPR. Abbreviation for *cardiopulmonary resuscitation*.

craze. A network of small cracks or fractures on or under the surface of a material such as enamel, metal, or plastic. In pacing, crazing usually refers to small cracks in the insulation of a pacing lead.

crista terminalis. Also referred to as the terminal crest. Portion of the right atrium on the lateral wall where the pectinate muscle terminates. The sinus node is located epicardially at the junction of the crista terminalis and the superior vena cava.

critically timed stimulus. An electrical impulse delivered with a specific coupling interval to induce or terminate an arrhythmia. In electrophysiologic testing and antitachycardia pacing, critically timed stimuli often are applied in pairs or triplets and may be delivered with unequal coupling intervals.

cross-programming. The accidental or intentional reprogramming of a pacemaker manufactured by one company by using a programmer manufactured by another company. Cross-programming may cause dysprogramming, pacemaker malfunction, or anomalous behavior of the pacemaker. Current safeguards make cross-programming virtually impossible. See also *dysprogramming, misprogramming, phantom programming*.

cross-sensing. See *crosstalk*.

cross-stimulation. Inappropriate stimulation of the heart chamber (atrium or ventricle) other than the one to which the pacemaker output pulse was delivered. For example, cross-stimulation occurs if a ventricular output pulse results in atrial stimulation.

crosstalk. In pacing, inappropriate sensing of a pacemaker output pulse or an intrinsic event by the pacemaker-sensing channel for the chamber other than the one in which the paced time or intrinsic event occurred. For example, crosstalk occurs when an atrial event is sensed on the ventricular-sensing channel of the pacemaker or if an intrinsic ventricular event or a ventricular output pulse is sensed by the atrial-sensing channel of the pacemaker. If crosstalk occurs in dual-chamber pacemakers, it may cause inappropriate inhibition of the other pacemaker channel. Blanking periods have been incorporated into the circuitry of dual-chamber pacemakers to help prevent crosstalk. See also *blanking period*.

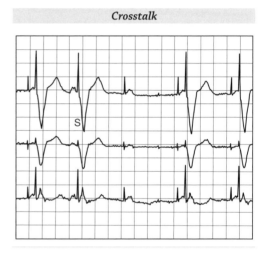

Crosstalk

crosstalk blanking. See *blanking period*.

crosstalk detection window. See *crosstalk sensing window*.

crosstalk sensing window. A short portion of the timing cycle that occurs immediately after the ventricular blanking period in some dual-chamber pacemakers. Any event that is sensed during this portion of the timing cycle results in a triggered ventricular stimulus at the end of an abbreviated atrioventricular interval. The abbreviated atrioventricular interval is known as safety pacing. Crosstalk sensing window is also referred to as crosstalk detection window. See the figure *AV interval*.

CRT. Abbreviation for *cardiac resynchronization therapy*.

CRT-D. Abbreviation used to designate *cardiac resynchronization therapy with defibrillation-cardioversion* capabilities.

cryoprobe. An instrument that delivers extreme cold to tissue. Cryoprobes sometimes are used in cryosurgery to destroy arrhythmogenic myocardial tissue. See also *cryosurgery, probe*.

cryosurgery. A surgical technique used to selectively destroy tissue by the application of an extremely low temperature (less than −60°C). The low temperature required for cryosurgery is achieved by controlled evaporation of liquid nitrogen, which is then delivered by means of a cryoprobe. Cryosurgery is used to destroy arrhythmogenic tissue during surgery for the correction of arrhythmias. See also *cryoprobe*.

Cs. Abbreviation for *cesium*.

CSM. Abbreviation for *carotid sinus massage*.

CSNRT. Abbreviation for *corrected sinus node recovery time*.

CTAF. See *Canadian Trial of Atrial Fibrillation*.

CTOPP. See *Canadian Trial of Physiologic Pacing*.

cupric sulfide. See *lithium-cupric sulfide*.

current (I). The transfer of electrical charge (electrons) through a cross-section of a conductor. In electrophysiology, current is the flow of ions that results in the movement of charge. Current is related to voltage (V) and resistance (R) as expressed by Ohm's law: $I = V/R$. Current is expressed in amperes. For specific ion currents, see I_x (e.g., I_{Na} for sodium current).

current density (J). The current (I) per unit of a cross-section area of a conductor. In pacing, current density commonly is measured as the amount of current at the electrode surface that is delivered to excitable tissue. The current density at the electrode surface is $J_a = I/A_a$, where A_a is equal to the surface area of the electrode. The current density at the closest excitable tissue is $J_c = I/A_c$, where A_c is equal to the surface area of the virtual electrode. See also *effective electrode*.

current drain. The average amount of current drawn from a battery by the external load of a system. In pacing, the current drain depends on many factors, including the circuitry; the percentage of paced events; programmed variables such as rate, amplitude, and pulse duration; the electrode material and surface area; and, in a constant voltage system, the impedance of the pacing system. Current drain occurs with each paced and sensed event. Current drain typically is lower for a sensed event than for a paced event.

current leakage. A reduction of deliverable charge to the cathode of an electrical circuit caused by a shunt within the system. Current is shunted from the primary circuit of the system through an accessory pathway of low resistance. Leakage of current into tissue surrounding a pacing system may occur if the hermetic seal of the pacemaker neck is incomplete or if there is a break in the lead insulation.

current of injury. In pacing, the elevation of the ST segment that corresponds to electrode contact with endocardium or epicardium during electrode implantation. The degree of ST-segment elevation is an indicator for optimal lead placement. The current-of-injury pattern that occurs as a result of pacing lead placement should not be confused with the current-of-injury pattern that occurs with cellular damage, such as that in an evolving myocardial infarction.

current threshold. Pacing threshold expressed in minimum milliamperage at which capture is maintained.

cutdown. In pacing, a surgical approach in which the venous entry point for insertion of a pacing lead is directly visualized.

CWS. Abbreviation for *chest wall stimulation*.

cycle length. The amount of time between one event and the next in a repetitive signal. Cycle length is a measurement of the interval between spontaneous intrinsic cardiac activity and the delivery of programmed electrical stimuli. Cycle length is a measurement of rate. It is expressed in milliseconds and is equal to 60,000 divided by the number of beats per minute. See also *beats per minute*.

cyclic adenosine monophosphate (cAMP). A second messenger that couples cell membrane receptors to a wide variety of cellular effectors such as ion channels. For example, it is responsible for mediating the effects of β-adrenergic stimulation in a wide variety of cells. Cyclic adenosine monophosphate is formed by the action of adenylyl cyclase on adenosine triphosphate. See also *adenylyl cyclase*.

cyclic guanine monophosphate (cGMP). A regulatory nucleotide that modulates the hydrolysis of cyclic adenosine monophosphate.

d

D (dual). Letter used in the NBG code for pacemakers. When used in the code's first position, it designates that a pacemaker model can pace in both the atrium and the ventricle; in the code's second position, it designates that a pacemaker can sense in both the atrium and the ventricle; and in the code's third position, it designates that a pacemaker can be triggered to pace by a sensed event in one chamber and inhibited by a sensed event in the other chamber. See the table *NBG code*.

DAC. Abbreviation for *digital-to-analog converter*.

Dacron pouch. See *pouch*.

DAD. The NBG code for a dual-chamber pacing mode in which pacing occurs in the atrium and the ventricle, sensing occurs only in the atrium, and the mode of response is inhibited or triggered. DAD also is an abbreviation for *delayed afterdepolarization*.

damping. A successive decrease in waveform amplitude. Damping is used to reduce the amplitude of intrinsic cardiac signals and applied electrical waveforms for representation on electrocardiograms and intracardiac electrograms.

Danish pacing trial. Prospective trial in 225 consecutive patients with sinus node dysfunction randomized to atrial (*n*=110) or ventricular (*n*=115) pacing and followed for up to 5 years. During follow-up, atrial pacing, compared with ventricular pacing, was associated with lower frequencies of atrial fibrillation and thromboembolic complications and a lower mortality rate. In a later follow-up study, the beneficial effect of atrial pacing was enhanced over time, being associated with a significantly higher survival rate, lower incidence of atrial fibrillation, fewer thromboembolic complications, lower incidence of heart failure, and a low-risk of atrioventricular block (Andersen HR, Thuesen L, Bagger JP, Vesterlund T, Thomsen PE. Prospective randomised trial of atrial versus ventricular pacing in sick-sinus syndrome. Lancet. 1994;344:1523-8; Andersen HR, Nielsen JC, Thomsen PE, Thuesen L, Mortensen PT, Vesterlund T, et al. Long-term follow-up of patients from a randomised trial of atrial versus ventricular pacing for sick-sinus syndrome. Lancet. 1997;350:1210-6).

DAO. Abbreviation for *dynamic atrial overdrive*.

DAPPAF. See *Dual-Site Atrial Pacing to Prevent Atrial Fibrillation*.

data storage. A function of pacemakers and implantable cardioverter-defibrillators by which patient information and device performance data are stored within the circuitry and retrieved through telemetry. See also *diagnostic data, event counter, pacemaker monitor, patient information storage*.

data transmission. The transfer of data or information from one device to another (e.g., between an implanted device to an external programmer). See also *telemetry*.

DAVID. See *Dual-Chamber and VVI Implantable Defibrillator trial*.

DAVID II. See *Dual-Chamber and VVI Implantable Defibrillator II trial*.

DBS. Abbreviation for *drawn-brazed strand*.

DBT. Abbreviation for *devise-based testing*.

DC. Abbreviation for *direct current*.

DCM. Abbreviation for *dilated cardiomyopathy*.

DDD. The NBG code for dual-chamber pacing. Pacing and sensing occur in both the atrium and the ventricle, and the mode of response is inhibited or triggered. See also *dual-chamber pacing, upper rate behavior*. •

DDDR. The NBG code for dual-chamber rate-adaptive pacing. Pacing and sensing occur in both the atrium and the ventricle, the mode of response is inhibited or triggered, and the pacemaker is capable of rate-adaptive pacing via a sensor that monitors a physiologic or nonphysiologic variable. See also *dual-chamber pacing, rate-adaptive pacing, upper rate behavior*. •

DDDRD. The NBG code representing DDDR pacing. The "D" in the fifth position indicates that there is multisite pacing in both atria and ventricles.

DDI. The NBG code for atrioventricular sequential dual-chamber inhibited pacing in which pacing and sensing occur in both the atrium and the

DDD Pacing

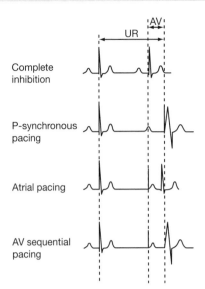

UR, upper rate. Modified from Hayes DL, Levine PA. Pacemaker timing cycles. In: Ellenbogen KA, editor. Cardiac pacing. Boston: Blackwell Scientific Publications; 1992. p. 263-308. Used with permission.

ventricle, and the mode of response is inhibited. Sensed atrial activity inhibits the atrial output pulse but does not reset the atrial timing cycle. In DDI pacing, the timing cycle of each channel typically is controlled by the ventricular channel of the pacemaker to maintain a constant RV or VV interval. DDI pacing is similar to DVI pacing; however, atrial sensing in DDI pacing reduces the possibility of atrial competition between the P wave and the atrial output pulse. See also *AV sequential pacing, AV sequential ventricular-inhibited pacing mode (DVI)*.

DDIR. The NBG code for atrioventricular sequential dual-chamber inhibited pacing in which pacing and sensing occur in both the atrium and the ventricle, the mode of response is inhibited, and the pacemaker is capable of rate-adaptive pacing via a sensor that monitors a physiologic or nonphysiologic variable. DDIR pacing is suitable for a patient with paroxysmal supraventricular rhythm disturbances that require dual-chamber rate-adaptive pacing. In the DDIR mode, the pacemaker will not be triggered by (will not track) the paroxysmal supraventricular tachycardia but still can provide rate-adaptive pacing via the sensor.

DDT. See *dual-chamber triggered pacing mode (DDT)*.

DDT/I. An obsolete designation for DDD pacing. See also *DDD*.

DDX. A device-specific code used to denote a DDD

pacing mode that has an option in which the pacemaker's atrial refractory period is automatically extended if a premature ventricular contraction is sensed. See also *postventricular atrial refractory period extension*.

dead-end pathways. 1. In patients with either atrial or ventricular tachycardia associated with a diseased substrate, portions of scarred tissue or peri-infarct regions may exhibit slow conduction but not be actively involved in the circuit and are referred to as dead-end pathways. 2. Portions of an arrhythmogenic substrate that can be regions wherein pacing captures local myocardium and resets reentrant atrial or ventricular tachycardia without change in the surface electrocardiographic morphology but not critical to the genesis of the arrhythmia (bystander pathway).

DEBUT. See *Defibrillator Versus β-Blockers for Unexplained Death in Thailand*.

deceleration-dependent aberration. Abnormal intraventricular conduction that occurs as heart rate decreases. Deceleration-dependent aberration may be due to enhanced phase 4 depolarization in one of the bundle branches, leading to slowed conduction, or to block that occurs when the bundle branches are activated. Deceleration-dependent aberration is much less common than acceleration-dependent aberration. See also *acceleration-dependent aberration, depolarization phases*.

DDD: Upper Rate Behavior

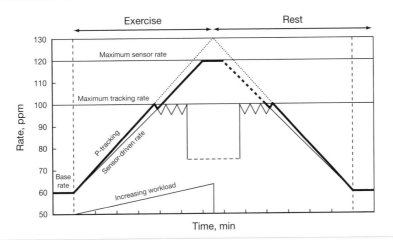

DDDR: Upper Rate Behavior

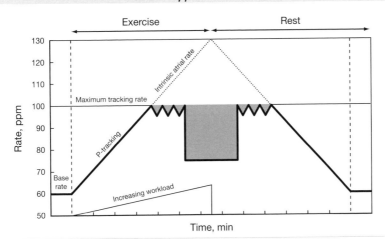

DDI Pacing

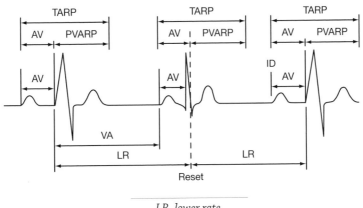

LR, lower rate.

deceleration-dependent bundle branch block. Infrahisian block in either the right or the left bundle branch that occurs with slowing of the supraventricular rate.

decode. See *demodulation*.

DECREASE-HF. See *Device Evaluation of CONTAK RENEWAL 2 and EASYTRAK 2: Assessment of Safety and Effectiveness in Heart Failure.*

decremental conduction. In cellular electrophysiology, progressive diminution of an action potential as it travels along a fiber and results in slower conduction. The term often is used in clinical electrophysiology to denote atrioventricular nodal-like conduction, in which conduction becomes progressively slower as extrastimuli become increasingly premature.

decremental pacing. A technique used during electrophysiologic testing to analyze antegrade or retrograde conduction through the atrioventricular node, the His-Purkinje system, or accessory pathways. The atrium or ventricle is paced at a cycle length just below the intrinsic rhythm, that is, at a rate just above the intrinsic rhythm. The paced cycle length is progressively shortened until block occurs or until a predetermined minimum cycle length is reached. Decremental pacing sometimes is referred to as incremental pacing because of the progressively increased pacing rate. However, the term *decremental pacing* focuses on cycle length rather than on pacing rate and thus is the preferred term. See also *atrial decremental pacing, ventricular decremental pacing.*

default. In pacing, the automatic selection of nominal values by a pacemaker programmer at the initiation of programming. The default position values are physiologic and usually are specific for different pacemaker models.

default value. See *default.*

defibrillation. Termination of atrial or ventricular fibrillation, usually by the delivery of a brief electrical shock to the head either directly or through two electrodes (two paddles) placed on the chest wall. The electrical shock is not synchronized with any element of the cardiac cycle. It depolarizes the entire myocardium simultaneously; when it is successful, it allows the sinus node to resume its control as the primary intrinsic pacemaker of the heart. Direct-current electrical shocks delivered via the chest wall to defibrillate the heart typically range from 50 to 400 J. Far less energy is required for direct cardiac defibrillation, and thus energy shocks delivered during open-chest surgery or by an implantable cardioverter-defibrillator typically range from 5 to 40 J. See also *implantable cardioverter-defibrillator.*

defibrillation circuit. In cardiac defibrillators, the programmed circuit for the shocking energy. This may involve one or more defibrillation coils and an electrically active can; at times, subcutaneous electrodes, subcutaneous patches, or coronary sinus coils may form part of the defibrillation circuit.

defibrillation lead. An electrical connector used to deliver shocks to the heart.

defibrillation patch electrode. An epicardial lead used to deliver energy for defibrillation.

defibrillation probability curve. The graph expressing the relationship between the energy, voltage, or current of a shock and the percentage of success in terminating ventricular fibrillation.

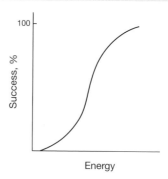

Defibrillation Probability Curve

defibrillation shock. An electrical discharge to the heart sufficient to depolarize large sections of the myocardium regardless of their previous state. Defibrillation shocks usually are intended to terminate episodes of ventricular tachycardia or ventricular fibrillation.

defibrillation threshold (DFT). The minimum electrical energy or voltage required to successfully terminate ventricular fibrillation. Use of the term *threshold* in this context is an oversimplification of fact because the defibrillation threshold is a probabilistic function and thus there is no discrete value that separates success from failure.

defibrillation threshold testing. A format of inducing fibrillation in a patient and evaluating the efficacy of varying shock strengths for defibrillation, both to ensure that the device can reliably rescue and to guide device programming. There are several protocols, but a main method of testing begins with a shock of a given energy and, if successful, "stepping down" to lower energies in subsequent defibrillation attempts in order to identify the minimum effective defibrillation threshold.

defibrillation waveforms. Waveforms of the shocking pulse for cardiac defibrillation. Shocking energy delivery in a single direction is referred to as monophasic. A reversal in the direction of electrical energy transfer during energy delivery is referred to as biphasic. See also *biphasic waveform, tilt.*

Defibrillator in Acute Myocardial Infarction Trial (DINAMIT). This was an open, multicenter, randomized, prospective study designed to assess the impact of implantation of a cardioverter-defibrillator and optimal medical therapy compared with optimal medical therapy alone on all-cause mortality in high-risk patients within 40 days after myocardial infarction. Other inclusion data included left ventricular ejection fraction of 35% or less, depressed standard deviation of sinus RR intervals 70 milliseconds or less or increased heart rate, and mean RR interval 750 milliseconds or less. The primary end point was all-cause mortality. The study found that therapy with an implantable cardioverter-defibrillator did not reduce mortality in high-risk patients in the early period after infarction. It did significantly reduce arrhythmic death by more than 50%, although this was offset by a significant increase in nonarrhythmic death (Hohnloser SH, Kuck KH, Dorian P, Roberts RS, Hampton JR, Hatala R, et al, DINAMIT Investigators. Prophylactic use of an implantable cardioverter-defibrillator after acute myocardial infarction. N Engl J Med. 2004;351:2481-8).

Defibrillators in Non-ischemic Cardiomyopathy Treatment Evaluation (DEFINITE). In this trial, patients with nonischemic dilated cardiomyopathy, left ventricular ejection fraction less than 36%, and premature ventricular complexes or nonsustained ventricular tachycardia were randomized to standard medical therapy or to standard medical therapy plus a single-chamber implantable cardioverter-defibrillator. In patients with severe, nonischemic dilated cardiomyopathy who were treated with

angiotensin-converting enzyme inhibitors and β-blockers, the implantation of an implantable cardioverter-defibrillator significantly reduced the risk of sudden death from arrhythmia and was associated with a reduction in the risk of death from any cause (not statistically significant). (Kadish A, Dyer A, Daubert JP, Quigg R, Estes NA, Anderson KP, et al. Defibrillators in Non-Ischemic Cardiomyopathy Treatment Evaluation [DEFINITE] Investigators. Prophylactic defibrillator implantation in patients with nonischemic dilated cardiomyopathy. N Engl J Med. 2004;350:2151-8).

defibrillator systems analyzer (DSA). A device used to assess variables and to deliver shocks of different energies for determination of the defibrillation threshold during implantation of an implantable cardioverter-defibrillator.

Defibrillator Versus β-Blockers for Unexplained Death in Thailand (DEBUT). This randomized clinical trial compared the annual all-cause mortality rates among patients with sudden unexplained death syndrome treated with β-blockers and those treated with an implantable cardioverter-defibrillator. The study found that treatment with an implantable cardioverter-defibrillator provides full protection from death related to primary ventricular fibrillation in a population with sudden unexplained death syndrome and is superior to β-blocker treatment (Nademanee K, Veerakul G, Mower M, Likittanasombat K, Krittayapong R, Bhuripanyo K, et al. Defibrillator Versus β-Blockers for Unexplained Death in Thailand [DEBUT]: a randomized clinical trial. Circulation. 2003 May 6;107:2221-6. Epub 2003 Apr 14).

DEFINITE. See *Defibrillators in Non-ischemic Cardiomyopathy Treatment Evaluation.*

deflectable catheters. A catheter in which the tip can be deflected to steer the catheter into certain vessels and areas of the heart. Technically, this maneuver may be much easier than trying to steer a straight catheter into the same vessel or region.

deformation. The gradual reversible decay of the oxide layer on the surface of the aluminum plates of an electrolytic capacitor and the consequent loss of insulation and capacitance. The oxide layer may be re-formed by the application of high voltage. The effect of deformation in an implantable cardioverter-defibrillator is lengthening of charge times.

delayed afterdepolarization (DAD). A secondary depolarization of the cell membrane that occurs after full recovery, that is, during phase 4. If the delayed afterdepolarization is of sufficient amplitude to attain threshold, a subsequent action potential may occur. Delayed afterdepolarizations and early afterdepolarizations compose the cellular mechanism that underlies triggered activity. Delayed afterdepolarizations may be the cause of arrhythmia due to digitalis toxicity. See also *depolarization phases, early afterdepolarization.*

Delayed Afterdepolarization

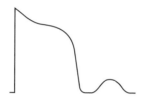

delayed longitudinal contraction (DLC). With tissue Doppler techniques, regional myocardial segments can be tracked to determine their degree of longitudinal systolic shortening. When there is dyssynchrony of the left ventricle, this technique may show delayed longitudinal contraction.

delayed rectifier. The potassium current predominantly responsible for repolarization. See also I_K.

delayed rectifier potassium channels. Cardiac ion channels responsible for repolarization that occurs during phase 2 and phase 3 of the action potential. Currents using these channels include I_{Kr} and I_{Ks}. Disorders related to the delayed rectifier potassium channel are responsible for some forms of the long QT syndrome.

deliverable battery capacity. The usable capacity of a battery. In pacing, deliverable battery capacity depends on self-discharge losses, pacing rates, declining voltage, and current drain. The typical usable capacity of a lithium-iodide battery is 70% to 80%. In a lithium-cupric sulfide battery, it is 90%. See also *battery capacity.*

delta wave. The slurring of the initial portion of the QRS complex, as seen on an electrocardiogram in preexcitation syndromes. See also *accessory pathway, Wolff-Parkinson-White syndrome.*

deltopectoral groove. Anatomic structure formed by the deltoid muscle and the clavicular head of the pectoralis major. In pacemaker and implantable cardioverter-defibrillator lead placement, this may serve as a major landmark when accessing the cephalic vein, which traverses the groove along with the thoracoacromial arteries and nerves.

demand pacing. Pacing in which the pacemaker output is inhibited in response to a sensed spontaneous depolarization, such as in VVI pacing. If no intrinsic activity is sensed before the end of the alert period of the timing cycle, the pacemaker delivers an output pulse. See also *inhibited pacing.*

demodulation. The separation of a coded electrical signal from a carrier signal; the process of retrieving information from a modulated carrier signal. In pacing, demodulation is used during programming or telemetry to separate the information that has been encoded onto and transmitted by the modulated carrier signal from that signal. See also *carrier signal, modulation.*

denervation. Interruption or destruction of nerve pathways. Regional cardiac denervation, either sympathetic or parasympathetic, may occur as a result of myocardial infarction. Partial

Delta Wave

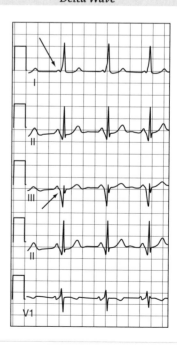

and nonuniform sympathetic denervation may be arrhythmogenic (e.g., atrial fibrillation, torsades de pointes).

denervation supersensitivity. An enhanced response to a neurotransmitter in tissue in which the nerve supply has been interrupted. For example, supersensitivity to norepinephrine occurs in myocardial tissue that is sympathetically denervated and exhibits exaggerated shortening of refractoriness and enhanced conduction.

depletion indicator. A device function that signals battery life is diminishing. Depletion indicators vary between different manufacturers and models of implantable devices. See also *battery depletion, battery status.*

depolarization. A shift of the membrane potential in the positive direction; that is, the tendency of the intracellular fluid to become positive relative to the extracellular fluid. In the heart, waves of depolarization spread from cell to cell and result in contraction of either both atria (in response to an atrial stimulus) or both ventricles (in response to a ventricular stimulus). In pacing, a stimulus depolarizes the membrane and results in an action potential if threshold is reached. See also *depolarization phases.*

depolarization phases. Components of an action potential that describe a recorded waveform that corresponds to specific biochemical changes across cell membranes. If a microelectrode is introduced into an atrial or ventricular cell, an intracellular resting potential of about −80 to −90 mV relative to the extracellular fluid is recorded; that is, the intracellular fluid has a negative charge relative to the extracellular fluid. Activation of a resting myocardial cell by an intrinsic or extrinsic stimulus (mechanical, chemical, or electrical) disrupts the transmembrane potential and produces an action potential, during which the intracellular resting potential shifts from negative to positive. In a recorded action potential, phase 0 is the upstroke in which membrane potential moves from a resting level of about −90 mV to about +30 mV. This phase is mediated by a rapid inward flow of sodium ions and a rapid outward flow of potassium ions across cell membranes. Phase 1 is visible as a slight movement of membrane potential in an outward current direction toward baseline. Phase 2 is called the plateau phase, because the membrane potential remains relatively constant. Phases 1 and 2 are mediated by a slow inward flow of sodium and calcium ions. Phase 3 represents repolarization and is mediated by an outward flow of sodium and an inward flow of potassium. This is the energy-consuming phase that is dependent on adenosine triphosphate. Phase 4 represents electrical diastole and requires just enough energy consumption to maintain the resting potential and ionic gradients across the cell membrane. In the specialized conduction system of the heart (unlike cells of the working myocardium), phase 4 is characterized by gradual depolarization that brings the tissue to threshold and leads directly to another depolarization. See also *resting potential.* •

Depolarization Phases

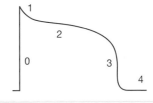

depolarization sequence. During the mapping of arrhythmias in the electrophysiology laboratory, the identified sequence of electrical activation from the earliest site to the remainder of the myocardium of either ventricle or atrium. See also *activation mapping, site of earliest activation.*

desethylamiodarone. An active metabolite of amiodarone.

DESIRE. See *DESynchronization as Indication for Resynchronization.*

desmoplakin right ventricular cardiomyopathy. Inherited disorder of right ventricular dysfunction with frequent occurrences of ventricular tachyarrhythmia and need for cardiac ablation or implantable defibrillators.

DESynchronization as Indication for Resynchronization (DESIRE). This trial will try to identify responders to cardiac resynchronization therapy as defined by electromechanical echocardiographic measurements and to determine whether dyssynchrony measurements can be used for patient selection. Patients included are those with severe heart failure with dilated cardiomyopathy of idiopathic or ischemic cause without any conventional pacing indication, but they must have an indication for

Depolarization and ECG Waveform

	Resting potential, mV	Conduction velocity, m/s	Action potential duration, ms	Waveform
Sinus node	-50 to -60	>0.05	100 to 300	
Atrial myocardium	-80 to -90	1.0	100 to 300	
AV node	-60 to -70	<0.05	100 to 300	
His bundle	-90 to -95	3.0	300 to 500	
Ventricular myocardium	-80 to -90	1.0	100 to 200	
				Surface ECG

cardiac resynchronization therapy. The protocol assesses cardiac resynchronization therapy by echocardiography and evaluates its effectiveness through a composite criterion combining mortality, morbidity, and functional status. It evaluates safety by reporting adverse events (Sorin Group: ELA Medical).

detection. Recognition of arrhythmia, or noise, by a pacemaker or implantable cardioverter-defibrillator. Detection occurs when the criteria for a detection algorithm are satisfied.

detection algorithm. The process by which sensed intervals are analyzed for evidence of tachycardias. Algorithms may, for example, test the proportion of detected intervals that are faster than a given rate cutoff, the change in intervals that occurs at onset, or the stability of the intervals. The detection algorithm is programmable in most devices.

detection criterion. The proportion of sensed cardiac intervals that are shorter than the detection interval required to detect a tachycardia.

detection enhancements. Term used to describe several programmable variables that help implantable cardioverter-defibrillators differentiate between types of tachycardias (e.g., supraventricular tachycardia from ventricular tachycardia). Variables analyzed include a tachyarrhythmia's stability, onset, sustained rate duration, ventricular electrogram width or morphology, and atrial-to-ventricular timing.

detection zones. During programming of implanted cardiac defibrillators, differing criteria may be programmed to allow detection of slower ventricular tachycardia, faster ventricular tachycardia, and ventricular fibrillation. Various discriminating criteria in addition to heart rate are used to define these detection zones.

device-based monitoring. Usually, the use of an implanted device to monitor cardiac rhythm. Devices with extended features also may monitor cardiac pressures, surrogates for myocardial function, impedance, and other markers for heart failure. Device-based monitoring may be associated with the capability for remote electronic surveillance via the Internet.

device-based testing (DBT). Testing for inducibility of arrhythmia and defibrillation thresholds, performed using the programmable functions of an implanted device.

device-based therapy. Generic term for the use of implanted devices and occasionally wearable external devices to either detect or treat (or both) tachyarrhythmias and bradyarrhythmias.

device-device interaction. Generic indication that device 1 can or has interacted or affected function of device 2. There are many types of such potential interactions. If a patient has a pacemaker implanted and subsequently has another device implanted, the two could interact. The second device could be another cardiac device, a spinal cord stimulator, any electrical device, or a device with mechanical interaction with the initial system. The definition also may relate to an implantable device that is interfered with by another device in an environment that produces electromagnetic interference.

Device Evaluation of CONTAK RENEWAL 2 and EASYTRAK 2: Assessment of Safety and Effectiveness in Heart Failure (DECREASE-HF). This is a randomized trial assessing the implications of V-V timing in patients with an implantable cardioverter-defibrillator and includes patients with standard indications for cardiac resynchronization therapy. The primary end point of the study is peak oxygen consumption. Patients are randomized to cardiac resynchronization therapy, cardiac resynchronization therapy with left ventricular offset, or left ventricular pacing only. Patient inclusion criteria include New York Heart Association class III or IV, left ventricular ejection fraction 35% or less, QRS duration 150 milliseconds or more, PR interval 320 milliseconds or less, P-wave duration less than 150 milliseconds, creatinine 2.5 mg/dL or less, and spontaneous, inducible, or at high risk for life-threatening ventricular arrhythmias (De Lurgio DB, Foster E, Higginbotham MB, Larntz K, Saxon LA. A comparison of cardiac resynchronization by sequential biventricular pacing and left ventricular pacing to simultaneous biventricular pacing: rationale and design of the DECREASE-HF clinical trial. J Card Fail. 2005;11:233-9).

device recall. A recall is an action taken to address a problem with a medical device that violates U.S. Food and Drug Administration law. Recalls occur when a medical device is defective, when it could be a risk to health, or when it is both defective and a risk to health. A recall sometimes means that the medical device needs to be checked, adjusted, or fixed. If an implanted device (e.g., a pacemaker or an artificial hip) is recalled, it does not always have to be removed. When an

implanted device has the potential to fail unexpectedly, physicians are encouraged to contact their patients to discuss the risk of removing the device compared with the risk of leaving it in service (U.S. Food and Drug Administration [homepage on the Internet]. Rockville: Center for Devices and Radiological Health [updated 2005 Dec 19; cited 2006 Dec 15]. Learn About Medical Device Recalls. Available from: http://www.fda.gov/cdrh/recalls/learn.html). See also *recall*.

Device Recalls

Class I

There is a reasonable probability that the use of or exposure to a product will cause serious adverse health consequences or death

Class II

Use of or exposure to a product may cause temporary or medically reversible adverse health consequences or the probability of serious adverse health consequences is remote

Class III

Use of or exposure to a product is not likely to cause adverse health consequences

Modified from U.S. Food and Drug Administration [homepage on the Internet]. Rockville: Center for Devices and Radiological Health [updated 2005 Dec 19; cited 2006 Dec 15]. Learn About Medical Device Recalls. Available from: http://www.fda.gov/cdrh/recalls/learn.html.

device-specific features. Certain programmable options and therapeutic features are nearly identical from device to device of the same manufacturer and between comparable devices of varying manufacturers. Some other functions, however, may be specific to a device or provided by a particular manufacturer, and these are referred to as device-specific features.

dexamethasone sodium phosphate (DSP). The corticosteroid most commonly used in steroid-eluting pacing leads. See also *hydrocortisone*.

DF-1. Designation for connectors of implantable cardiac rhythm management devices, such as defibrillators and defibrillator leads, that conform to the international standard (ISO 11318). DF-1 connectors are unipolar and are for high-voltage applications such as defibrillation. The major portion of the lead connector is 3.2 mm in diameter. O-ring seals are located on the lead connector.

DFT. Abbreviation for *defibrillation threshold*.

diagnostic data. In pacing, information that is monitored, recorded, and stored by a pacemaker and describes the function of the pacemaker. Diagnostic data may, for example, include the frequency of paced and sensed events in each chamber, the frequency of sensed premature ventricular contractions, and the response of a rate-adaptive sensor over time. Such information may be retrieved through telemetry. See also *data storage, event counter, pacemaker monitor*.

diaphragmatic pacing. Stimulation of the diaphragm by pacing stimuli. Diaphragmatic pacing may be therapeutic (e.g., paralyzed diaphragm). However, diaphragmatic pacing as it relates to implanted devices implies a complication in which the diaphragm is stimulated. Clinically, this may manifest as a rhythm "spasm" or "jerking" sensation. Rarely, it may manifest as hiccups. Diaphragmatic pacing may be correctable by lowering the output of the device, but at times it requires lead repositioning.

diaphragmatic stimulation. Intermittent contractions of the diaphragm caused by stimulation of the diaphragm or phrenic nerve by pacemaker output pulses. Diaphragmatic stimulation may indicate perforation of the myocardium by an endocardial pacing lead or placement of an epicardial or endocardial lead on, or too close to, the phrenic nerve. Diaphragmatic pacing also may be purposeful to create a respiratory assist.

diastole. The period of dilatation of the heart, especially the ventricles. Diastole is the resting and filling stage of the cardiac cycle.

diastolic dysfunction. Diastole encompasses the period during which the myocardium no longer generates force and shortens and as a result returns to an unstressed length and force. Diastolic dysfunction occurs when this return to the unstressed length and force is slowed, prolonged, or incomplete. It is usually defined by echocardiographic variables.

diastolic mitral regurgitation. Regurgitation through the mitral valve which occurs during diastole. This may occur when atrial contraction is not followed by adequately synchronized left ventricular contraction, such as during atrioventricular block. It also may be due to significant increases of left ventricular end-diastolic filling pressures, such as in the presence of severe aortic regurgitation and restrictive ventricular hemodynamics.

diathermy. The passage of localized heat through body tissues by use of a high-frequency electrical current, such as short waves or microwaves. The response of an implanted pacemaker to diathermy is unpredictable. The pacemaker may be inhibited or triggered, depending on its preset or programmed mode, or it may change to its noise reversion mode. Damage to the pacemaker circuitry or tissue adjacent to the pacing system is improbable.

differential amplifier. An amplifier designed to measure voltage as it is applied to two separate input terminals and to reject any voltage that has the same measured amplitude at both terminals. The difference between the voltages measured at the terminals is amplified as it is processed through the differential amplifier circuit. The ground of the differential amplifier is common to both inputs. In pacing, the principle of the differential amplifier is applied to differential bipolar sensing to minimize inappropriate sensing by the pacemaker. See also *common-mode rejection ratio, differential bipolar sensing, differential input*.

differential AV interval. A function of most dual-chamber pacemakers which permits a longer atrioventricular interval after a paced atrial event than after a sensed atrial event. See also *rate-variable AV interval*.

differential bipolar sensing. In pacing, a sensing configuration in which the anode and cathode of a bipolar lead are used for sensing and the pacemaker case serves as the remote reference electrode. Differential bipolar sensing measures differential input, and thus signals that occur simultaneously at the anode and cathode of the lead are rejected. Differential bipolar sensing minimizes inappropriate sensing of electromagnetic interference and myopotentials. See also *common-mode rejection ratio, differential input*.

differential input. In a differential amplifier, the difference in the voltage as measured between the two input terminals. Differential input is unique in the manner in which it is measured. Most amplifiers measure the voltage difference between the input terminals of the amplifier and the ground of the circuit rather than between the two terminals of the amplifier. In pacing, differential input is the basis for common-mode rejection and differential bipolar sensing that is used in the sensing circuitry of the pacemaker to distinguish intrinsic cardiac events from extraneous noise. See also *common-mode rejection ratio, differential amplifier, differential bipolar sensing*.

digital electrocardiography. Electrocardiography performed using a digital acquiring system. Pacemaker spikes may be less well seen in a digitally sampled electrocardiographic system. Automated measurements and remote monitoring using a Web-based system are facilitated with digital monitoring systems.

digitalis. A cardiac glycoside that prolongs sinus node and atrioventricular nodal refractoriness, decreases conductivity through the atrioventricular node, decreases heart rate, and increases contractility. Digitalis does not significantly affect pacing thresholds. Clinical preparations are digoxin and digitoxin.

digitalis toxicity. The condition that results from an overdose of digitalis. Although digitalis toxicity may cause any arrhythmia, the classic (but not the most common) arrhythmias are nonparoxysmal junctional tachycardia and bidirectional ventricular tachycardia. Digitalis toxicity predisposes to potentially lethal arrhythmias after cardioversion, whereas digitalis use itself does not. Nausea is the most common side effect of digitalis toxicity.

digital signal. A signal that consists of numbers in a given base numbering system, which in computers usually is binary, to represent the quantified variables that occur in a problem or calculation. In pacing, digital signals are used to transmit programming and telemetry information. See also *analog signal, binary code*.

digital-to-analog converter (DAC). A circuit or device that changes a digital signal, such as a binary code, into a proportional analog signal, such as an electrical voltage signal. In pacing, a digital-to-analog converter is used to convert digital signals from the pacemaker circuitry into analog signals of different amplitudes, such as the output pulse conducted through the lead to the heart.

digoxin. A digitalis preparation with a half-life of about 36 hours. Digoxin is excreted by the kidneys. See also *digitalis, digitalis toxicity*.

dilated cardiomyopathy (DCM). A condition characterized by left ventricular dilatation and markedly reduced left ventricular function.

Left bundle branch block is common in patients with dilated cardiomyopathy. Currently, dilated cardiomyopathy is not an accepted indication for permanent right ventricular pacing. Dilated cardiomyopathy also is referred to as idiopathic cardiomyopathy.

dilator. A plastic tube, the distal end of which is used to dilate a vessel opening for insertion of a pacing lead. See also *lead introducer*.

dilator-sheath technique. Technique for gaining access to the vascular system for both ablation and pacing procedures. A dilator is used to widen the subcutaneous entry site and as a guide for a sheath that is passed over the dilator and remains in the vasculature.

diltiazem. A class IV antiarrhythmic, calcium-channel–blocking agent that prolongs atrioventricular nodal refractoriness and conduction and slightly decreases sinus node automaticity but does not affect refractoriness in atrial, ventricular, or accessory pathway tissue. Diltiazem has efficacy in the treatment of supraventricular arrhythmias and has electrophysiologic properties similar to those of verapamil. Diltiazem is metabolized in the liver and has a plasma half-life of about 3.5 hours.

DINAMIT. See *Defibrillator in Acute Myocardial Infarction Trial*.

diode. An electronic component with two leads that characteristically passes current in only one direction and has a fixed characteristic voltage drop. Diodes are used in rectifiers, logic circuits, and voltage protection circuits. See also *diode drop*.

diode drop. The characteristic voltage drop across a conducting diode, for example, 0.6 V for a silicone diode.

diphenylhydantoin. See *phenytoin*.

direct angiotensin receptor antagonists. Important drugs in the pharmacotherapy for congestive heart failure. In distinction to angiotensin-converting enzyme inhibitors, these drugs act at the level of the angiotensin receptor and are not associated with troublesome cough, which sometimes occurs with angiotensin-converting enzyme inhibitors. See also *angiotensin-converting enzyme inhibitors*.

direct current (DC). A type of electrical current that does not vary in voltage over time. Direct current is the type supplied by pacemaker batteries. In cardioversion-defibrillation, direct current is used for defibrillation shocks.

direct-current ablation. 1. The destruction of tissue by application of a direct-current shock. Lesions caused by direct current are larger (1-2 cm) and less well demarcated than those caused by radiofrequency energy. Because direct-current shocks are painful, patients must be anesthetized when the shocks are delivered. Further, if the direct-current energy is delivered during the arrhythmia that is to be treated, the rhythm frequently terminates regardless of whether the circuit has been affected. 2. A method of treating arrhythmia by ablating via both thermal injury and barotrauma using direct current. Historically, direct-current ablation was the first transvenous method used for ablation. Inadvertent collateral injury to both myocardial and extramyocardial tissue and the frequent complication of ventricular fibrillation during ablation limited its utility.

direct-current cardioversion. The use of direct current via transcutaneous patches to terminate an arrhythmia. Frequently used in the electrical treatment of atrial fibrillation or emergency treatment of hemodynamically unstable ventricular tachycardia. The energy delivery is synchronized to a cardiac signal, usually the QRS complex.

directional catheter. Electrophysiologic mapping or ablation catheter or a catheter used to facilitate coronary sinus interventions which are capable of being deflected in one or two directions, usually in a single plane.

directional guide. Preformed guiding sheath with the ability to be torqued or deflected independent of any deflecting mechanism of the inserted lead or catheter.

direct lead delivery. Replacement of a lead in the coronary sinus, endocardium, or epicardial surface without the use of a guiding sheath.

disabled. As it pertains to implantable device therapy, *disabled* refers to rendering some aspect of the device or therapeutic aspect of the device ineffective or unavailable. For example, in a DDD pacemaker, the device could be programmed to the AAI mode, which would, in effect, disable ventricular pacing and sensing. In an implantable cardioverter-defibrillator, the tachyarrhythmia therapies could be turned off or disabled at the patient's request or temporarily during a procedure if there is concern about electromagnetic interference that could cause false detection of a tachyarrhythmia.

discrete component. Previously, a separate and distinct hardware component of a circuit, such as a transistor, a resistor, or a capacitor. Each discrete component required a manually soldered electrical interconnection, which made the circuit more susceptible to sudden failure from faulty components or inadequate attachment. Early pacemaker circuits were composed of traditionally defined discrete components, which limited pacemaker size and longevity. The term *discrete component* now refers to individual components such as integrated circuits, which may contain large numbers of transistors, resistors, and capacitors. See also *hybrid circuit, integrated circuit.*

discriminant P-wave sensing. The ability to discriminate between retrograde and antegrade P waves. Pacemaker-mediated tachycardia theoretically could be prevented with discriminant P-wave sensing. See also *pacemaker-mediated tachycardia.*

discrimination algorithm. With implanted defibrillators, detection in a ventricular tachycardia or ventricular fibrillation zone from high rates may be caused by a ventricular arrhythmia or a rapidly conducted atrial arrhythmia. A discrimination algorithm is a programmed hierarchy that uses criteria other than the cycle length or rate, including beat-to-beat variability, rapidity of onset of rapid rates, or electrogram morphology, to distinguish between supraventricular and ventricular arrhythmias.

dislodgement. The displacement of an endocardial lead. If the movement of the lead is apparent radiographically, it is called macrodislodgement. If there is no apparent radiographic movement of the lead but the clinical findings are compatible with dislodgement, it may be called microdislodgement. Dislodgement may be indicated by changes in the pacing or sensing thresholds, including a transient or complete loss of sensing or capture. Dislodgement may be confirmed by radiographic studies. See also *displacement, macrodislodgement, microdislodgement.*

disopyramide. A class IA antiarrhythmic agent that prolongs refractoriness in atrial, ventricular, and accessory pathway tissue. Refractoriness in atrioventricular nodal tissue does not respond in a predictable manner. Disopyramide is excreted by the kidneys and has a half-life of 4 to 10 hours. Anticholinergic side effects occur

Dislodgement of Lead

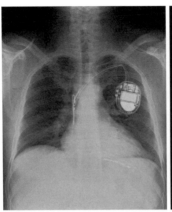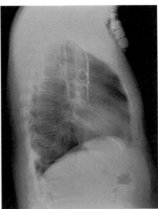

in approximately 25% of patients, but they can be managed with pyridostigmine. Other side effects induce proarrhythmia and congestive heart failure.

dispersion of refractoriness. Variability in repolarization throughout the myocardium such that at a given time some cells are fully recovered and may conduct normally, other cells are in their period of absolute refractoriness and cannot conduct at all, and others are partially repolarized and can conduct with various degrees of slowing. This situation may lead to conditions that support reentrant rhythms. Dispersion of refractoriness also is known as nonuniform recovery of excitability.

dispersion of repolarization. Spatial differences in the myocardium in the rate and magnitude of repolarization. Increased dispersion of repolarization may give rise to certain ventricular arrhythmias.

displacement. In pacing, a change in the position of a lead. Displacement may refer to dislodgement, penetration, or perforation of the myocardium by a lead. Displacement usually is indicated by changes in the pacing or sensing thresholds, including a transient or complete loss of sensing or capture. Displacement may be confirmed by radiographic studies. See also *dislodgement, perforation.*

dissection. As it pertains to implantable device therapy, a vascular complication that could occur as a result of transvenous lead placement. For example, a potential complication of placing a coronary sinus lead is dissection of the coronary vein.

dissociated pulmonary vein rhythm. During radiofrequency ablation of atrial fibrillation, circumferential ablation is performed around the pulmonary vein ostia. After successful ablation, either complete electrical silence (entrance block) in the vein is noted or spontaneous depolarizations (pulmonary vein rhythm) within the pulmonary vein demonstrate exit block to the atrium and are dissociated with atrial activation. •

dissociation. In cardiac physiology, separate rhythms occurring simultaneously in different parts of the myocardium.

distal. Farther from the given point of reference. For example, in anatomy, if the shoulder is used as the point of reference, the wrist is distal to the elbow, and the elbow is proximal to the wrist. In pacing, the pacemaker case typically is used as the point of reference. For example, the terminal pin of a pacing lead is located at the proximal end of the lead, and the stimulating electrode is located at the distal tip of the lead. In an endocardial bipolar lead, the cathode typically is located at the distal tip of the lead and the anodal ring is located several millimeters proximal to the lead tip. Thus, the cathode is referred to as the distal-tip electrode and the anode is referred to as the proximal-ring electrode, even though the two electrodes are located only a few millimeters apart and both are some distance from the pacemaker case.

distal-tip electrode. An electrode located at the end of an endocardial pacing lead which is at the farthest point from the lead terminal pin. The distal-tip electrode usually is the cathode

Dissociated Pulmonary Vein Rhythm

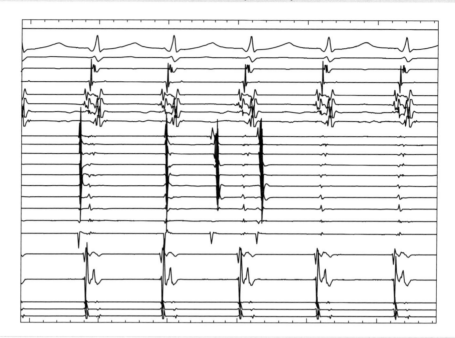

of the pacing circuit. To complete the pacing circuit after the delivery of a pacemaker output pulse, current flows between the distal-tip electrode and the pacemaker case in a unipolar system and between the distal-tip electrode and the proximal-ring electrode in a bipolar system. See also *electrode*.

DLC. Abbreviation for *delayed longitudinal contraction*.

dofetilide. A class III antiarrhythmic agent used primarily for the maintenance of sinus rhythm in patients with atrial fibrillation and flutter

and for the chemical cardioversion to sinus rhythm from atrial fibrillation and flutter.

DOO. The NBG code for dual-chamber asynchronous pacing. The atrium and ventricle are paced sequentially at a fixed rate, and neither chamber is sensed. DOO pacing is a common magnet-mode response in DDD pacing. See also *dual-chamber asynchronous pacing mode (DOO)*.

DOOR. The NBG code for dual-chamber asynchronous pacing with rate modulation.

dopamine. A naturally occurring catecholamine that is the direct precursor in the formation of

Double-Counting

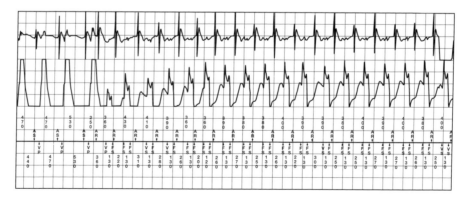

norepinephrine. Dopamine is transformed into norepinephrine by the action of the enzyme dopamine β-hydroxylase.

Doppler echocardiography. 1. Use of the Doppler principle to measure velocity of red blood cells. Doppler measurements of blood velocities are integral to the diagnosis of valve disorders. 2. Use of Doppler principles to measure tissue velocity. Doppler tissue echocardiography is commonly performed for assessment of ventricular dyssynchrony to identify optimal sites for left ventricular lead placement and cardiac ablation.

Doppler tissue imaging (DTI). Doppler tissue imaging filters velocities obtained from blood flow and measures velocity of myocardial and anular tissue. Doppler tissue imaging is useful in the diagnosis of myocardial infarction, myocardial ischemia, ventricular dyssynchrony, and ventricular or atrial compliance. See also *Doppler echocardiography*.

dose-response curve. Curve showing the clinical response or response in a measured laboratory value with changing dosage of a particular drug or intervention. Also may refer to the relationship defining the effects of radiation exposure.

Dotter basket. See *Dotter retriever*.

Dotter basket snare. See *Dotter retriever*.

Dotter retriever. A retractable wire basket that is passed within a sheath through the vascular system. A Dotter retriever may be used for extracting hardware, such as a retained pacing lead, from within the circulation.

double-counting. 1. In earlier generations of biventricular pacing systems, sensing of activation on the right ventricular lead and sensing of activation on the left ventricular lead were sometimes counted as two separate ventricular events. This phenomenon is more likely to occur when significant delay in intraventricular conduction is present. Double counting in this situation could give rise to inappropriate detection and treatment of ventricular arrhythmia. 2. General term referring to the detection of a local myocardial signal and a delayed signal or signal from neighboring myocardial tissue as two separate signals.

double tachycardia. More than one tachycardia may exist in a patient at a given time. In one example, an atrial tachycardia may exist along with a ventricular tachycardia. More rarely, two different atrial tachycardias or two different ventricular tachycardias may exist simultaneously. For double tachycardias to occur in a given chamber, entrance block to prevent suppression or termination, usually from prior cardiac surgery or infarction, is required. Double tachycardias may occur with digitalis toxicity.

double-wave reentry in atrial flutter. An unusual arrhythmia in a single atrial flutter circuit, such as that associated with the cavotricuspid isthmus in which two simultaneous waves of reentry that are out of phase with each other may occur. This phenomenon usually transiently occurs during pacing maneuvers used to define the circuit of atrial flutter.

downward rate smoothing. A programmable variable in some pacemakers and implantable cardioverter-defibrillators which controls the largest decrease in pacing rate when the intrinsic or sensor rate interval is decreasing. See also *rate smoothing*.

dP/dt. The maximum rate of increase of ventricular pressure, that is, the derivative of pressure with respect to time.

dP/dt sensing. Measuring changes in dP/dt as a method of rate adaption in permanent pacing systems. Such a system requires incorporation of a pressure transducer in the permanent pacing lead.

drawn-brazed strand (DBS). In pacing, a lead conductor made of several small wires that, during manufacturing, have been drawn and soldered together with silver. Drawn-brazed strands are used to achieve low resistances and to minimize the external load of the pacing system on the battery. See also *braided conductor*.

drive cycle. The amount of time, usually constant, between consecutive output pulses in a burst stimulation sequence. The drive cycle is used in electrophysiologic testing and is designated on an intracardiac electrogram as S_1. The drive cycle is expressed in milliseconds. See also *burst stimulation*.

drive stimulus. See *drive cycle*.

drive train. See *pacing train*.

dromotropic. Having an effect on the electrical conductivity of a nerve fiber. *Dromotropic* usually is used in reference to the effects of drug therapy on atrioventricular nodal conduction. A drug that has a negative dromotropic effect diminishes conductivity, whereas one that has a positive dromotropic effect increases conductivity.

drug. See name of individual drug and *antiarrhythmic agent*.

drug-device interactions. Any of several interactions whereby administration of a drug may affect the function of a pacemaker or implantable cardioverter-defibrillator, or vice versa. An example is administration of a class IC drug to a pacemaker-dependent patient, which could result in significant increases in pacing threshold and potential loss of capture.

drug-eluting lead. A permanent pacing lead that provides time-released delivery of a drug, typically a corticosteroid, to the tissue immediately adjacent to the pacing electrode. The purpose of the drug is to minimize the acute trauma caused by the lead and thus improve the pacing threshold. There are multiple designs or mechanisms by which the drug is delivered. See also *pacing threshold, sensing threshold, steroid-eluting lead, threshold maturation*.

drug-induced channelopathies. Acquired forms of ion-channel disorders triggered by or entirely caused by the use of certain drugs. Often, patients with a drug-related channel disorder resulting in arrhythmia have an underlying inherited channelopathy (e.g., macrolide antibiotic-related torsades de pointes).

dry battery. A battery composed of dry cells in a common housing. Such a battery provides desired voltage or current values without the production of gas from internal chemical reactions. Dry batteries can be sealed hermetically to protect the pacemaker circuitry from battery chemicals. The lithium-based batteries used in implantable pacemakers are examples of dry batteries.

dry pocket. An uncommon condition of the pacemaker pocket which may occur after implantation of a pacemaker in a preexisting pocket during pacemaker replacement. The presence of a dry pocket indicates that the pacemaker case is in contact with relatively dry materials such as dense fibrotic tissue, air, or remnants of a woven mesh pouch. These materials cause excessive resistance and are poor conductors of electrical current. Dry pocket thus may cause intermittent failure to output in a unipolar pacing system. Dry pocket usually can be eliminated by application of pressure to the pocket. In rare cases, it may be necessary to inject sterile isotonic saline into the pocket. These invasive techniques increase the risk of pocket infection. See also *air entrapment*.

DSA. Abbreviation for *defibrillator systems analyzer*.

D-sotalol. Enantiomer of the racemic DL-sotalol mixture. D-Sotalol, a class III antiarrhythmic drug, has mainly potassium channel blocking effects and, compared with the DL mixture, is relatively proarrhythmic in patients with myocardial dysfunction.

DSP. Abbreviation for *dexamethasone sodium phosphate*.

DTI. Abbreviation for *Doppler tissue imaging*.

dual atrioventricular conduction. Atrial inputs to the atrioventricular node are anatomically discrete. Inputs superior to the tendon of Todaro occur with shorter conduction times and are referred to as the fast pathway. Posterior inputs have longer conduction times and are referred to as the slow pathway. Patients who have discrete changes in conduction from atrial pacing or sinus rhythm through the atrioventricular node have dual atrioventricular conduction.

dual AV nodal pathways. See *dual AV nodal physiology*.

dual AV nodal physiology. The occurrence of two pathways, one fast and one slow, within or near the atrioventricular node. These two pathways compose the substrate that supports atrioventricular nodal reentrant tachycardia. The fast pathway has rapid conduction and a relatively long refractory period, whereas the slow pathway has prolonged conduction and a relatively short refractory period. Typically, atrioventricular nodal reentrant tachycardia occurs when an atrial premature complex blocks in the fast pathway, conducts in the antegrade direction over the slow pathway, and then returns to the atria via the fast pathway. The atrial origin of the slow pathway is extranodal and usually is located posteriorly in the region of the entrance to the coronary sinus. The fast pathway may be the normal atrioventricular node. Dual atrioventricular nodal pathways also are described as dual AV nodal physiology. Patients may have dual AV nodal physiology in the antegrade or retrograde direction without necessarily having atrioventricular nodal reentrant tachycardia.

Dual-Chamber and VVI Implantable Defibrillator (DAVID) trial. This single-blind, parallel-group, randomized clinical trial was designed to determine the efficacy of dual-chamber pacing compared with backup ventricular pacing in patients with standard indications for implantation of an implantable cardio-verter-defibrillator but without indications for antibradycardia pacing. All patients received an implantable cardioverter-defibrillator with dual-chamber, rate-responsive pacing capability. Patients were randomly assigned to have the devices programmed to ventricular backup pacing at 40 beats per minute (VVI-40; n=256) or dual-chamber rate-responsive pacing at 70 beats per minute (DDDR-70; n=250). For patients with standard indications for implantable cardioverter-defibrillator therapy, no indication for cardiac pacing, and a left ventricular ejection fraction of 40% or less, the trial found that dual-chamber pacing has no clinical advantage over ventricular backup pacing and may be detrimental by increasing the combined end point of death or hospitalization for heart failure (Wilkoff BL, Cook JR, Epstein AE, Greene HL, Hallstrom AP, Hsia H, et al, Dual Chamber and VVI Implantable Defibrillator Trial Investigators. Dual-chamber pacing or ventricular backup pacing in patients with an implantable defibrillator: the Dual Chamber and VVI Implantable Defibrillator [DAVID] Trial. JAMA. 2002;288:3115-23).

patients needing an implantable cardioverter-defibrillator but without overt indications for pacing, AAI pacing with maximal concomitant drug therapy will not increase the rate of the combined end point of mortality or hospitalization for new or worsened heart failure when compared with patients with ventricular backup pacing (ClinicalTrials.gov [homepage on the Internet]. Bethesda: U.S. Department of Health and Human Services National Institutes of Health [updated 2005 Sep 10; cited 2006 Dec 15]. DAVID II [Dual Chamber and VVI Implantable Defibrillator [DAVID] Trial II]. Available from: http:www.clinicaltrials.gov/ct/show/NCT00187187).

dual-chamber asynchronous pacing mode (DOO). The dual-chamber pacing mode in which the atrium and ventricle are paced at a preset or programmed rate independent of any intrinsic electrical or mechanical activity. The ventricular output pulses sequentially follow the atrial output pulses after a preset atrioventricular interval. In dual-chamber asynchronous pacing, intrinsic cardiac electrical activity is not sensed, and thus competition with intrinsic rhythm may occur. In unstable cardiac

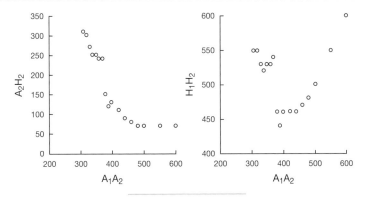

Dual AV Nodal Physiology

Graphic example of dual AV nodal physiology showing A_1A_2 versus A_2H_2 (left) and A_1A_2 versus H_1H_2 (right). Note the sudden prolongation of AV nodal conduction at A_1A_2 (370 milliseconds). This is consistent with block in the fast pathway (fast pathway ERP) and conduction down the slow pathway.

Dual-Chamber and VVI Implantable Defibrillator (DAVID) II trial. This study (in progress) randomizes patients with an implantable cardioverter-defibrillator to either VVI (ventricular demand) pacing at 40 beats per minute or AAI (atrial demand) pacing at 70 beats per minute, will evaluate the hypothesis that, in

conditions, an asynchronous atrial spike during the vulnerable period may initiate arrhythmias. See also *asynchronous pacing.*

dual-chamber demand pacing. See *dual-chamber pacing.*

dual-chamber pacing. Pacing in both the atrium and the ventricle to mimic the natural atrioventricular contraction sequence of the heart. Dual-chamber pacing requires the use of two leads, one in the atrium and one in the ventricle. Dual-chamber pacing encompasses many modes, including DDD, DDDR, DVI, DVIR, DDI, DDIR, VDD, and VDDR.

dual-chamber rate-adaptive pacing mode (DDDR). The dual-chamber pacing mode in which pacing and sensing occur in the atrium and the ventricle, and the mode of response is inhibition or ventricular tracking of an atrial event. The pacemaker also is capable of rate-adaptive pacing via a sensor that monitors some physiologic or nonphysiologic variable and adjusts the heart rate accordingly.

dual-chamber rate-modulated pacing. See *DDDR*.

dual-chamber triggered pacing mode (DDT). Pacing in which a pacemaker output pulse is delivered synchronously with each sensed intrinsic atrial and ventricular event. Dual-chamber triggered pacing can be used temporarily for diagnostic and therapeutic purposes under direct clinical observation to evaluate the integrity of the leads in terms of their ability to sense. It also can be used to determine whether inappropriate sensing of noise or myopotentials is occurring, to terminate supraventricular or ventricular tachycardia, and to perform noninvasive electrophysiologic studies.

dual-sensor rate-adaptive pacing. See *dual sensors*.

dual sensors. The pairing of a physiologic sensor and an activity sensor in a single rate-adaptive device in an attempt to balance the strengths of the sensors (e.g., minute ventilation sensor integrated with an accelerometer).

dual-site atrial pacing. Pacing the atria in two sites. This term could represent pacing the right atrium in two sites, pacing a right atrial site and a coronary sinus location that would stimulate the atria, or pacing a right atrial site and a left atrial epicardial site.

Dual-Site Atrial Pacing to Prevent Atrial Fibrillation (DAPPAF). This was a randomized trial assessing the safety, tolerance, and effectiveness of overdrive high right atrial, dual-site right atrial, and support (DDI or VDI) pacing in patients with symptomatic atrial fibrillation and bradycardias. Patients were randomized to the three groups in a crossover trial. Investigators concluded that dual-site right atrial pac-

ing is safe and better tolerated than high right atrial and support pacing. In patients taking antiarrhythmic agents, dual-site right atrial pacing prolonged the time to recurrent atrial fibrillation and high right atrial pacing tended to prolong the time to recurrent atrial fibrillation compared with support pacing. Dual-site right atrial pacing provided superior symptomatic and asymptomatic prevention of atrial fibrillation compared with high right atrial pacing in patients with symptomatic atrial fibrillation at a frequency of 1 episode or less per week (Saksena S, Prakash A, Ziegler P, Hummel JD, Friedman P, Plumb VJ, et al, DAPPAF Investigators. Improved suppression of recurrent atrial fibrillation with dual-site right atrial pacing and antiarrhythmic drug therapy. J Am Coll Cardiol. 2002;40:1140-50).

dual-site (multisite) pacing. Generally used to represent pacing in either the atria or the ventricles in two (dual) or more (multi) sites.

dual-site right atrial pacing. Pacing the right atria in two sites. The most common sites used include the high right atrial appendage and near the ostium of the coronary sinus. One technique advocates pacing both sites simultaneously, and in another technique one site is paced first and then triggers pacing from the other site.

Duchenne muscular dystrophy. A type of muscular dystrophy; one of the most common sex-linked lethal diseases in humans. In addition to the musculoskeletal manifestations, there may be associated cardiac conduction abnormalities.

DVI. The NBG code for atrioventricular sequential ventricular-inhibited pacing. Pacing occurs in the atrium and the ventricle, sensing occurs only in the ventricle, and the mode of response is inhibited. See also *AV sequential pacing, AV sequential ventricular-inhibited pacing mode (DOO)*.

DVIR. The NBG code for atrioventricular sequential, ventricular-inhibited, rate-adaptive pacing. Pacing occurs in the atrium and ventricle, sensing occurs only in the ventricle, and the mode of response to sensed events is inhibited. The pacemaker also is capable of rate-adaptive pacing via a sensor that monitors some physiologic or nonphysiologic variable.

dye extravasation. During angiography, the appearance of contrast material outside the vessel lumen. The contrast material may extravasate into the vessel wall or completely free of the lumen.

Dual-Site Atrial Pacing

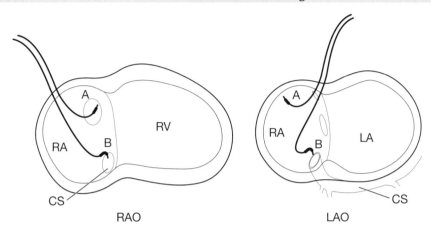

CS, coronary sinus; LA, left atrium; LAO, left anterior oblique; RA, right atrium;
RAO, right anterior oblique; RV, right ventricle.

DVI Pacing

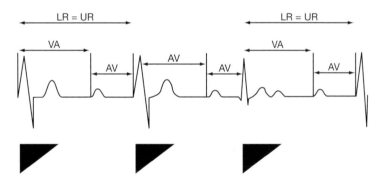

Modified from Hayes DL, Levine PA. Pacemaker timing cycles. In: Ellenbogen KA, editor. Cardiac pacing. Boston: Blackwell Scientific Publications; 1992. p. 263-308. Used with permission.

dynamic atrial overdrive (DAO). A pacing algorithm for the prevention of atrial arrhythmias. The algorithm alters the atrial pacing rate so it remains slightly above the patient's intrinsic rate. DAO algorithm was evaluated in the ADOPT-A Trial. See also *Atrial Dynamic Overdrive Pacing Trial*.

dysprogramming. The unexpected and incorrect programming of a pacemaker due to an extraneous electrical field, such as from arc welding, or the use of a programmer from a manufacturer other than that of the implanted pacemaker. See also *misprogramming, phantom programming*.

dysrhythmia. An abnormal rhythm. Cardiac dysrhythmia denotes a disturbance in which heart rhythm varies from the accepted normal rhythm in terms of rate, regularity, or the propagation of a wave of depolarization as it passes through the cardiac conduction system.

dyssynchronous contraction. Left ventricular contraction that is not synchronous (i.e., temporal heterogeneity of left ventricular wall motion occurs).

dyssynchrony. Temporal heterogeneity of left ventricular wall motion. The most common presentation is that of septal inward motion appearing early in the cardiac cycle and free-wall motion appearing delayed.

E. Abbreviation for *electrical field strength, energy.*

EAD. Abbreviation for *early afterdepolarization.*

EAR. Abbreviation for *electrogram amplitude reduction.*

early activation site. In an electrophysiologic study, point-to-point mapping with an electrode-tipped catheter is performed. The site that shows the earliest electrogram typically preceding the surface P wave (atrial tachycardia) or QRS complex (ventricular tachycardia) is called the early activation site. In automatic arrhythmias, this site is the target for ablation. In reentrant arrhythmias, this site represents the exit from the slow zone responsible for the tachycardia. See *site of earliest activation.*

early afterdepolarization (EAD). Spontaneous depolarizations that occur during phase III of the action potential. This is the mechanism of arrhythmia in patients with polymorphic ventricular tachycardia.

Early Afterdepolarization

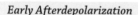
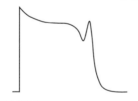

Ebstein's anomaly. Abnormal apical displacement of the tricuspid valve leaflets. A portion of the myocardium above the tricuspid valve is right ventricular myocardium because of this displacement. This anomaly is associated with accessory pathways.

eccentricity. Deviation from expected performance. In pacing, eccentricity refers to a pseudomalformation in which unusual or unexpected operation of a pacemaker may occur with design specifications. Eccentricity should not be confused with pacemaker malfunction. See also *pseudomalfunction.*

eccentric retrograde atrial activation. During electrophysiologic study in patients with an accessory pathway, ventricular pacing is performed to assess the mechanism of ventriculoatrial activation. If, during ventricular pacing, the site of earliest atrial activity is not in the septal region, eccentric retrograde atrial activation is present. This is usually a manifestation of an accessory pathway not located on the septum. See also *concentric retrograde atrial activation.*

ECG. Abbreviation for *electrocardiogram.*

ECG filter. Filter settings on standard electrocardiographic machines to allow appropriate filtering of noise and high-frequency noncardiac signals.

echo beat. During atrial or ventricular pacing, the occurrence of a spontaneous recurrent atrial or ventricular nonpaced complex. Echo beats occurring repetitively constitute tachycardia. The provocation of an echo beat signifies the presence of a dual mechanism of conduction. See also *reentrant circuit.*

echo-derived intraventricular (interventricular) dyssynchrony. Tissue echocardiography can be used to define the presence of and extent of interventricular (right ventricle to left ventricle) and intraventricular dyssynchrony. Various factors, including tissue velocity temporal variation, strain rates, and combined tissue and standard Doppler measurements, are used to define interventricular and intraventricular dyssynchrony.

echo-Doppler imaging. Use of the Doppler principle to evaluate velocity of either the red blood cells or the myocardial tissue (tissue Doppler) for identifying ideal left ventricular lead placement sites and patients likely to benefit from resynchronization therapy.

echogenicity. The echocardiographic appearance of tissue is dependent on the specific properties of a particular tissue and the differences between that tissue and surrounding structures. The degree of reflectance of ultrasound waves of the sampled tissue is referred to as its echogenicity. Infarcted myocardium, ablated tissue, and fibrous tissue are highly echogenic.

echo zone. The range of coupling intervals of extrastimuli that produces echo beats. For example, zone 4 in the sinoatrial conduction time plot is an echo zone.

ectopic atrial tachycardia. A common form of supraventricular tachycardia resulting from abnormal automaticity of atrial myocardial cells. Common sites of origin for ectopic atrial tachycardia include the pulmonary vein, superior vena cava, crista terminalis, and coronary sinus.

ectopic beat. Depolarization originating earlier than expected from a focus outside the sinus node. Ectopic beats may be atrial, junctional, or ventricular in origin. This is in distinction to an escape beat, which occurs later than the expected sinus beat.

ectopic focus. A focus located in the atrium, junction, or ventricle responsible for single ectopic beats, nonsustained automatic tachycardia, or sustained automatic tachycardia.

ectopic impulse generation. Sinus nodal and atrioventricular nodal tissue has a unique action potential that enables ectopic impulse generation. Phase 4 of depolarization, which is typically flat and in a polarized state in myocardial cells, shows a drift toward baseline and eventual reaching of a threshold potential in nodal tissue. The absence of I_{K1} and the presence of I_f currents are among the factors enabling ectopic impulse generation in nodal tissue.

ectopic rhythm. See *ectopic focus*.

edrophonium. A rapid-acting cholinergic agent that has been used to manage supraventricular tachycardias or to transiently cause atrioventricular block during atrial tachycardias. Edrophonium acts as a reversible anticholinesterase. It may cause sinus bradycardia, cardiac standstill, or hypotension in some patients. Edrophonium has been supplanted by newer medications such as adenosine.

EDVI. Abbreviation for *end-diastolic volume index*.

effective electrode. In pacing, the distal-tip electrode of a pacing lead. The surface area of the effective electrode is defined by the surface area of the lead electrode and the surface area of the fibrotic tissue between the lead electrode and the nearest excitable tissue. The effective electrode size is determined by the thickness of fibrotic encapsulation and is inversely related to the electrical field strength at the electrode-myocardial interface. The effective electrode also is referred to as the virtual electrode. See also *electrical field strength*.

effective refractory period (ERP). The longest cycle length during pacing from one cardiac chamber during which conduction block to the other cardiac chamber occurs. For example, if conduction occurs to the ventricle during pacing the atrium at 370-millisecond cycle length but not at 360 or shorter cycle lengths, then 360 milliseconds is the effective refractory period of the atrioventricular node. See also *atrial effective refractory period, AV conduction system effective refractory period, AV nodal effective refractory period, His-Purkinje system effective refractory period, VA conduction system effective refractory period, ventricular effective refractory period*.

efferent nerves. Autonomic nerves that innervate distal myocardium. These nerve fibers may originate in an autonomic ganglion or the sympathetic chain or central vagal nuclei.

EGM. Abbreviation for *electrogram*. See *intracardiac electrogram*.

EHR. Abbreviation for *extended high rate*.

ejection fraction. The percentage of blood volume ejected from the ventricle during systole. Depending on the laboratory and the method used to measure ejection fraction, the normal value is usually 50% to 60%. Ejection fraction is calculated by dividing the stroke volume by the end-diastolic volume.

EKG. Abbreviation for *electrocardiogram*.

elastomer. A synthetic material that, at room temperature, can be stretched under low stress to at least twice its original length and on immediate release of the stress readily returns to approximately its original length. Typical elastomers are synthetic rubbers or plastics, such as silicone rubber. In pacing, elastomers frequently are used as the insulation material of pacing leads.

elective replacement indicator (ERI). Indicator signifying that the pulse generator is nearing the end of battery life. Battery voltage in pacemakers and time to charge capacitor in defibrillators are the primary determinants of elective replacement indicator status. See also *end of life, end-of-life indicators*.

elective replacement time. See *elective replacement indicator*.

electrical activation. Cell-to-cell activation in atrial and ventricular myocardium which defines the depolarization wave front, intracardiac electrical activation sequence, and surface electrocardiogram.

electrical alternans. Electrocardiographic phenomenon in which there is alternating amplitude of P waves (QRS alternans or T-wave alternans). This occurs in patients with large pericardial effusions or with rapid supraventricular tachycardia.

electrical anisotropy. Conduction from one myocardial site to another is partly dependent on the myocardial tissue architecture. Electrical conduction times are shorter across parallel myocardial fibers. When fiber orientation changes abruptly, anisotropy is present and conduction velocity decreases. When electrical anisotropy is extreme, reentrant arrhythmias may result.

electrical atrial remodeling. Process in which the genesis and maintenance of arrhythmia are changed by the repeated presence or continued absence of that arrhythmia. In atrial fibrillation, the ease of induction and persistence of atrial fibrillation are increased by the presence of prior atrial fibrillation.

electrical cardioversion. The use of electrical energy to restore normal cardiac rhythm. In electrical cardioversion, the converting electrical field is applied synchronous with the QRS to avoid genesis of fibrillation.

electrical field strength (E). In pacing, the distribution of applied voltage (V) across the radius of an electrode (Ro) and the effective electrode size (r). Electrical field strength decreases as the effective electrode size increases and is usually expressed in millivolts per millimeter. See also *effective electrode*.

electrical heterogeneity. Myocardial tissue that conducts the electrical wave front in a differing and nonuniform pattern is electrically heterogeneous. Electrical heterogeneity is common in ischemic cardiomyopathy and infiltrative cardiac disorders and after cardiac surgery.

electrical impulse propagation. Once a cell or group of cells has been depolarized, the wave front propagates to other myocardial cells. This impulse propagation is dependent on the amplitude of the initial depolarizing signal, myocardial architecture, and gap junction between myocardial cells.

electrical interference. In pacing, the disruption of normal pacemaker function. Electrical waveforms that have frequency characteristics similar to spontaneous intrinsic cardiac activity may be misinterpreted by the pacemaker sensing circuit and may be processed through the pacemaker circuitry. See also *electromagnetic interference*.

electrical remodeling. Process of electrical changes induced by the continued presence or sustained absence of an arrhythmia. In the ventricle, initially difficult to induce ventricular fibrillation may become easier to induce and more sustained once ventricular fibrillation has been induced. Electrical remodeling also occurs in the reverse direction, that is, maintenance of an arrhythmia-free state for a significant amount of time may make further spontaneous induction of that arrhythmia less likely to occur.

electrical stimuli. Stimuli capable of inducing depolarization of a single myocardial cell or group of myocardial cells. Electrical stimuli may be artificial, such as from a pacemaker or during an electrophysiologic study, or from normally spontaneously depolarizing tissue, such as the sinus node or atrioventricular junction.

electrical storm. Highly malignant disorder in which episodes of ventricular tachycardia, ventricular fibrillation, and polymorphic ventricular tachycardia occur in close succession. A frequent example of the vicious cycle responsible for electrical storms is ventricular fibrillation occurring as a result of myocardial ischemia, provoking further ischemia and further induction of ventricular fibrillation. Without urgent intervention, electrical storm is fatal despite the presence of a normally functioning cardiac defibrillator.

electroanatomic mapping. 1. Generally, the defining of electrical activation times in various anatomic locations. Electroanatomic mapping is performed in one form or another in all ablation procedures, traditionally with point-to-point mapping under fluoroscopic guidance. 2. Specifically, the use of a system (CARTO; Biosense Webster, Inc., Diamond Bar, California) of triangulation to define and tag catheter movements along with the recorded electrograms in three dimensions.

electroanatomic remodeling. See *electrical remodeling*.

electroanatomic substrate mapping. With certain arrhythmias, traditional point-to-point mapping to define the arrhythmia circuit or activation sequence is not possible. Examples include hemodynamically unstable arrhythmias or difficult-to-induce arrhythmias. The myocardium can be mapped in the absence of arrhythmia-defining anatomic sites of electrically abnormal tissue. Thus, myocardial scar, diseased myocardium, and normal myocardium can be defined. In some instances, ablation can be performed targeting the electrically abnormal anatomic sites as a treatment for tachyarrhythmias.

electrocardiogram (ECG, EKG). Typically obtained with 12 leads, including precordial, limb, and augmented leads, the electrocardiogram represents the sum of electrical potentials and activation in the atrium (P wave) and ventricle (QRS complex) and ventricular repolarization (T wave). See also *P wave, QRS complex, T wave.*

Electrocardiogram: Basic Intervals

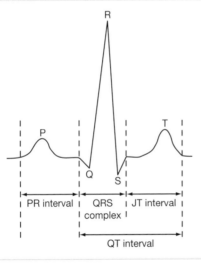

electrocardiographic guidance. The use of surface or intracardiac tracings to guide lead placement. This technique may be particularly useful when placing an atrial lead and trying to achieve an atrial site that minimizes interatrial conduction times. It also may be useful for locating the coronary sinus and for finding a "best" coronary venous position based on QRS morphology and width.

electrocautery. A process used to destroy tissue by passing an electrical current through it. The electrical current is delivered to the tissue through a small wire, which frequently is made of platinum. Electrocautery is a common

source of electromagnetic interference in the hospital environment and has several potential adverse effects, including permanent damage to the pulse generator; inhibition of the pulse generator; reversion for a fall-back mode, noise reversion mode, or electrical rest; and myocardial thermal damage due to transmission of electrical discharge to the heart via the lead(s), resulting in myocardial infarction or ventricular fibrillation or both.

electroconvulsive therapy. Application of an electrical field to the brain as a therapy for certain psychiatric disorders (severe intractable depression, catatonic stupor). Implantable cardiac devices may require programming before and reprogramming after electroconvulsive therapy.

electrode. The portion of an electrical conductor through which current enters or leaves the conductor. In pacing, the electrode is the conductive portion of a pacing lead. Ideally, the electrode transfers electrical stimuli, such as charge, current, power, and energy, in excess of the endocardial pacing threshold and causes cardiac depolarization. The electrode also is the portion of the pacing system by which intrinsic cardiac activity is sensed. See also *ball-tip electrode, distal-tip electrode, porous electrode, porous-surface electrode, proximal-ring electrode, totally porous electrode.*

electrode catheter. An extruded plastic or woven catheter used in transvenous endocardial mapping. An electrode catheter can have 2 to 12 electrodes for bipolar stimulation or recording. A typical electrode catheter has two to four electrodes and is 4F to 7F in diameter. The primary type of electrode catheter is designed specifically for intracardiac electrographic recording and pacing. Electrode catheters can be used to deliver energy for ablation. See also *endocardial mapping catheter, temporary lead.*

electrode configuration. The geometric configuration of the electrodes that are used to pass current through the heart or to sense spontaneous electrical events in the heart. In a bipolar electrode system, the two electrodes are external to the pulse generator and usually are located close to each other on or within the heart. In a unipolar electrode system, the stimulation electrode, usually the cathode, is located on or in the heart, and the reference electrode (indifferent electrode), normally the anode, is all or part of the metal pacemaker case. Bipolar and unipolar systems have similar stimulation thresholds (the stimulus amplitude and duration required for reliable capture in electrical diastole), but bipolar systems are less susceptible to far-field sensing of extraneous electrical signals and are less likely to produce extracardiac stimulation. See also *bipolar electrode system, unipolar electrode system*.

electrode dislodgement. See *dislodgement*.

electrode fracture. A term used incorrectly to describe conductor fracture. See also *conductor fracture, insulation failure*.

electrode impedance. See *transitional electrode impedance*.

electrode-myocardial interface. The point at which an endocardial or epicardial pacing electrode and the myocardium are in contact. Also referred to as electrode-tissue interface. This interface defines the transition zone between ionic conduction in the tissues and ohmic conduction through the electronic circuitry. It is the site of electron accumulation when an output pulse is delivered; the magnitude of the electronic accumulation determines the degree of polarization. Contact of the electrode against the tissue results in an inflammatory response that is responsible for the increase in pacing thresholds in the early post-implantation period.

electrode temperature (T$_E$). In ablation procedures, the temperature of the ablating electrode with myocardial contact is monitored to allow titration of energy delivery. Low electrode temperatures suggest more tissue contact, whereas high electrode temperatures suggest insufficient cooling of the surrounding tissue and risk for coagulum formation.

electrode tip. The tip of electrical mapping, ablation, or pacemaker-defibrillator lead electrode. Contact of the electrode tip to myocardial tissue is vital for device function and delivery of ablation energy.

electrode-tissue interface. See *electrode-myocardial interface*.

electrogram (EGM). The summed local action potentials obtained through an electrode catheter, unipolar or bipolar, typically making contact with the ventricular or atrial myocardium. These waveforms represent local myocardial activation. Variables that are measurable from this graphic representation of depolarization include amplitude, slew rate, and, in some cases, the profile of the ST segment. An electrogram is also referred to as an intracardiac electrogram and should not be confused with a surface electrocardiogram. See also *sinus node electrogram*.

electrogram amplitude reduction (EAR). During ablation, the local epicardial electrogram

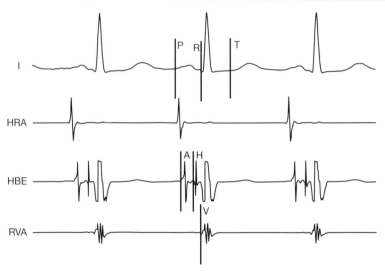

Electrogram (Intracardiac)

Surface and intracardiac lead intervals. Marks are placed for measurement of the AH, HV, PR, and QT intervals. Measurements in this case were as follows: AH = 75 ms; HV = 40 ms; PR = 150 ms; QT = 350 ms.

decreases in amplitude. This reduction in electrogram amplitude is a marker for tissue necrosis. The reduction in electrogram amplitude of 25% of amplitude at starting energy delivery can be used as an end point for ablation at that site. The lack of electrogram amplitude reduction is a marker for poor tissue contact.

electrogram morphology. The local electrogram, either unipolar or bipolar, from an electrode at the tip of a pacemaker lead or electrophysiologic catheter has a specific morphology depending on the wave front of electrical activation. In implanted devices, this morphology can be used to distinguish ventricular arrhythmias from rapidly conducted supraventricular arrhythmias.

electrolyte. Any substance that, when in solution, is dissociated into ions and thus is capable of carrying electrical current by ionic conduction. For example, electrolytes may be specific chemical compounds such as those used in a battery or capacitor or the ions in body fluids. Electrolyte abnormalities in a patient with a pacemaker may result in pacing or sensing abnormalities. See also *hyperkalemia*.

Electrolyte Concentrations in Millimeters

	Extracellular	Intracellular
Na$^+$	140	10
K$^+$	4	140
Ca^{2+}	2	1×10^{-4}
Cl$^-$	140	30

electrolytic capacitor. A type of capacitor technology used to achieve high values needed in high-energy applications such as cardioversion-defibrillation. Electrolytic capacitors generally are composed of tightly wound spiral rolls of aluminum foil, known as plates, separated by an electrolytic solution or gel. The aluminum possesses an oxide layer that insulates the plates from one another and gives the capacitor its charge-storing ability. See also *deformation*.

electromagnetic field (EMF). A region in which magnetic or electrical potentials exist. These potentials may arise from many sources and may interfere with the function of an implanted device.

electromagnetic interference (EMI). In pacing, the interference or disruption of normal pacemaker function by electromagnetic activity in the environment. Electromagnetic signals may be misinterpreted by the pacemaker circuitry, pass through the sensing amplifier of the pacemaker, and interfere with pacemaker function. The pacemaker may be inhibited or triggered, depending on the pacing mode, thus causing temporary unexpected behavior. Some forms of electromagnetic interference cause the pacemaker to operate in its interference or noise mode. For example, electromagnetic interference may cause a pacemaker to switch from its programmed mode and rate to fixed-rate or asynchronous pacing at a different rate. Potential sources of electromagnetic interference include equipment in the hospital environment such as that used for magnetic resonance imaging, electrocautery, and defibrillation. Potential sources of electromagnetic interference outside the hospital environment include welding equipment and electrical motors. Household appliances rarely are a source of electromagnetic interference. See also *noise*.

electromechanical coupling. 1. Once a myocardial cell, or group of cells, has been depolarized, it begins to contract. There is a finite interval between electrical activation and mechanical contraction called the electromechanical coupling interval. This electromechanical coupling may vary from one myocardial site to another, resulting in mechanical dyssynchrony despite the presence of normal electrical activation. 2. Predictable sequence of myocardial contraction (mechanical) that follows and is caused by electrical activation of the myocardium.

electromechanical delay. Despite normal electrical activation, there may be delays in the timing of mechanical contraction from inappropriately long electromechanical coupling intervals. See also *electromechanical coupling*.

electromechanical dissociation. 1. Electrical activation of the myocardium typically precedes mechanical contraction by a relatively constant amount. In diseased hearts, particularly cardiomyopathy, varying and unpredictable amounts of delay may occur between electrical activation and contraction; this delay is termed electromechanical dissociation. 2. The continuation of intrinsic cardiac electrical impulses in the absence of contraction when the heart has failed mechanically. Electromechanical dissociation can be verified when electrical impulses are present on an electrocardiogram even though the patient has no pulse. Electromechanical dissociation is a life-threatening condition. It may be the result of many causes, including pericardial tamponade, tension pneumothorax, and massive pulmonary embolism.

electromyographic interference. Alterations in pacemaker function to myopotential interference. See also *myopotential*.

electronic article surveillance equipment. Antitheft equipment used by, for example, retail businesses and libraries. A tag that is electronically detectable is connected to the merchandise; if the tag is not removed or deactivated, it sets off an alarm when it passes through a detector. Detectors usually are located at exits. Certain types of this equipment are capable of causing clinically significant electromagnetic interference in implantable devices.

electronic circuitry. See *circuitry*.

electropharmacology. The pharmacology relevant to the treatment of arrhythmias. This is usually used in reference to membrane-active antiarrhythmic agents that alter ion channel physiology. See also *antiarrhythmic agent, programmed electrical stimulus*.

electrophysiologic alternans. Marked variation in the amplitude of the surface electrocardiographic waves (T wave, QRS complex, or P wave) occurs in certain clinical disorders, including rapid supraventricular tachycardia and large pericardial effusion. Alternans in the T wave may be a marker for ventricular arrhythmogenicity.

electrophysiologic remodeling. Several electrophysiologic changes, including in refractoriness, action potential duration, and conduction, that occur after termination of a chronic arrhythmia which make reinitiation or sustaining of that arrhythmia less likely.

electrophysiologic stimulation. During electrophysiologic study and ablation procedures, stimulation with either incremental pacing or extrastimulus placement to provoke arrhythmias.

electrophysiologic stimulator. A device that produces different programmed electrical stimuli for application to the myocardium at specified coupling intervals during electrophysiologic testing.

electrophysiologic study (EPS). Electrical recording and stimulation used to evaluate the cardiac conduction system and the formation of cardiac arrhythmia. Such studies usually require the use of electrodes to record responses to stimuli delivered to the myocardium. Electrical stimulation, particularly incremental pacing or the introduction of extrastimuli, may be used. Specific applications of electrophysiologic studies include identification of the exact location of block in patients with atrioventricular conduction disorders, identification of the exact origin of ectopic impulses in various tachycardias, and assessment of drugs and devices for the treatment of cardiac arrhythmias. Results of electrophysiologic studies indicate the most appropriate antiarrhythmic treatment, which may be surgery or drugs or any combination thereof.

Electrophysiologic Study Versus Electrocardiographic Monitoring (ESVEM). This trial was designed to determine whether electrophysiologic study or Holter monitoring more accurately predicts the efficacy of antiarrhythmic agents in patients with aborted sudden death or sustained ventricular tachyarrhythmias. Investigators concluded that Holter monitoring more frequently predicted drug efficacy than electrophysiologic study (The ESVEM Investigators. Determinants of predicted efficacy of antiarrhythmic drugs in the electrophysiologic study versus electrocardiographic monitoring trial. Circulation. 1993;87:323-9).

electrophysiology (EP). Area of cardiology involved with the diagnosis, treatment, and study of the underlying mechanisms responsible for tachyarrhythmias and bradyarrhythmias. See also *electrophysiologic study*.

electrophysiology laboratory. 1. Laboratory in which electrophysiologic procedures, including electrophysiologic studies, and radiofrequency and other ablative procedures are performed. Typically consist of fluoroscopy, electrical mapping systems, electrical stimulators, and a fluoroscopic table. 2. Research laboratory in which basic electrophysiology procedures, including optical mapping, voltage clamp, and microelectrode studies, are performed.

electrotonus. Passive conduction of electrical activity across a nonexcitable region. Electronic conduction can reset or modulate protected foci.

Elgiloy. Trademark for a hypoallergenic, biocompatible alloy of cobalt, nickel, iron, chromium, molybdenum, and manganese. In pacing, Elgiloy was at one time widely used as the conductor coil for some pacing leads.

ELT. Abbreviation for *endless-loop tachycardia*.

embolism. Downstream migration via the bloodstream to a more distal vascular site or organs from a source of thrombus, tissue, or air. Embolism producing stroke or end-organ damage may occur during left atrial or left ventricular ablation procedures. Air embolism may occur during right-sided ablation procedures or device implantation. Embolization of foreign materials, including portions of implanted leads or electrophysiologic catheter, also may occur.

embolization. See *embolism*.

emergency pacing. Temporary external pacing used during resuscitation to correct asystole. Emergency pacing can be used until transvenous temporary pacing can be initiated. This method of pacing potentially can be accomplished via esophageal pacing, but it is not a recommended approach.

EMF. Abbreviation for *electromagnetic field*.

EMI. Abbreviation for *electromagnetic interference*.

EMIAT. See *European Myocardial Infarct Amiodarone Trial*.

encainide. A class IC antiarrhythmic agent that prolongs refractoriness in atrial, atrioventricular nodal, ventricular, and accessory pathway tissue. In the Cardiac Arrhythmia Suppression Trial (CAST), encainide was associated with an increase in mortality compared with use of a placebo. The drug has been withdrawn from the market by the manufacturer.

encapsulation. 1. Physiologically, an inflammatory tissue response followed by the formation of fibrous tissue around an implanted foreign material, such as a pacing lead or pacing electrode. Electrode encapsulation increases the effective electrode surface area and affects the electrical field strength at the electrode-myocardial interface. 2. In pacemaker design, encapsulation refers to the encasement of pacemaker components with epoxy resin to provide a hermetic seal. Pacemaker encapsulation prolongs battery life and prevents damage to the electronic circuitry. See also *effective electrode, hermetic seal*.

encircling cryoablation. Cryoablation performed encircling either the pulmonary veins for atrial fibrillation or ventricular or atrial myocardial scars to prevent recurrence of reentrant arrhythmia. See also *ablation, cryosurgery*.

encode. See *modulation*.

Encor retention wires. The Encor J-shaped atrial pacing lead (Telectronics, Inc., Englewood, Colorado) had a retention wire similar to that of the Accufix J lead. Like the Accufix lead, the Encor lead retention wire was subject to fracture and potential clinical complications. The lead was placed on advisory in 1995.

end-diastolic volume index (EDVI). The end-diastolic volume divided by the body surface area.

endless-loop tachycardia (ELT). See *pacemaker-mediated tachycardia*.

endocardial activation maps. Maps obtained during electrophysiologic procedures using an endocardial catheter. The endocardial activation sequences may be different from those obtained from the mid myocardium or epicardially obtained maps.

endocardial catheter mapping. Electrophysiologic mapping accomplished by use of a catheter or lead, with multiple electrodes at its distal tip, positioned within the heart via a transvenous approach. Endocardial catheter mapping is used to locate the origin of supraventricular or ventricular tachycardias. The location of the focus or foci of the tachycardia often can be identified within 4 mm. See also *electrode catheter, endocardial surface mapping*.

endocardial coagulum. Coagulum formed on the endocardial surface of the atrium or ventricle, often also found on the ablation catheter during cardiac ablation procedures. Coagulum formation may be the result of the direct denaturation of fibrinogen and thus not entirely prevented with heparin use.

endocardial defibrillation. Defibrillation for malignant ventricular arrhythmias performed with catheters placed endocardially, typically in the right ventricle. See also *endocardial defibrillation lead*.

endocardial defibrillation lead. A lead designed to deliver high voltage to the myocardium by an endocardially placed lead. An endocardial defibrillation lead also is referred to as a nonthoracotomy lead. See also *nonthoracotomy lead system*.

endocardial electrogram. Electrogram obtained when contact with myocardium is made with an endocardial catheter. In contradistinction, epicardial electrograms are obtained epicardially. See also *electrogram*.

endocardial encircling ventriculotomy. Procedure for treatment of ventricular tachycardia, usually in patients with ischemic cardiomyopathy. Ablative lesions are placed around existing scars in regions of peri-infarct slow conduction. Sometimes refers to surgical incision around ventricular scars.

endocardial lead. Pacing or defibrillator lead placed endocardially, usually in the right ventricle or right atrium. Leads placed in the coronary sinus for left ventricular pacing or via thorocotomy are considered epicardial pacing leads. See also *active fixation, atrial J lead, coronary sinus lead, endocardial defibrillation lead, endocardial screw-in lead, passive fixation.*

endocardial left ventricular pacing. Transvenous stimulation of the left ventricle. This technique has been performed to achieve permanent biventricular pacing. To date, experience with this technique is very limited. Concerns are thromboembolic phenomenon that could result with a permanent catheter in the system circulation.

endocardial mapping. Electrophysiologic mapping with endocardial catheters to diagnose abnormalities in the conduction system and induce arrhythmia. See also *epicardial mapping.*

endocardial mapping catheter. Electrode catheters used via the venous or atrial system to map the endocardium of the ventricles and atria and myocardium in venous structures. See also *endocardial catheter mapping.*

endocardial mapping techniques. The use of endocardial catheters to define the activation sequence during arrhythmia. Endocardial mapping techniques may not define the intra-myocardial and epicardial portions of complex reentrant circuits and epicardial automatic arrhythmia.

endocardial pacing. Pacing for bradyarrhythmia via the venous system with the pacing lead typically placed in the right ventricle or right atrium.

endocardial potential maps. Electrophysiologic maps obtained typically during sinus or paced rhythm (not during tachycardia). The unipolar or bipolar voltage (potential) is mapped to try to define areas of abnormal myocardium that may form portions of an arrhythmogenic reentrant tachycardia circuit. In addition to the local electrogram amplitude, the conduction velocity also may be approximated to identify the slow zone of the tachycardia circuit.

endocardial resection. A surgical procedure for the treatment of ventricular tachycardias, especially those initiated at sites of prior myocardial infarction. The arrhythmogenic focus or circuit is excised by peeling away from the healthy tissue. An endocardial resection may be limited to the tissue region from which the tachycardia originates, or it may include the entire area of visible endocardial scarring.

endocardial right ventricular pacing. Pacing of the right ventricle with leads placed transvenously onto the endocardial surface of the right ventricle.

endocardial screw-in lead. An active fixation lead with a fixed or deployable screw device at the distal tip of the lead. The degree of penetration of the corkscrew tip into the myocardium varies with the specific lead design. Many screw-in lead tips are retractable to facilitate transvenous insertion and minimize vascular damage. Depending on the design, either the screw or the distal rim of the lead may function as the active electrode.

endocardial signal. A spontaneous intrinsic atrial or ventricular event sensed and recorded via an atrial or ventricular lead or via a specially designed catheter. Endocardial signals are recorded as intracardiac electrograms. See also *electrode catheter, electrogram.*

endocardial surface mapping. A technique used in electrophysiologic studies to locate the site of origin of atrial or ventricular tachycardia. Areas of delayed or fragmented potentials are evaluated during normal sinus rhythm and during tachycardias. The site of origin of the tachycardia and its conduction pathway can be identified after induction of the arrhythmia through electrical stimulation. See also *endocardial catheter mapping.*

endocarditis. Inflammation, usually infections, of the endocardial surface of the heart, particularly the valves. Valvular endocarditis may complicate pacemaker lead infection. Conduction abnormalities necessitating pacemaker implantation may occur in endocarditis of the aortic valve.

endocardium. Innermost layer of the heart lining the myocardium and cardiac valves. See also *epicardium, myocardium.*

end of life (EOL). In pacing, the point at which the usable energy of a pacemaker battery is greatly reduced and replacement of the pacemaker is mandatory. In most pacemakers, the approach of end of life is indicated by an alteration in magnet rate or pulse duration. In other pacemakers and in cardioverter-defibrillators, end-of-life status is evaluated by the circuitry and is included in telemetered information. End-of-life characteristics differ among devices and manufacturers. Therefore, when the battery status of a given pacemaker or cardioverter-defibrillator model is assessed, it is imperative to know the end-of-life indicators specified by the manufacturer. See also *elective replacement indicator, magnet rate*.

end-of-life indicators. The alteration of magnet rate or pulse duration measurements, or a telemetered indicator, that occurs when a pacemaker battery reaches a critical point of depletion. When end-of-life indicators are reached, plans should be made to replace the pulse generator. See also *end of life*.

end of service (EOS). A term not commonly used to indicate battery depletion. The term is not specific as to the degree of battery depletion.

endoplasmic reticulum. Intracytoplasmic structure important in intracellular transport and protein synthesis.

energy (E). The amount of work a system is capable of doing. In an electrical system, energy is the product of the voltage applied, the current delivered, and the amount of time for which the voltage and current are applied. In pacing, energy may be used to evaluate the output of both constant-current and constant-voltage pacing systems. The energy delivered from the pacemaker to the electrode-myocardial interface is defined as the product of the pulse duration, the voltage, and the current. In pacing systems, energy is expressed in microjoules. In implantable cardioverter-defibrillators, shocks delivered for cardioversion or defibrillation are expressed in joules. Other examples are radiofrequency energy, cryoenergy, and ultrasound energy.

energy density. The ratio of available battery energy to battery volume or battery weight, that is, the energy within a battery per unit volume or unit weight. High-energy density is the basis for a large amount of available energy contained within a small battery.

energy output pacemaker programming. The use of calculated energy (taking into account output voltage and pulse width) in programming an adequate (2 or 3:1) safety margin for pacing output.

enhanced automaticity. One of the primary mechanisms for arrhythmia in which there is increased frequency of automaticity. This is the mechanism of arrhythmia in sinus tachycardia and most atrial tachycardia. See also *abnormal automaticity*.

EnSite system. Trademark for a mapping system that does not require electrode-myocardial contact (St. Jude Medical, St. Paul, Minnesota). Laser-etched electrodes on an intracavitary basket-like catheter use the inverse solution principle to calculate (virtual) electrograms on the endocardial surface of the chamber in which the mapping catheter is placed.

entrainment. Continuous resetting of a reentrant circuit by pacing drive faster than the tachycardia cycle length. Four criteria exist, each of which is sufficient to diagnose entrainment: 1) constant fusion occurs except in the first complex after termination of pacing, which is unfused and occurs at the pacing cycle length; 2) progressive fusion occurs at different pacing cycle lengths; 3) tachycardia termination occurs during pacing, the stimulus-to-electrogram interval shortens, and the morphology of the electrogram changes; and 4) pacing at two different cycle lengths yields a shorter stimulus-to-electrogram interval and a change in electrogram morphology at the shorter pacing cycle length, but the tachycardia is not terminated. Only reentrant rhythms can truly be entrained. See also *concealed entrainment, resetting*.

entrance block. Inability of a depolarization wave front to enter a region of myocardium. Entrance block to a site that exhibits enhanced automaticity results in failure of overdrive suppression. See also *exit block*.

entry port. See *aperture*.

environmental stress cracking (ESC). A form of deterioration that occurs on some polyurethane pacing leads. Environmental stress cracking is characterized by rough-walled cracks that appear to be due primarily to tearing. The tears occur in patterns related in depth and orientation to some strain vector in the material. See also *insulation failure*.

EOL. Abbreviation for *end of life*.

EOS. Abbreviation for *end of service*.

EP. Abbreviation for *electrophysiology*.

ephedrine. A sympathomimetic agent that increases blood pressure and can be used as an alternative drug for the treatment of vasodepressor carotid sinus hypersensitivity or neurocardiogenic syncope.

epicardial breakthrough. Traditionally, arrhythmias have been mapped endocardially. However, certain automatic arrhythmias and exit sites of reentrant circuits may be epicardial in location. Such sites are referred to as the epicardial breakthrough sites for the arrhythmia.

epicardial lead. Pacing or defibrillator lead placed epicardially. Epicardial leads may be used in temporary pacing or permanent pacing or with an implantable cardioverter-defibrillator. See also *endocardial lead.*

epicardial left ventricular pacing. Usually refers to pacing the left ventricle by placement of epicardial leads via thoracotomy or other pericardial access. Stimulation of the left ventricle with leads placed in the ventricular branches of the coronary sinus also paces the left ventricle epicardially. See also *endocardial left ventricular pacing.*

epicardial mapping. 1. Defining a focus for circuit of arrhythmia using catheters placed on the epicardial surface of the heart at thoracotomy or via pericardial access. 2. Mapping at open surgical procedures, traditionally using a series of electrodes (sock) and defining the arrhythmogenic substrate targeted for surgical excision or ablation.

epicardial pacing. Pacing either the ventricle or the atrium from the epicardium either by a thoracotomy or using the coronary venous system. Epicardial pacing also is referred to as myocardial or epimyocardial pacing. See also *endocardial pacing.*

epicardial patch. Defibrillator patch placed epicardially, usually through a limited thoracotomy. See also *defibrillation patch electrode.*

epicardial potentials. Electrograms obtained on the epicardial surface of the heart either with catheters placed through the coronary veins at open chest surgery or via pericardial access.

epicardial screw-in lead. A sutureless epicardial lead. An epicardial screw-in lead has a corkscrew that is used to penetrate the myocardium and to embed the lead into the tissue. A portion of the screw-in lead tip often is insulated to decrease the effective surface area and increase the impedance. The screw may or may not function as the electrode. Epicardial screw-in leads available currently are unipolar. Epicardial

screw-in leads also are referred to as epimyocardial leads.

epicardial steroid lead. An epicardial pacing lead that allows chronic elution of a steroid substance at the electrode-epicardial interface in an effort to achieve lower chronic thresholds.

epicardial ventricular mapping. Method of mapping for ventricular arrhythmias either via the coronary venous system or the pericardial surface or utilizing the pericardial space to identify the site of epicardial foci or to define reentrant circuits.

epicardial ventricular tachycardia. Ventricular tachycardia that has either the focus of origin or critical components of the reentrant circuit of ventricular tachycardia located on the epicardial surface of the ventricle.

epicardium. The outermost of the three layers of the heart wall. The epicardium covers the external surface of the myocardium and is the innermost of the two layers of the pericardium, the fibroserous sac that surrounds the heart. In epicardial pacing, the electrodes are attached by sutures or a fixation device directly to the pericardial surface of the heart. See also *endocardium, myocardium.*

epimyocardial lead. Lead used for epimyocardial pacing. See also *epicardial lead.*

epimyocardial pacing. See *epicardial pacing.*

epinephrine. Hormone secreted by the adrenal gland (synonym, adrenaline). One of the principal catecholamines typically increasing heart rate and conduction velocities in the atrium and ventricular myocardium.

episode. In implantable cardioverter-defibrillators, the sequence from the onset of an arrhythmia through its detection and treatment to termination of the arrhythmia.

episode diagnostics. Stored electrograms and other event data, usually retrievable, that help elucidate the details of a stored event.

epoxy resin. A high-strength, biocompatible polymer used for coating, adhesion, or casting. In pacing, epoxy resin is used to encapsulate pacemaker components by coating and to form the pacemaker connector block.

EPROM. Abbreviation for *erasable programmable read-only memory.*

EPS. Abbreviation for *electrophysiologic study.*

epsilon wave. Epsilon waves, rarely observed in clinical practice, result from late potentials favoring the development of ventricular rhythm disorders by reentry. Epsilon waves are a clinical feature of right ventricular arrhythmogenic dysplasia.

erasable programmable read-only memory (EPROM). A form of memory used to store software programs. Erasable programmable read-only memory can be erased and reprogrammed for modification or revisions of the programs. See also *read-only memory*.

ERI. Abbreviation for *elective replacement indicator*.

erosion. Deterioration of tissue over an implanted pulse generator or movement of a lead toward or through the skin. Smaller and more contoured pacemakers are less susceptible to erosion. If any portion of the pulse generator completely erodes through the skin, the site should be considered infected and appropriate surgical intervention should be performed. In the context of lead or pulse generator erosion, erosion also is referred to as extrusion. See also *extrusion*.

ERP. Abbreviation for *effective refractory period*.

ESC. Abbreviation for *environmental stress cracking*.

escape beat. Occurs during bradyarrhythmias with failure of the primary automatic focus. The escape beat from sinus arrest may arise from the atrial myocardium, atrioventricular nodal junction, fascicles, or ventricular myocardium. See also *escape rhythm*.

escape interval. 1. Interval between the normal beat and an escape beat. A prolonged escape interval suggests high-grade block or disease of the primary automatic focus and a poor escape rhythm. 2. The time between a paced or sensed cardiac event and the subsequent pacing stimulus. The escape interval is measured in milliseconds. See also *atrial escape interval, ventricular escape interval*.

escape rate. See *escape interval*.

escape rhythm. When the primary automatic focus (e.g., sinus node) fails, either asystole or an escape rhythm occurs. The escape rhythm may be from the atrium, atrioventricular junction, His-Purkinje system, or ventricular myocardium. An escape rhythm from the atrioventricular node is evidenced on an electrocardiogram by a narrow QRS complex with a rate of 40 to 60 beats per minute. Escape rhythms from the ventricle are evidenced by a wide QRS complex with a rate of 20 to 30 beats per minute.

esmolol. Intravenous β-blocker with a short half-life frequently used in the acute treatment of atrioventricular node-dependent arrhythmia.

esophageal electrode. Electrode placed via the pharynx into the esophagus to better define atrial activity when the surface P waves are difficult to distinguish.

esophageal electrogram. A recording of cardiac electrical activity via a catheter placed in the esophagus. See also *esophageal pacing and recording*.

esophageal fistulization. Typically, fatal complications of surgical and endocardial ablation procedures for atrial fibrillation. A fistula is formed between the posterior left atrium and esophagus, resulting in permanent endocarditis and sepsis, air embolization, and bleeding.

esophageal lead. A catheter used for recording or pacing the left atrium via the esophagus. An esophageal electrode or pill electrode. See also *esophageal pacing and recording*.

esophageal pacing and recording. The diagnostic and therapeutic use of catheter electrodes, usually bipolar, in the esophagus to deliver electrical stimuli to the atria or ventricles or to record electrical activity from the atria. Placement of the electrodes in the esophagus does not require fluoroscopy or cardiac catheterization. Esophageal pacing requires a higher current output and pulse duration than endocardial pacing. Esophageal pacing is rarely used temporarily to treat sinus bradycardia or to terminate atrial flutter. In electrophysiologic testing, esophageal pacing may be used to initiate or terminate atrial arrhythmias, to determine sinus node recovery time, and to record ventriculoatrial intervals during supraventricular tachycardia. It also may be useful in recording atrial activity to aid in the diagnosis of a wide complex tachycardia.

ESVEM. See *Electrophysiologic Study Versus Electrocardiographic Monitoring*.

ESWL. Abbreviation for *extracorporeal shock-wave lithotripsy*.

ethanol ablation. Injection of ethanol into a coronary artery to create a small myocardial infarct and thus cure or control an arrhythmia. Ethanol has been used to create atrioventricular block, to destroy the focus or critical part of the circuit of ventricular tachycardia, and to create septal necrosis in patients with hypertrophic cardiomyopathy.

ethmozine. See *moricizine*.

ethylene oxide (ETO). A gas used for sterilization. Ethylene oxide is used for sterilization of the implantable components of a pacemaker or implantable cardioverter-defibrillator system, including the device itself, leads, and adaptors.

ETO. Abbreviation for *ethylene oxide*.

European Myocardial Infarct Amiodarone Trial (EMIAT). This was a cardiac morbidity and mortality trial that compared the use of amiodarone with implanted devices. Study investigators concluded that amiodarone could not be justified prophylactically for all patients with depressed left ventricular function. However, for patients in whom antiarrhythmic therapy is indicated, amiodarone was not proarrhythmic and reduced arrhythmic death (Julian DG, Camm AJ, Frangin G, Janse MJ, Munoz A, Schwartz PJ, et al, European Myocardial Infarct Amiodarone Trial Investigators. Randomised trial of effect of amiodarone on mortality in patients with left-ventricular dysfunction after recent myocardial infarction: EMIAT. Lancet. 1997;349:667-74. Erratum in: Lancet. 1997;349:1180. Lancet. 1997;349:1776).

eustachian ridge. Amphibological remnant of the valve of the inferior vena cava. In fetal life, the eustachian ridge and associated eustachian valve direct inferior venal caval blood to the fossa ovalis. The coronary sinus and compact atrioventricular node are located between the eustachian ridge and the tricuspid valve.

eustachian valve. See *eustachian ridge*.

event counter. A mechanism of pacemaker circuitry that counts pacemaker or intrinsic cardiac events. The information compiled by the event counter is stored in the pacemaker and may be obtained via telemetry. Events that may be counted include the number of heart beats; the derived mean heart rate; the percentage of paced activity; the number of beats classified as premature ventricular contractions, depending on the pacemaker's criteria for premature ventricular contractions; and, in rate-adaptive pacemakers, sensor activity. The event counter in an implantable cardioverter-defibrillator stores the number of detected episodes of ventricular tachycardia or ventricular fibrillation. It also may tally other events, such as the number of times each type of therapy was successful. See also *data storage, pacemaker monitor*.

event histogram. A diagnostic feature that summarizes all cardiac activity in terms of intrinsic versus paced activity in atrium and ventricle (e.g., PR, PV, AR, AV events). It may also indicate the number of premature ventricular complexes as defined by the pulse generator.

event marker. A function in most pacemakers which generates a graphic record that shows, for example, when either chamber is being paced or sensed and when the refractory periods begin and end. Implantable cardioverter-defibrillators also can transmit marker channels to show various functions such as the type of sensed event, the beginning or end of capacitor charging, or the fulfillment of detection criteria. The data provided by the marker channels are obtained via telemetry from the implanted pulse generator. The marker channel recording may be superimposed on a surface electrocardiogram or may be recorded as an independent tracing. Event markers are useful for troubleshooting or routine follow-up. See also *marker pulse*.

event monitor. See *event recorder*.

event recorder. A patient-activated continuous loop of tape used for recording a rhythm strip during symptoms such as syncope or lightheadedness. Event recorders are useful for brief or sudden episodes because the wearer can activate the device and save the recorded information after the event has occurred. Event recorders may be used continuously for months at a time. See also *Holter monitoring*.

event snapshot. Another term for a triggered event recording available in some devices that have the ability to capture a specific event for future retrieval. The event displays paced and sensed events when the event is triggered; event triggering occurs with magnet application in some pulse generators when the feature is programmed "on."

evoked QT interval. Interval calculated by analysis of the evoked response to pacing of the evoked depolarization and repolarization signals. Evoked QT interval is used in certain devices for sensor-driven pacing. The evoked QT interval is shorter during exercise or other catecholamine stress and would be programmed to result in an increased pacing rate.

evoked response safety margin. The ratio of the evoked response signal amplitude to the evoked response programmed sensitivity. This is typically programmed in such a way to allow for adequate discrimination between the evoked response signal and polarization signal. See also *polarization*.

evoked response sensitivity. Measurement used in devices with autocapture function or algorithms requiring sensing of the evoked response signal. If the evoked response sensitivity does not allow for a safety margin sufficient to reproducibly detect evoked response potentials as distinct from the polarization potentials, autocapture cannot be turned on. See also *polarization*.

evoked response sensitivity test. In certain devices with an automated capture feature, the evoked response sensitivity test is performed to check whether an adequate margin can be maintained between the amplitude of the polarization signal and the evoked response signal. If an evoked response sensitivity cannot be programmed with adequate safety margin for both the polarized signal (sensitivity above the polarization single amplitude) and the evoked response signal (programmed sensitivity sufficiently below the evoked response single amplitude), autocapture cannot be programmed on evoked response. It may also be referred to as the evoked response signal.

excimer laser. Laser system used in laser-aided extraction of an implanted pacemaker and implantable cardioverter-defibrillator leads. A modified excimer laser system can be used instead of radiofrequency ablation for ablative procedures.

excitability. A property of cardiac cells that allows them to depolarize and generate an action potential in response to a stimulus. The excitability of cardiac cells varies in different periods of the cardiac cycle. For example, excitability is absent during the absolute refractory period. Pacing is ineffective if tissue is nonexcitable.

excitable cells. Myocardial cells capable of being depolarized by either a pulse generator output pulse or a neighboring depolarized cell.

excitable gap. In a reentrant arrhythmia circuit, a portion of myocardium in the circuit has recovered from refractoriness and can be excited by a second wave front or pacing stimulus. The presence of an excitable gap allows entrainment, termination, or induction of a double reentrant circuit in reentrant arrhythmia. A large excitable gap allows entrainment, resetting, or termination of a tachycardia with late coupled extrastimuli.

excitable tissues. Groups of myocardial cells or conduction system cells capable of being depolarized by either a depolarizing wave front or output from a pulse generator.

excitation. Phenomenon wherein cardiac tissues are depolarized by either pacing stimuli or a depolarization wave front.

excitation-contraction coupling. Electrical stimulation causing depolarization of a myocardial cell results in a cascade of events that eventually produces shortening of the cellular myofilaments and results in contraction. This process linking excitation to contraction is excitation-contraction coupling and is an important determinant of the integrity of the myocardial synchrony.

excitation waves. Waves of depolarization originating either from spontaneous depolarization in tissue capable of inherent automaticity or from stimulation via a pacemaker or implantable cardioverter-defibrillation lead. Excitation waves travel from cell to cell mostly through gap junctions.

exclusion. A surgical technique used in the treatment of ventricular tachycardia. In exclusion, a fibrous barrier is created around the area of the arrhythmogenic tissue to prevent tachycardia formation or propagation beyond the scarred area. Exclusion is intended to isolate the arrhythmogenic tissue.

exercise capacity. Determined at exercise testing, usually with a standardized protocol (e.g., Bruce, chronotropic assessment exercise protocol, Naughton) and considers a patient's symptoms, heart rate, response to exercise, blood pressure response to exercise, and, in certain instances, level of oxygenation. See also *chronotropic assessment exercise protocol*.

exercise-induced arrhythmia. Certain arrhythmias are more frequent during exercise than at rest. These arrhythmias are often catecholamine-sensitive. Typical examples are right ventricular outflow tract tachycardia and catecholamine-sensitive polymorphic ventricular tachycardia.

exit block. Failure of an impulse to be conducted from its site of origin to adjacent tissue. Cardiac electrical phenomenon in which an automatic focus or site of exit from a reentrance circuit is unable to depolarize surrounding myocardium. A similar phenomenon also may occur within the cardiac conduction system. In pacing, exit block is one explanation for the failure of a pacing stimulus to capture the heart. The most common cause of exit block is thought to be an increased pacing threshold due to an excessive inflammatory response at the electrode-myocardial interface. Other causes of exit block include endocarditis, electrolyte imbalance, myocardial infarction, and tissue damage from defibrillation. See also *entrance block*.

explantation. Surgical removal of a device or component of a pacing or defibrillation system.

extendable-retractable lead. An active-fixation pacing lead in which the helix can be extended for anchoring to the myocardium and then retracted to free the lead from the myocardial surface. Such extension and retraction can be done repetitively if the lead must be repositioned multiple times.

extended high rate (EHR). In implantable cardioverter-defibrillators, the heart having maintained a rate that is equal to or farther than the programmed rate for a programmed duration.

extender. An additional length of pacing lead that can be used to extend the lead. The need for a lead extender is uncommon, but an extender may be used, for example, if a pacing lead is placed via the subclavian or cephalic vein and the pulse generator is implanted in the abdomen or flank.

external cardioversion. Application of an electrical field via cutaneous patches placed on the chest to convert tachyarrhythmias to sinus rhythm. In external cardioversion, monophasic or biphasic waveforms may be used and the electrical field is applied synchronous with the electrocardiographic signal. See also *defibrillation, internal cardioversion*.

external load. The resistance or impedance within the pacing system, that is, the sum of the impedances of the lead system, the electrodes, and the electrode-myocardial interface.

external overdrive. A type of chest wall stimulation in which electrical pulses are delivered to the chest wall at a rate faster than that of the implanted pacemaker or the intrinsic heart rate. The electrical impulses are sensed by the implanted pacemaker and may be used to test its sensing circuit, to approximate refractory periods, and to perform therapeutic or diagnostic testing. External overdrive is used most commonly for the delivery of triggered output pulses to control heart rate. For example, external overdrive may be used to terminate a supra-ventricular or ventricular tachycardia. See also *chest wall stimulation, overdrive pacing*.

external pacemaker. A pacemaker designed for placement outside the body. External pacemakers are used primarily for temporary pacing. See also *temporary pacemaker*.

external pacing. Temporary pacing via an external device. The term most frequently is used to describe transcutaneous temporary pacing but also is used to describe any method of temporary pacing in which the pacemaker is external to the body.

external pacing pads. Cutaneously placed patches linked to a pulse generator for temporary transcutaneous pacing in the emergency treatment of symptomatic bradyarrhythmia.

extracardiac signals. Electrograms identified in implanted device systems or during electrophysiologic study not originating from the heart. Examples include skeletal myopotential, diaphragmatic myopotentials, noise related to the lead, or external electromagnetic interference.

extracardiac stimulation. Electrical stimulation of noncardiac structures such as the phrenic nerve, diaphragm, or intercostal muscles from implanted devices and leads or during electrophysiologic study. During pacing system implantation, 10-V stimulation is performed to assess for the presence of extracardiac stimulation. However, extracardiac stimulation may not be obvious until the patient is no longer in a supine position or sedated state. Extracardiac stimulation may be managed in some patients by lowering the energy output of the device, but in other patients it may require lead repositioning.

extracorporeal shock-wave lithotripsy (ESWL). A noninvasive treatment used primarily for nephrolithiasis or cholelithiasis, in which an underwater spark gap is used to generate a shock wave focused on a kidney stone. Because the shock waves are capable of producing ventricular extrasystoles, the lithotriptor is designed to deliver pulses only when the ventricular myocardium is refractory. If extracorporeal shock-wave lithotripsy is used in patients with pacemakers, the following guidelines should be considered: 1) program the pacemaker to the VVI or VOO mode, 2) keep the focal point of the lithotriptor no closer than 6 inches from the pacemaker, and 3) use cardiac monitoring throughout the procedure. Extracorporeal shock-wave lithotripsy is relatively contraindicated in patients with implantable cardioverter-defibrillators.

extraction. 1. Method of removing a previously implanted pacemaker or implantable cardioverter-defibrillator leads. Extraction methods include traction, use of locking stylus, and laser- or radiofrequency energy-guided removal. 2. Removal of inadvertently placed catheter or stent fragments during ablative procedures.

extraction registry. A registry of lead extraction data is recommended as part of the North American Society of Pacing and Electrophysiology (NASPE) guidelines on lead extraction. The guidelines recommend that the registry should include all patients who undergo transvenous lead extraction techniques, patient statistics of clinical characteristics, success and complications of the procedure, 30-day follow-up, data analysis on an annual basis (at a minimum) with review of individual physician's data, and submission of all data to a national registry.

extrastimulus. An extrinsic electrical impulse, usually delivered at a preset or programmed coupling interval. In electrophysiologic studies, the first extrastimulus usually is indicated by S_2, and the subsequent stimuli as S_3, S_4, and so on. See also *programmed electrical stimulus*.

extrastimulus pacing. During electrophysiologic study, stimulation of the myocardium (atrial or ventricular) in a manner to simulate the spontaneous occurrence of premature ventricular complexes. Typically, a train of eight paced beats at a constant cycle length is followed by a ninth extra stimulus beat at a shorter coupling interval than the cycle length of the previously paced beat. With subsequent trains of stimulation, the coupling interval of the extrastimulus beat is shortened.

extrastimulus testing. Induction of arrhythmias with extrastimulus pacing suggests a re-entrant mechanism and is frequently used in ablative procedures and risk stratification for defibrillator placement. See also *extrastimulus pacing*.

extrasystole. Premature depolarization from atrial myocardium, ventricular myocardium, or the conduction system. An extrasystolic beat may exhibit entrance or exit block. A series of extrasystolic beats give rise to automatic tachycardia.

extrinsic activation. The creation of an action potential by external electrical stimulation. For a response to occur, the transmembrane potential must be reduced from the resting potential to threshold.

extrusion. In manufacturing, a process by which a material is forced through small holes to make continuous fibers. In pacing, many multifilar lead conductors are composed of extruded fibers and many lead insulators are made of extruded polymers. In pacing, extrusion also refers to erosion of a pacemaker or lead.

f

f. Abbreviation for *frequency*.

failure to capture. Failure of a pacemaker output stimulus to cause cardiac depolarization. See also *acute pacing threshold, chronic pacing threshold, pacing threshold, stimulation threshold, threshold maturation*.

failure to sense. Failure of a pacemaker to sense an intrinsic cardiac event. See also *acute sensing threshold, chronic sensing threshold, sensing threshold, threshold maturation*.

fallback. A programmable upper rate response of some dual-chamber pacemakers. Fallback occurs when the intrinsic atrial rate exceeds the rate at which ventricular output pulses can occur in 1:1 synchrony with intrinsic atrial events, that is, at the maximum tracking rate or upper rate limit. The ventricular paced rate decelerates to, and is maintained at, a programmable fallback rate that is lower than the original programmed maximum tracking rate. In some pacemakers, atrioventricular synchrony is lost when the fallback response is initiated because the ventricular channel immediately begins independent VVI pacing at the programmed initial fallback rate. In other pacemakers, some degree of atrioventricular synchrony is maintained when the upper rate limit is reached and the fallback response is initiated. Fallback also may indicate a post–mode-switch response whereby the device gradually decreases the paced ventricular rate. Depending on the fallback algorithm, the rate will decrease to either the sensor-indicated rate or the lower rate limit. The characteristics of the fallback response should be known so that its presence is not confused with malfunction of end of life. See also *fallback deceleration, pseudo-Wenckebach response, upper rate response*.

fallback deceleration. A programmable value of the fallback upper rate response. Fallback deceleration controls the amount of paced ventricular cycle (VV) lengthening by a constant, predetermined value between each successive VV interval as ventricular rate decreases from the upper rate limit to the fallback rate. Fallback deceleration is expressed in milliseconds per cycle. See also *fallback*.

fallback rate. See *fallback*.

false signals. Any signal that is interpreted by a pulse generator as intrinsic cardiac activity when it is not.

far-field blanking. A programmable interval in some pulse generators which begins with either

Failure to Capture

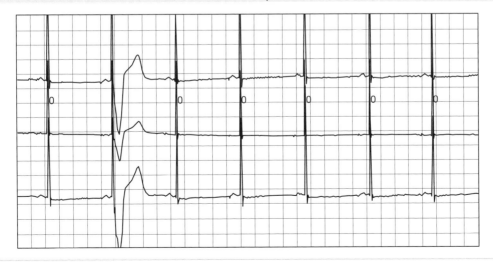

sensed or paced events and "sees" the sensed or paced far-field event on the atrial channel but does not use the event to fulfill criteria to meet mode-switching or to alter pacemaker timing cycle.

far-field electrogram. See *far-field signal, near-field electrogram.*

far-field endless-loop tachycardia. Type of endless-loop tachycardia occurring when the atrial channel detects a far-field ventricular electrogram or a delayed atrial electrogram. This detected signal is then tracked to the ventricle, setting up an endless-loop tachycardia.

far-field potential. An intrinsic electrical signal, visible on an intracardiac electrogram, that originates from myocardial cells distant to the distal-tip electrode of an endocardial catheter or pacing lead, often from a different cardiac chamber. An example of a far-field potential is ventricular activity on an atrial electrogram.

far-field R wave (FFRW). 1. When an R wave is sensed on an atrial channel, typically when the atrial lead has been placed in the anular region or deep in the right atrial appendage, it is referred to as a far-field R wave. Far-field R-wave sensing may cause inappropriate inhibition of pacing or double counting of atrial events. 2. During ventricular tachycardia ablation, a catheter placed at one myocardial site may sense electrograms (R waves) from the contralateral ventricle or sites distal to a scar.

far-field sensing. Phenomenon in which an electrophysiologic catheter or pacemaker lead senses an electrogram different from the electrogram generated at the site of myocardial contact with the lead.

far-field signal. Electrogram sensed by a pacemaker lead or electrophysiologic catheter different from electrogram at the electrode myocardial interface. See also *far-field sensing.*

fascicular block. Typically refers to either conduction block in the left anterior or left posterior fascicle of the left bundle branch. More generally can refer to conduction slowing or block at any infrahisian site.

fascicular premature depolarizations. Extrasystoles or premature depolarizations occurring in the infrahisian fascicular system. These beats resemble premature ventricular contractions but often have a sharp near-field initial deflection, suggesting an origin in the fascicular system.

fascicular rhythms. Sustained or nonsustained rhythm resulting from repeated fascicular premature depolarizations. See also *fascicular premature depolarizations.*

fascicular tachycardia. A fascicular rhythm with a rate more than 100 beats per minute. Fascicular tachycardia may be automatic, triggered, or reentrant. Fascicular tachycardia arising from the left posterior fascicle is a common form of ventricular tachycardia in young, healthy patients. See also *fascicular rhythms.*

fasciculoventricular accessory pathway. Normally the His bundle and proximal right and left bundles are electrically insulated from anular fibrous ensheathment. When there is a breach in this insulation, there is early exit from either the His bundle or proximal bundle branches to the ventricle, termed a fasciculoventricular tract. Fasciculoventricular accessory pathways are not associated with tachycardia.

Far-Field Sensing

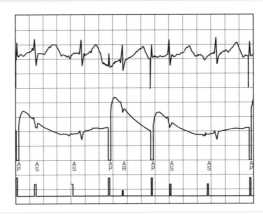

fasciculoventricular bypass tract. Fasciculoventricular bypass tracts present with preexcitation, short PR interval, and delta wave but electrophysiologic study does not show evidence of an atrioventricular bypass tract. Fasciculoventricular bypass tracts are not true bypass tracts but represent loss of the usual electrical insulation of the His and proximal bundle branches. See also *fasciculoventricular accessory pathway*.

fasciculoventricular fiber. A type of Mahaim fiber that connects the His bundle or bundle branches to the ventricle. By preexciting the ventricle, fasciculoventricular fibers cause small constant delta waves on the surface electrocardiogram. Fasciculoventricular fibers are not known to participate in tachycardias.

fast pathway conducts more rapidly but has a longer refractory period than the slow pathway. Also known as the beta pathway.

f channels. Specific type of sodium channel that is important in the normal automaticity in sinus nodal and atrioventricular nodal tissue.

FDA. Abbreviation for the United States *Food and Drug Administration*.

feedthrough wire. A conductor, surrounded by an insulator, that allows the passage of electricity between circuit components separated by a nonconductive partition. In pacing systems, feedthrough refers to the insulated electrical poles of the pacing circuit which connect the internal circuitry of the pacemaker within the pacemaker case to the connector block. The

Far-Field and Near-Field Electrograms

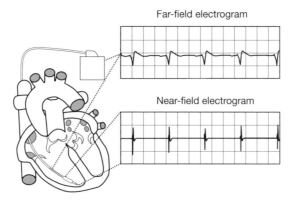

Modified from Hayes DL, Lloyd MA, Friedman PA. Cardiac pacing and defibrillation: a clinical approach. Armonk: Futura Publishing Company, Inc; 2000. p. 541-85. Copyrighted and used with permission of Mayo Foundation for Medical Education and Research.

fasciculoventricular pathway. See *fasciculoventricular bypass tract*.

fast channel. The ion channel that carries sodium and is responsible for the rapid upstroke of phase 0 in atrial, His-Purkinje, and ventricular cells. See also *depolarization*.

fast Fourier transform (FFT). A mathematic method that allows efficient computer-based frequency analysis of a signal. Fast Fourier transform analysis has been applied to the signal-averaged electrocardiogram in an attempt to avoid some of the intrinsic limitations of time domain analysis, but it has not gained widespread acceptance.

fast pathway. One of the limbs of the reentrant circuit in atrioventricular nodal reentry. The

conductor insulation creates a hermetic seal to prevent short circuiting. Glass and ceramic materials commonly are used as insulators. A feedthrough is required for each electrode connection point.

FFRW. Abbreviation for *far-field R wave*.

FFT. Abbreviation for *fast Fourier transform*.

Fibber. Trademark for a proprietary method to induce ventricular fibrillation (St. Jude Medical, St. Paul, Minnesota) during noninvasive electrophysiologic study at the time of implantation to determine defibrillation thresholds.

fibrillating wave fronts. During atrial or ventricular fibrillation, multiple wave fronts occurring as either circular reentrant circuits or spiral waves propagating three dimensionally in the myocardium responsible for the maintenance of fibrillation.

fibrillation. A cardiac arrhythmia characterized by continuous, uncoordinated activity of the atria or the ventricles. Unsynchronized electrical activity in the myocardium causes individual myofibrils to contract independently. The resulting rapid, tremulous, and ineffective activity of the atria or ventricles is characterized by quivering and twitching of the myocardium. Atrial fibrillation may be asymptomatic, but ventricular fibrillation typically is fatal if not corrected quickly. See also *atrial fibrillation, ventricular fibrillation*.

fibrillation induction. Methods to induce ventricular fibrillation, typically related to defibrillation threshold testing during implantation of cardioverter-defibrillators. Fibrillation induction methods include extrastimulus placement, shock on T wave, rapid ventricular pacing, direct-current shock, and, rarely, alternating-current shock.

fibrous capsule. A tough fibrous coating that forms, for example, around a pulse generator, as a result of the body's reaction to a foreign body such as an implantable pulse generator. Once the capsule is entered, it usually can be opened with relative ease with electrocautery or blunt dissection.

fib zone. Detection zone in defibrillators for detection of ventricular fibrillation. This zone is usually set at 180 beats per minute or more and may detect rapid ventricular tachycardias, ventricular flutter, or ventricular fibrillation.

field correction. See *recall*.

field effect transistor (FET). A type of transistor used for high-voltage switching, as in implantable cardioverter-defibrillators.

figure-eight reentry. The shape of the reentrant circuit thought to be responsible for most ventricular tachycardias associated with coronary artery disease. The central region contains the zone of slow conduction and is the critical portion of the circuit.

Fibrillation Induction

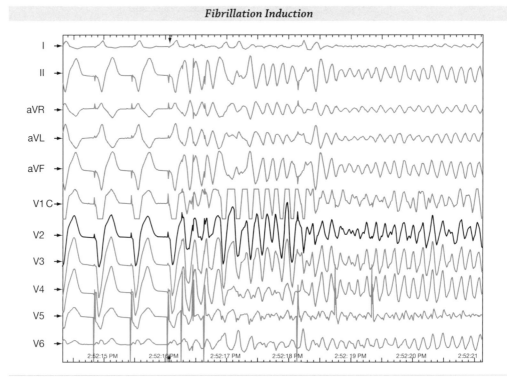

fibrillatory wave. Either two-dimensional reentrant waves or three-dimensional spiral waves responsible for the initial propagation and maintenance of atrial or ventricular fibrillation.

filter. An electronic component used to reject, attenuate, or deemphasize parts of frequency of the input signal. Applications include the rejection of high-frequency noise or unwanted direct-current signals. Filters usually are named according to the range of frequencies admitted, for example, high-pass filters, low-pass filters, and band-pass filters. Band-pass filters filter out both high and low frequencies. Pacemakers and implantable cardioverter-defibrillators use band-pass filters centered on a physiologic range of frequencies (20-60 Hz).

filtering of signals. Local electrograms sensed from electrode myocardial interfaces may be contaminated with background noise and far-field potentials. Filtering below and above a certain frequency allows better definition of the local myocardial electrogram.

fin. A passive fixation endocardial lead tip configuration, predominantly of historical interest. The fin is a triangular flat that projects axially from the lead. Fins usually are made of silicone rubber and often have apertures with the silicone rubber structure to facilitate tissue ingrowth. Three fins, spaced equidistant from each other, usually are used at the distal end of the lead just proximal to the distal-tip electrode. The fins are anchored in the trabeculae and secured by the ingrowth of fibrous tissue between the silicone structures. See also *endocardial lead, passive fixation*.

finger probe. A device used during intraoperative electrophysiologic mapping to sense intrinsic activity for the recording of an intracardiac electrogram. The probe fits onto the finger of the surgeon, and the outer surface of the probe contains unipolar or multipolar electrodes. The electrodes are placed in contact with the different regions of the cardiac tissue by movement of the finger probe. Finger probes most frequently are used for left ventricular mapping during aneurysmectomy with concomitant subendocardial resection for treatment of ventricular tachycardia.

first-degree atrioventricular block. See *first-degree AV block*.

first-degree AV block. Prolongation of the PR interval on a surface electrocardiogram to more than 200 milliseconds. This can be due to delay of conduction in the right atrium, atrioventricular node, His-Purkinje system, or any combination thereof. Intracardiac recordings can distinguish the site of conduction delay. See also *second-degree AV block, third-degree AV block*.

first-degree heart block. See *first-degree AV block*.

first-degree sinus node exit block. Prolongation of sinus node conduction time. Because sinoatrial conduction is electrically silent on the surface electrocardiogram, first-degree sinus node exit block can be diagnosed only from an intracardiac electrogram with recording of sinus node depolarization. See also *second-degree sinus node exit block, sinus node exit block, third-degree sinus node exit block*.

510(K). Section 510(K) of the Medical Device Amendments to the United States Food, Drug, and Cosmetic Act, which contains a premarket notification requirement. The premarket notification is used to introduce a device into commercial distribution when it is substantially equivalent to a device that was marketed in the United States before May 18, 1976, and the device does not meet the requirements for a Premarket Approval Application.

fixation mechanisms. The way in which a pacing, defibrillation, or coronary sinus lead becomes affixed to the surface where it is intended to stay. The most common fixation mechanisms for transvenous leads are active (i.e., a screw-in mechanism) or passive (e.g., tined). (Other non-tined passive-fixation mechanisms have been used, but tines are by far the most common.) Epicardial leads may be fixed in place with a screw-in (coil) mechanism or sewn in place. Coronary sinus leads most commonly have some cant configuration that occurs once the stylet is removed, and this is intended to wedge the lead into place.

fixed rate pacing. Pacing from either the atrium or the ventricle, typically in an asynchronous mode or without sensor-associated changes in pacing rate.

fixed tilt. Defibrillation voltage waveform characteristic in which the ratio of the final voltage to the initial voltage is fixed.

flange. A passive-fixation endocardial lead tip configuration, predominantly of historical interest. Flanges are truncated, cone-shaped structures attached around the distal end of the lead just proximal to the distal-tip electrode. Flanges anchor the lead tip within the trabeculae. A flange also may be referred to as a cuff. A flanged lead also is referred to as a wedge-tip lead. See also *endocardial lead, passive fixation*.

flecainide. A class IC antiarrhythmic agent that prolongs refractoriness in atrial, atrioventricular nodal, ventricular, and accessory pathway tissues. Flecainide has efficacy in the treatment of supraventricular and ventricular arrhythmias. Flecainide is metabolized by the liver, and 40% also is excreted unchanged by the kidneys. The plasma half-life of flecainide is 11 hours. Side effects of flecainide include a negative inotropic effect and proarrhythmia. In the Cardiac Arrhythmia Suppression Trial (CAST), flecainide was associated with an increase in mortality compared with a placebo in patients with coronary artery disease. Flecainide can increase pacing and sensing thresholds.

flex circuit. A flexible printed circuit typically used to interconnect circuit modules within tight spaces. See also *printed circuit board*.

flex life. A measure of material strength or, more specifically, a measure of fatigue resistance. Flex life is the number of cycles a material can be bent to a specified radius of curvature before failure, that is, before cracking or breaking occurs. In pacing, flex life is used to define the fatigue resistance of the lead and the conductor.

floating bipolar electrodes. See *orthogonal sensing*.

fluorescent imaging. An electrophysiologic method of imaging the wave front of depolarization and possible repolarization using fluorescent light.

fluoroscopy. Examination of deep structures with low-dose x-rays. In pacing, fluoroscopy is used primarily to visualize the passage of leads through venous channels and to verify lead placement.

flutter. A repetitive, regular, rapid arrhythmia occurring in the atria or ventricles at a rate of 250 to 350 beats per minute. Atrial flutter

Fontan Procedure

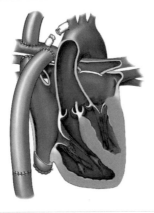

exhibits varying degrees of atrioventricular block. Ventricular flutter is life-threatening. See also *atrial flutter, ventricular flutter*.

flutter isthmus. 1. The arrhythmogenic substrate for most common forms of atrial flutter include the atrial tissue between the tricuspid valve and inferior vena cava. Also referred to as cavotricuspid isthmus. 2. A zone of slow conduction between two scars or two otherwise electrically inert structures forming the substrate for rapid tachycardias.

flutter wave (f wave). The flutter waves typically associated with atrial flutter give important clues to the specific circuit responsible for flutter. See *f waves*.

focal ablation. Ablation of either atrial or ventricular tissue for automatic or triggered automatic tachycardias, typically within a 3- to 5-mm radius of the earliest site of electrical activation during an arrhythmia.

focal atrial fibrillation. Mechanism or initiation and sometimes maintenance of atrial fibrillation from a rapidly discharging focus, typically in a venous structure such as the pulmonary veins, coronary sinus, or superior vena cava.

focal atrial tachycardia. Atrial tachycardias arising because of a localized repetitive discharge from either abnormal automaticity or triggered activity. Frequent sites of focal atrial tachycardia include the crista terminalis, coronary sinus, pulmonary vein, and inter-atrial septum. Focal discharge refers to a highly localized site of repetitive depolarization of either atrial or ventricular myocardial cells.

focal tachycardias. Generic term for arrhythmias arising from either the atrium or the ventricle as a result of abnormal automaticity or triggered activity.

Fontan procedure. A surgical procedure that creates a conduit to bypass the morphologic right ventricle (i.e., blood is diverted from the right atrium to the pulmonary arteries). It originally was used as a surgical approach for congenital tricuspid atresia. The incidence of both atrial flutter and atrial fibrillation is increased after the procedure. When patients require a permanent pacemaker or implantable cardioverter-defibrillator after the Fontan procedure, a common approach has been to place an epicardial ventricular lead at the time of the Fontan procedure and postoperatively to place an atrial transvenous lead if dual-chamber configuration is needed. Both leads are connected to the pulse generator at the time the atrial lead is placed. If no atrial lead is intended, then the device can be placed at the time of the Fontan procedure if an indication already exists. If not, the epicardial lead can be capped and left in a position where it can be easily accessed should the need for permanent pacing develop.

Food and Drug Administration (FDA). A section of the United States Department of Health and Human Services which regulates the manufacture, sale, and distribution of food, drugs, biologicals, cosmetics, and radiation-emitting products. The Food and Drug Administration is the principal federal agency in the United States responsible for protecting the public against unapproved and defective foods, cosmetics, drugs, and medical devices.

foramen ovale. In utero, this interatrial connection allows the flow of blood from the inferior vena cava to the left atrium. At birth, when the pressure in the left atrium exceeds that in the right atrium, physiologic closure occurs. In many persons, the forman ovale may remain patent.

fossa ovalis. Remnant of the fetal interatrial connection. The fossa ovalis is the site targeted for transseptal puncture and is bounded superiorly by the superior limbus and inferiorly by the inferior limbic continuation of the eustachian ridge. See also *eustachian ridge, oval fossa, superior limbus.*

fractionated electrograms. Prolonged, low-amplitude, high-frequency myocardial recordings thought to be related to the zone of slow conduction in a reentrant circuit. Fractionated electrograms usually are recorded in late diastole or throughout diastole.

fractionation. During catheter mapping of tachycardias, multiple low-amplitude electrograms sensed with no clear intervening isoelectric period.

fracture. See *conductor fracture.*

Frank lead system. Vectorcardiographic mapping system with seven electrodes arranged in three planes to allow three-dimensional mapping.

free running mode. The mode in which a pacemaker functions when it is not in the magnet mode, backup mode, or noise-reversion mode.

free wall accessory pathway. Atrioventricular bypass tracts located on the right or left free wall. Not septal accessory pathway.

French (gauge). A scale (abbreviated F) whose numbers correspond to the circumference, in millimeters, of the designated catheter or article. A 9-French catheter is 3 mm in circumference (1F = 0.33 mm).

frequency (f). The number of times a repetitive signal fluctuates in 1 second. Frequency correlates inversely with the interval from one leading edge of the signal to the next. In pacing, the pacemaker sensing circuit is tuned to recognize signals over a certain frequency range for further processing within the pacemaker circuitry. Frequency is expressed in hertz (Hz) or cycles per second.

frequency analysis. See *frequency domain analysis.*

frequency domain analysis. Breaking down the signal obtained from the signal-averaged electrocardiogram into its component wave frequencies by techniques such as fast Fourier transform. This technique presents amplitude (decibels) as a function of frequency. In contrast, time domain analysis assesses the amplitude of the signal as a function of time.

frequency modulation. A method of converting an analog signal into a tone of varying pitch. The tones created by frequency modulation can be transmitted over radio. In pacing, frequency modulation is used for transtelephonic monitoring. The pitch is modulated according to the deflections apparent from the electrocardiogram.

friction rub. A cardiac auscultatory finding that most commonly occurs with pericarditis. In pacing, a friction rub occasionally may be heard after lead placement. It may be caused by the tricuspid valve opening and closing against a ventricular lead that passes through the tricuspid valve. A rub also may represent pericarditis caused by perforation of the myocardium by an endocardial lead.

frontal plane (QRS) axis. In the 12-lead electrocardiogram, the primary QRS vector. The axis of the QRS complex typically is described in four quadrants (southwest, southeast, northeast, northwest). The normal axis is a southeast axis.

FRP. Abbreviation for *functional refractory period.*

fulguration. An ablative procedure used for the treatment of arrhythmias. Fulguration requires the use of an electrode catheter to deliver electrical current to the myocardium. The current is delivered to destroy the site from which an arrhythmia originates or a critical portion of the reentrant circuit. See also *ablation, electrode catheter*.

functional noncapture. Failure of an output pulse to depolarize the chamber in which the output pulse is delivered because it is delivered at a time when the myocardium is physiologically refractory.

functional reentry. Mechanism of arrhythmia or reentry occurs around an obstacle that is not anatomic. Functional reentry is an important mechanism of arrhythmogenesis, initiating several forms of ventricular arrhythmia in nonischemic cardiomyopathy.

functional refractory period (FRP). The minimum period of time between two consecutively conducted impulses. See also *atrial functional refractory period, AV conduction system functional refractory period, AV nodal functional refractory period, His-Purkinje system functional refractory period, VA conduction system functional refractory period, ventricular functional refractory period*.

functional-status questionnaires. A type of questionnaire sometimes used to assess individuals before and after device implantation. It is an assessment that is self-administered and is used to provide information on the psychological and physical state and social functions of a patient.

functional undersensing. Failure to sense an appropriate signal because it occurs during a refractory period of the pacemaker.

funny current. Sodium channel current important in the genesis of automaticity in sinus and atrioventricular nodal tissue.

Furman, Seymour (July 12, 1931-February 20, 2006). One of the pioneers of cardiac pacing who, in the late 1950s, developed the first pacemaker, which led directly to today's devices.

fusion beat. 1. A cardiac contraction that occurs when two intrinsic depolarizations of a particular heart chamber are initiated from separate initiation sites and the two depolarizations merge. In pacing, fusion beats may occur when an intrinsic cardiac depolarization of a particular chamber (atrium or ventricle) merges with a pacemaker output pulse within that chamber. Electrocardiographically, fusion beats have varying morphologic findings. The merging depolarizations usually do not contribute evenly to the total depolarization. 2. With biventricular pacemakers or defibrillators, a resulting QRS complex from both right and left ventricular pacing vectors is a type of fusion and can be used to judge the extent of electrical synchrony. 3. A surface QRS or P wave resulting from two separate automatic arrhythmia exit sites or an arrhythmia exit site and a paced site. See also *pseudofusion beat, pseudopseudofusion beat*.

f waves. Atrial activity in atrial fibrillation and sometimes atrial flutter. These waves may appear regular in some leads (V_1) and irregular in other leads during atrial fibrillation.

g

gain. The degree of magnification or amplification applied by an amplifier, expressed in decibels or as a ratio.

galvanic interference. A type of electromagnetic interference produced by a closed current pathway from any current or voltage source. In pacing, galvanic interference may occur when two electrodes make contact within the body. This contact can create a closed current pathway and inhibit pacemaker output. See also *electromagnetic interference*.

gap junction. Low-resistance channels that connect cardiac cells and allow for intercellular communication by passive flow of current. See also *connexin, connexon*.

gap phenomenon. Prolongation of conduction at a site proximal to the region of block which allows the blocked area to recover and conduct impulses. This typically occurs when the distal area of the conduction system has a longer refractory period than a more proximal area. Gap phenomenon is one possible explanation for unexpected conduction of an impulse at a shorter coupling interval than an impulse that had blocked at a longer coupling interval. This phenomenon may occur in either the antegrade or the retrograde direction.

gating. Phenomenon allowing spatial and temporal differences in cationic or anionic currents crossing the plasma membrane. May refer to ionic-channel–regulating mechanisms.

gating current. See *gating*.

gauge pins. Used in choosing the correct locking stylet. Tools used to measure the inner coil diameter. Measured inner diameter should be matched to corresponding locking stylet.

GCV. Abbreviation for *great cardiac vein*.

generator. See *pulse generator*.

glossopharyngeal nerve. Cranial nerve IX, which may serve as the main afferent nerve pathway in episodes of vasovagal syncope.

glucocorticoids. A class of steroid hormones that possess anti-inflammatory response. Glucocorticoids, usually dexamethasone, are used to reduce pacing thresholds by incorporating a small amount of the drug in the tip of the lead, allowing the drug to be eluted slowly.

G proteins. Guanine nucleotide-binding proteins that act as second messengers, linking stimulation of cell membrane receptors with cellular effector systems such as enzymes or ion channels. The actions of sympathetic and parasympathetic receptors on ion channels are dependent on G proteins. G proteins may be stimulatory or inhibitory.

great cardiac vein (GCV). Vein formed by the confluence of several ventricular veins distal to the posterolateral vein. The great cardiac vein joins the posterolateral vein to form the coronary sinus.

ground. A conductor used in an electrical current to establish an arbitrary zero potential reference for the rest of the circuitry. In pacing, the body may be used as the ground for testing the electrical variables of the pacing leads at the time of implantation.

grounding. The intentional connection of an electrical circuit to a ground. Grounding is recommended whenever line-powered equipment, such as electrocautery equipment, is used near a patient with an implanted pacemaker. Grounding minimizes the chances of extraneous electrical currents from reaching the heart via the pacemaker, lead, and electrode. See also *ground*.

guidewire. A coiled wire spring, of a defined length, designed to fit within a percutaneous catheter. Guidewires facilitate the insertion and positioning of a catheter within a blood vessel. They also facilitate the insertion of a lead introducer. Guidewires usually are stainless steel and are coated with polytef for lubricity and biocompatibility. The stainless steel core may be fixed or movable, and the shape of the guidewire may vary (i.e., the guidewire may be straight at both ends or one end may be J-shaped).

guiding catheter. A catheter that is used to provide support to ease or enhance the navigation of another catheter or interventional device. During placement of a coronary sinus lead, a guiding catheter may be helpful when the coronary venous anatomy is challenging.

guiding sheath. A sheath used for the introduction of intravascular catheters into a specific cardiac chamber or cardiac location.

h

H₁. During extrastimulus testing, the His-bundle deflection associated with the atrial paced beats (non-extrastimulus).

H₂. The His-bundle deflection associated with or produced by an atrial extrastimulus (A₂) after an atrial paced train.

HA. See *HA interval*.

HA interval. Retrograde conduction through the atrioventricular node. Typically measured from the end of the His-bundle deflection to the earliest atrial deflection. The HA interval is the primary driver for the atrioventricular node reentrant circuit.

halo catheter. Widely spaced multielectrode catheter usually placed along the tricuspid anulus during right-sided accessory pathway and atrial flutter ablation procedures.

hardware. The electrical and mechanical components of an electronic system, such as microprocessors, resistors, and capacitors. In pacing, hardware also refers to accessory equipment such as the programmer and the pacing systems analyzer. Unlike software, hardware cannot be altered after manufacturing is complete. See also *software*.

hard-wired. The permanent interconnection of circuit functions for a specific purpose, formed either on an integrated circuit or from manufactured circuits. Hard-wired connections are unalterable after manufacturing is complete.

HBE. Abbreviation for *His-bundle electrogram*.

HCM. Abbreviation for *hypertrophic cardiomyopathy*.

HDE. Abbreviation for *humanitarian device exemption*.

H deflection. Also known as the His-bundle electrogram. This deflection may be seen after the atrial electrogram in sinus rhythm and most supraventricular tachycardias. The H deflection may occur after the atrial electrogram in junctional tachycardia and atrioventricular nodal reentrant tachycardia.

header. The superior portion of a pacemaker or implantable cardioverter-defibrillator. The header houses the receptacles into which the lead connectors are inserted. See also *connector block, lead connector, lead terminal pin*.

head-up tilt-table testing. See *tilt-table testing*.

Health Care Financing Administration (HCFA). See *Centers for Medicare and Medicaid Services*.

heart block. A disruption in the propagation of electrical impulses through the atrioventricular conduction system. Heart block is most common in the atrioventricular conduction system. However, it also may occur in the His bundle or bundle branches. It can be caused by acute tissue damage, such as myocardial infarction, or, more commonly, by degenerative disease of the cardiac conduction system as a result of senescence. Heart block is subclassified as first-degree block, type I and type II second-degree block, and third-degree block. See also *first-degree AV block, second-degree AV block, third-degree AV block*.

heart rate. The rate at which the heart contracts, measured in beats per minute. See also *bradycardia, intrinsic heart rate, tachycardia*.

heart rate histogram. Monitoring and display by an implantable device of the heart rate trend over a period of time. See the figure *Bin*.

heart rate variability. The variance in sinus cycle length over a period of time, usually assessed over 24 hours. Heart rate variability is used as a measure of parasympathetic tone. Persons with diminished heart rate variability have reduced vagal tone and probably are at increased risk of death after myocardial infarction.

Heart Rhythm Society (HRS). Professional society dedicated to the evaluation, treatment, and management of cardiac rhythm disturbances and education of caregivers about heart rhythm disturbances. Formerly the North American Society of Pacing and Electrophysiology. The Heart Rhythm Society is the international leader in science, education, and advocacy for cardiac arrhythmia professionals and patients and the primary information resource on heart rhythm disorders. Its mission is to improve the care of patients by promoting research, education, and optimal health care policies and standards.

heavyweight guidewires. In over-the-wire left ventricular pacing lead systems, less pliable, relatively stiffer wires may be used to overcome tortuous venous segments or to subselect intramyocardial vessels.

HEI. Abbreviation for *hysteresis escape interval*.

hematoma. A collection of blood that occurs outside a blood vessel. A hematoma is caused by a leak or injury and can be a complication of placement of a pulse generator if there is poor hemostasis or if the patient is receiving anticoagulants or antiplatelet agents.

hemiblock. Delayed or blocked conduction through either the anterior or the posterior fascicle of the left bundle branch.

hemodynamic monitoring. A broad term for monitoring many potential variables that indicate a patient's hemodynamic status (e.g., cardiac output, pulmonary capillary wedge pressure, pulmonary artery pressure, blood pressure). Temporary (percutaneous) hemodynamic catheters also may have the capability of temporary pacing. Hemodynamic monitoring relates to permanent device placement in that contemporary devices, investigational as of the writing of this text, are capable of long-term hemodynamic monitoring.

hemopericardium. A collection of blood within the pericardial space. This may be a complication of lead perforation.

hemopneumothorax. Pneumothorax with associated hemorrhagic effusion. Hemopneumothorax is a potential complication of subclavian puncture.

hemothorax. A collection of blood within the thoracic cavity. This may occur in combination with a pneumothorax (i.e., hemopneumothorax), which may be a complication of subclavian puncture.

HERG. See *HERG (human ether-a-go-go) channel*.

HERG (human ether-a-go-go) channel. Channel associated with the delayed rectifier potassium current (I_{Kr}). So-named because a homologous channel in fruit flies is associated with ether-induced leg movement.

HERG gene. Gene coding for the HERG channel. See also *HERG channel*.

hermetic seal. A fluid-impermeable seal of the pacemaker case or pacemaker circuitry that protects the circuitry from fluid invasion. Initially, epoxy resin was used to encapsulate pacemaker circuitry components and the pacemaker case. Currently, metallic pacemaker cases more frequently are sealed hermetically by welding. See also *epoxy resin*.

heteromeric gap junctions. Intracellular ion channel junctions located at the nexus or intercalated disk. Each gap junction is made up of two connexons, which in turn are made up of several peptide chains.

H-gate binding. Binding on the intracellular inactivation gate.

H₁-H₂ interval in refractory periods. The interval measured between the His-bundle deflection associated with atrial paced beats in the pacing train and the His-bundle deflection associated with the atrial extrastimulus beat.

H-H intervals. Intervals between two consecutive His-bundle deflections with or without intervening atrial depolarization or paced beats. H-H intervals may be antegrade, retrograde, or measured during His-bundle tachycardias.

HIFU. Abbreviation for *high-intensity focused ultrasonography*.

high defibrillation threshold. A defibrillation threshold more than 10 J less than the maximal energy output of the device is considered high.

high-energy implantable cardioverter-defibrillator. Device capable of delivering higher energy, usually more than 40 J. It is typically large and is used in patients with high defibrillation thresholds.

high-frequency stimulation. Rapid rate pacing used to terminate an arrhythmia or to initiate an arrhythmia during electrophysiologic testing.

high-intensity focused ultrasonography (HIFU). A newer method for ablation utilizing focused ultrasound delivered via a catheter not necessarily making contact with the myocardium to be ablated.

high-pass filter. An electronic filter that allows the passage of frequencies above a given cutoff. A high-pass filter acts mathematically as a differentiator, that is, it emphasizes high slew rates in the input signal.

high-rate atrial activity. A monitoring feature that relates to the programmed criteria that define high rate, such as the atrial tachycardia and atrial fibrillation zones. Activity implies sporadic, inconsistent detection (random single events), and events imply that, at minimum, the detection criteria were met.

high-rate atrial events. See *high-rate atrial activity*.

high-rate episodes. A monitoring feature. Detection of high-rate atrial episodes can be triggered either from mode switching (if enabled) or the programmed detection criteria. Detection of high-rate ventricular episodes also is based on programmed detection criteria. The key variables of this diagnostic data are event date and time, duration of the episode, and maximum rate during the episode.

high-rate timeout. In specific devices, a feature that ensures that sustained high ventricular rates are managed with tachytherapy by limiting the time that detection criteria for supraventricular tachycardia can withhold detection. When the timeout period expires, ongoing episodes can be detected and treated.

high right atrial electrogram (HRA). The endocardial recording obtained from the lateral right atrium near the junction with the superior vena cava.

high right atrium (HRA). The area of the atrium that has been the most common anatomic site for right atrial lead placement.

high thoracic left sympathectomy. A surgical procedure used to treat long QT syndrome. In this procedure, left sympathetic nerve innervation of the first five thoracic ganglia. The stellate ganglion is not interrupted, and thus Horner's syndrome usually is avoided.

high voltage (HV). Higher voltage in comparison with that required for pacing used in defibrillators to deliver energy for cardioversion or defibrillation.

high-voltage charging. Charging in defibrillators before high-voltage therapy, such as cardioversion or defibrillation.

high-voltage (high-energy) therapy. See *high voltage*.

His bundle. That portion of the specialized cardiac conduction system that transmits electrical impulses from the atrial myocardium to the ventricular myocardium. The His bundle extends from the lower end of the atrioventricular node and passes through the right fibrous trigone along the posterior edge of the muscular interventricular septum. The lower boundary of the His bundle, as it enters and descends into the ventricular myocardium, is marked by the division of the conduction fibers into the left and right bundle branches. The His bundle is also referred to as the common atrioventricular bundle.

His-bundle deflection. The deflection indicated on a His-bundle electrogram that corresponds to the propagation of an impulse through the bundle. The His-bundle deflection usually is recorded with a bipolar catheter placed across the tricuspid valve. See also *His-bundle electrogram*.

His-bundle electrogram (HBE). The intracardiac electrogram of the His bundle recorded with the use of endocardial bipolar or multipolar catheters. His-bundle electrograms are used in the assessment of wide complex rhythms, atrioventricular conduction, and preexcitation syndromes. His-bundle electrograms allow evaluation of the AH interval, atrioventricular nodal conduction time, and the HV interval. See also *electrogram*.

His-bundle pacing. Stimulating the heart at or very near the His bundle. This may be done via a temporary pacing catheter during an electrophysiologic study, and permanent His-bundle pacing also has been reported. The theoretical advantage of His-bundle pacing is that pacing from this point allows more normal ventricular depolarization and may minimize or obviate the deleterious effect of right ventricular apical pacing. His-bundle pacing has been shown to result in higher pacing thresholds than septal or apical pacing in some patients.

His deflection. Electrogram associated with conduction through the His bundle. His deflections may be antegrade or retrograde or from automatic His-bundle discharges. See *His-bundle deflection*.

His potential. See *His-bundle deflection*.

His-Purkinje conduction delay. Conduction delay that occurs below the level of the compact atrioventricular node. This term includes intrahisian delay and bundle branch delay but typically is used in describing patients with nonspecific conduction abnormality in the His-Purkinje system.

His-Purkinje system. That portion of the specialized cardiac conduction system which extends from the His bundle through the left and right bundle branches to the Purkinje network within the walls of the ventricles. The His-Purkinje system conducts impulses from the atrioventricular node to the ventricular myocardium.

His-Purkinje system effective refractory period. In antegrade conduction, for a given cycle (A_1-A_1), the shortest V_1-V_2 generated in response to any H_1-H_2 interval. In retrograde conduction, for a given cycle (V_1-V_1), the shortest H_1-H_2 interval generated in response to any V_1-V_2 interval. See also *functional refractory period*.

His-Purkinje system functional refractory period. In antegrade conduction, for a given cycle (A_1-A_1), the shortest V_1-V_2 generated in response to H_1-H_2 interval. In retrograde conduction, for a given cycle (V_1-V_1), the shortest H_1-H_2 interval generated in response to any V_1-V_2 interval. See also *functional refractory period*.

His-Purkinje system relative refractory period. In antegrade conduction, the longest H_1-H_2 interval at which the H_2-V_2 interval exceeds the H_1-V_1 interval. See also *relative refractory period*.

His-synchronous premature ventricular complex. During narrow complex tachycardia, a premature ventricular complex delivered during the time of His bundle refractoriness. His-synchronous premature ventricular complexes are used to differentiate atrioventricular reentrant tachycardia from atrioventricular nodal reentrant tachycardia. In atrioventricular reentrant tachycardia, a His-synchronous premature ventricular complex is able to reset atrial activation or terminate tachycardia without activation of the atrium.

His-to-atrial (HA) interval. See *HA interval*.

histogram. See *event histogram, heart rate histogram*.

His-to-ventricular (HV) interval. See *HV interval*.

His-ventricular block. Conduction block occurring distal to the bundle of His usually in the His-Purkinje system or both bundle branches.

Hodgkin-Huxley scheme. Explanatory scheme devised by Drs. Hodgkin, Huxley, and Katz explaining activation, inactivation, and resting states of ion channels.

Holter monitoring. Noninvasive ambulatory electrocardiographic recording used for the assessment of rhythm disorders. Holter monitoring allows continuous observation of cardiac rate and rhythm during normal activity or during selected diagnostic procedures such as stress testing. Intermittent and transient arrhythmias are recorded and correlated with clinical symptoms reported by the patient. Holter monitoring can be used for the detection of episodic

or asymptomatic arrhythmias. Cardiac activity is most commonly recorded for a period of 24 hours. See also *event recorder*.

housekeeping current. The amount of current used for ongoing tasks such as monitoring the intrinsic rhythm and logging data. The average housekeeping current, or static current drain, is usually about 10 μA. The housekeeping current is $\approx$8 μA for single chambers, $\approx$10 μA for dual chambers, and $\approx$12 μA for cardiac resynchronization therapy devices.

HRA. Abbreviation for *high right atrial electrogram, high right atrium*.

HRS. See *Heart Rhythm Society*.

H spikes. His-bundle electrograms, particularly when noted in the setting of junctional tachycardia, are referred to as H spikes.

HUD. Abbreviation for *humanitarian use device*.

human ether-a-go-go–related gene. See *HERG (human ether-a-go-go) channel*.

humanitarian device exemption (HDE). Regulated by the U.S. Food and Drug Administration, a humanitarian device exemption is an exemption for use of a device that has not been approved. This is necessary for conditions that are so unusual that it would be difficult, if not impossible, for a manufacturer to demonstrate clinical safety and efficacy in a large number of patients. In these cases, a humanitarian device exemption may be granted if the device is not believed to pose a significant or unreasonable risk of injury or illness; the probable benefit to the patient's health outweighs the risk of injury or illness. The exemption for a specific patient must be approved by a facility's Institutional Review Board, and the Board must supervise subsequent clinical assessment of the device.

humanitarian use device (HUD). A device that is intended to benefit patients in the treatment and diagnosis of diseases or conditions that affect or are manifested in fewer than 4,000 individuals in the United States per year.

HUT. Abbreviation for *head-up tilt*. See *tilt-table testing*.

HV. Abbreviation for *high voltage*. See *HV interval*.

HV interval. The amount of time required for a wave of depolarization to travel from the His bundle to the ventricles. In electrophysiologic studies, the HV interval is measured from the beginning of the His bundle deflection to the earliest ventricular activity in any lead (surface or intracardiac). Normal values of the HV interval range from 35 to 55 milliseconds. See also *His-bundle electrogram*.

H₂-V₂ interval. The interval between the His-bundle deflection and the ventricular electrogram associated with or produced by an atrial extrastimulus delivered after an atrial paced train.

HV refractory. Paced ventricular beats delivered at a time of infrahisian refractoriness. The HV conduction system is refractory when atrial pacing results in infrahisian refractoriness before compact atrioventricular nodal refractoriness.

hybrid circuit. A circuit with a combination of integrated circuits and discrete components. Some of the electronic components of a hybrid circuit are affixed directly to the hybrid substrate at the time of manufacture, as in the integrated circuit, whereas others are connected to the circuit board after its manufacture, as in a discrete circuit. See also *discrete component, integrated circuit*.

hydrocortisone. The major glucocorticoid secreted by the adrenal cortex. Hydrocortisone may lower acute pacing thresholds when given systemically. However, pacing thresholds again increase when use of the medication is discontinued. Another glucocorticoid, dexamethasone sodium phosphate, is incorporated into the distal tip of some pacing leads as a method of maintaining low pacing thresholds. See also *dexamethasone sodium phosphate, steroid-eluting lead*.

hyperbaric pressure recommendations. Patients with implantable devices may inquire about activities in which hyperbaric pressure is increased, especially scuba diving. Scuba diving to a depth of 30 feet has been the usual restriction. A patient with a device who scuba dives needs to discuss with his or her physician the potential risks of being 30 feet under water and having the implantable cardioverter-defibrillator deliver a shock for any reason. The recommendations are based on a qualification testing process. Exposure to such depths narrows the safety margin of protection from any external trauma (i.e., the patient may reach the limit of protection diving to the stated limits, and then, if the device is hit by something else, such as another diver or a stone, this otherwise relatively

minor trauma and the added stress on a device result in damage to it and altered function).

hyperkalemia. An increase of serum potassium levels. In the paced patient, hyperkalemia may result in sensing and pacing abnormalities. This occurs most commonly in the permanently paced patient who is undergoing hemodialysis.

hyperpolarization-activated. See *hyperpolarization-activated ion channels*.

hyperpolarization-activated ion channels. Most ion channels exhibit activation with cellular depolarization; however, certain ion channels (chloride, stretch) may be activated when the intracellular potential is more negative than the extracellular potential into the depolarized state (less than –100 mV).

hyperpolarized. The lowering of intracellular voltage below the typical polarized state (–80 to –100 mV).

hypersensitive carotid sinus syndrome. See *carotid sinus hypersensitivity*.

hypertrophic cardiomyopathy (HCM). A cardiomyopathic condition characterized by hypertrophic changes in the left or right ventricle with no known cause. The ventricles may be concentrically involved, or the changes may be regional. Dual-chamber permanent pacing was at one time advocated as a treatment to reduce refractory symptoms. Randomized clinical trials have failed to show that dual-chamber pacing is a viable therapy for this condition. A patient with hypertrophic cardiomyopathy is prone to ventricular arrhythmias and may have syncope or sudden cardiac death and may be a candidate for primary prevention with implantation of a cardioverter-defibrillator.

hypertrophic obstructive cardiomyopathy. See *hypertrophic cardiomyopathy*.

hypervagotonia. Overactivity of the cardiac parasympathetic system which results in sinus bradycardia or atrioventricular nodal Wenckebach at a relatively long cycle length.

hypoallergenic. Causing little or no allergic reaction. Hypoallergenic materials are used for pacemaker and defibrillator cases, leads, and electrodes.

hysteresis. In pacing, the extension of the escape interval after a sensed intrinsic event. Hysteresis increases the pacing interval after an intrinsic event to allow more time for intrinsic activity to be sensed by the circuitry of the implanted pacemaker. If no intrinsic event occurs before the end of the hysteresis period, the pacemaker delivers an output pulse. See also *rate-variable AV interval*.

hysteresis escape interval (HEI). The amount of time (in milliseconds) of the longer interval after an intrinsic beat when hysteresis is programmed "on." For example, if the pacemaker is programmed to a lower rate of 70 beats per minute with a hysteresis escape rate of 50 beats per minute, the hysteresis escape rate interval is 1,200 milliseconds.

hysteresis escape rate. The programmed rate at which the pacemaker escapes after an intrinsic event; after the hysteresis escape rate interval, the pacemaker returns to pacing at the programmed lower rate.

Hysteresis

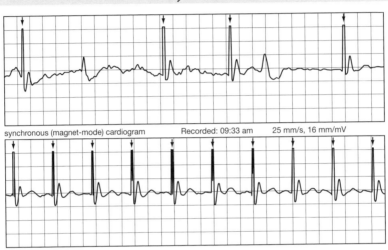

synchronous (magnet-mode) cardiogram   Recorded: 09:33 am   25 mm/s, 16 mm/mV

i

I. 1. Used in the third position of the NBG code for pacemaker nomenclature to designate the mode of response; indicates inhibited (i.e., if intrinsic activity is sensed in a given chamber, pacemaker output will be inhibited). 2. The abbreviation for *current*. See the table *NBG code*.

IAB. Abbreviation for *intra-atrial block*.

IART. Abbreviation for *intra-atrial reentrant tachycardia*.

ibutilide. Class III antiarrhythmic agent. Intravenous administration and rapid onset of action allow its use for acute cardioversion of atrial fibrillation. Also can be used for the acute cardioversion of atrial flutter. Ibutilide carries the risk of prolonging the QT interval and subsequent polymorphic ventricular tachycardia (torsades de pointes).

ibutilide fumarate. See *ibutilide*.

I_{Ca}. Calcium current.

$I_{Ca,L}$. Calcium current referred to as L-type calcium current.

I_{Ca-L}. The slow calcium current responsible for phase 0 in sinus and atrioventricular nodal cells. I_{Ca-L} also is present in atrial and ventricular cells, where it contributes less to phase 0 because of the dominant role that I_{Na} plays, but it affects the plateau phase and triggers calcium release from the sarcoplasmic reticulum. I_{Ca-L} is blocked by verapamil, diltiazem, and the dihydropyridines, and it is enhanced by β-adrenergic agonists.

$I_{Ca,T}$. Calcium current referred to as T-type calcium current.

I_{Ca-T}. A calcium current that may contribute to spontaneous phase 4 depolarization in cells that have intrinsic automaticity. I_{Ca-T} is not affected by verapamil, diltiazem, dihydropyridines, or β-adrenergic blockers.

ICD. Abbreviation for *implantable cardioverter-defibrillator*. ICD is the accepted generic abbreviation for all implantable cardioverter-defibrillators.

ICD Registry. Also referred to as the CMS National ICD Registry, this is a registry mandated by the Centers for Medicaid and Medicare Services (CMS) to follow Medicare beneficiaries who receive primary prevention therapy with an implantable cardioverter-defibrillator. The ICD Registry is a partnership of the American College of Cardiology and the Heart Rhythm Society and is administered by the American College of Cardiology-National Cardiovascular Data Registry. This is the leading example of a new approach to coverage by the CMS, termed Coverage with Evidence Determination (CED). The goal is to determine how newly approved therapies, in this case implantable cardioverter-defibrillators, perform in patient populations and for providers outside the confines of a randomized clinical trial.

ICD II trial. See *Multicenter InSync ICD Randomized Clinical Evaluation II*.

ICE. Abbreviation for *intracardiac echocardiography*.

ICEG. A seldom-used abbreviation for *intracardiac electrogram*. See *electrogram*.

ice mapping. The use of cryoenergy to aid the mapping of various arrhythmias. With this technique, moderate amounts of cryoenergy (typically temperatures at about −30°C) are delivered via a cryocatheter at various intercardiac sites. When such energy is delivered at a site that represents the source of an automatic tachycardia or the slow zone of a reentrant tachycardia, the tachycardia terminates (mapped to the site with Ice).

ice water immersion. A technique used historically to abort supraventricular tachyarrhythmias.

ICHD code. The first accepted system of abbreviations used to describe pacing modes. The Intersociety Commission on Heart Disease (ICHD) Resources devised this code, which was based on five letters: the first letter represented the heart chamber(s) being artificially paced, the second letter represented the heart chamber(s) being sensed by the pacemaker, the third letter represented the mode of response of the pacemaker to sensed events, the fourth letter represented pacemaker programmability, and the fifth letter represented any special antitachycardia function. This code has been replaced by the NBG code. See also *NBG code*.

I_{Cl}. An outward current caused by the inward flow of chloride ions. I_{Cl} may play a role in shortening action potential duration in ventricular cells in response to catecholamines.

ICV. Abbreviation for *inferior caval vein*.

ID. Abbreviation for *intrinsic deflection*.

IDE. Abbreviation for *investigational device exemption*.

idiopathic cardiomyopathy. See *dilated cardiomyopathy*.

idiopathic left ventricular tachycardia. A sustained ventricular tachycardia that occurs in patients with structurally normal hearts. Idiopathic left ventricular tachycardia morphology shows right bundle branch block with left-axis deviation. It frequently responds to verapamil, but it does not respond to β-blockers. Idiopathic left ventricular tachycardia is entrainable and can be initiated and terminated using programmed ventricular stimulation, a suggestion that reentry is the underlying mechanism.

idiopathic left ventricular tachycardias (ILVT). Group of closely related disorders presenting with a right bundle branch morphology, superior axis, QRS complex, and ventricular tachycardias. The most common form of this group of tachycardias occurs in young patients with normal hearts and arises from the region of the left posterior fascicle. Idiopathic left ventricular tachycardias respond to both medical therapy with calcium channel blockers or β-blockers and radiofrequency ablation.

idiopathic monomorphic ventricular tachycardia. Single-morphology ventricular tachycardia that occurs in normal hearts, such as idiopathic left ventricular tachycardia and certain right ventricular tachycardias, including those that arise from the outflow tract or the region of the moderator band.

idiopathic ventricular tachycardia. See *idiopathic monomorphic ventricular tachycardia*.

idioventricular rhythm. A ventricular escape rhythm characterized by a rate of 20 to 40 beats per minute and wide QRS complexes. Idioventricular rhythms often occur in patients with third-degree atrioventricular block.

IECG. Abbreviation for *intracardiac electrogram*. See *electrogram*.

IEGM. Abbreviation for *intracardiac electrogram*. See *electrogram*.

I_f. The pacemaker current in Purkinje fibers and possibly in sinus node cells. I_f is an inward current that is carried by sodium, enhanced by catecholamines, and suppressed by acetylcholine.

IHR. Abbreviation for *intrinsic heart rate*.

I_K. The delayed rectifier. I_K is the potassium current that contributes to phase 3 repolarization.

I_{K1}. Type of potassium current. See also *potassium currents, repolarization*.

$I_{K,ACh}$. The acetylcholine-activated potassium current that hyperpolarizes the sinus node, the atrioventricular node, and atrial cells. $I_{K,ACh}$ slows the rate of the sinus node, slows conduction through the atrioventricular node, and shortens the action potential duration in atrial cells. $I_{K,ACh}$ is activated by adenosine and thus sometimes is called $I_{K,Ado}$.

$I_{K,Ado}$. Adenosine-activated potassium current. See also *potassium currents*.

$I_{K,ATP}$. The adenosine triphosphate (ATP)-dependent potassium current that is activated by a decrease in intracellular ATP levels and thus may reduce energy consumption during ischemia by shortening action potential duration. See also *potassium currents*.

I_{KI}. The inward rectifier. I_{KI} is the potassium current that plays a major role in maintaining resting potential (phase 4) in atrial, Purkinje, and ventricular cells. It is not present in sinus nodal cells.

I_K **potassium current.** See *potassium currents*.

I_{Kr}. Important potassium current associated with normal cardiac repolarization.

I_{Ks}. Important repolarizing potassium current in cardiac myocytes. Slowly acting repolarizing potassium current. See also I_{Kr}.

$I_{K,slow}$. Slow-type potassium current. Important potassium current associated with repolarization. See also *potassium currents, repolarization*.

I_{Kur}. Ultrarapid form of potassium current in atrial myocytes.

IkV. Voltage-gated potassium channel–associated current. See also *potassium currents*.

iliac vein approach. A surgical approach used for placement of temporary pacing leads. The iliac vein approach has been used successfully for the placement of permanent pacing leads.

ILR. Abbreviation for *implantable loop recorder*.

ILVT. Abbreviation for *idiopathic left ventricular tachycardias*.

immediate recurrence. Usually refers to the immediate recurrence of atrial fibrillation after cardioversion. Immediate recurrence as a phenomenon can be used for mapping sites of origin of atrial fibrillation initiation.

Immediate Risk Stratification Improves Survival (IRIS). This is a large-scale, prospective, randomized trial to evaluate the benefit of implantable cardioverter-defibrillator therapy for reduction of total mortality in patients considered at high risk of sudden death early after acute myocardial infarction (Steinbeck G, Andresen D, Senges J, Hoffmann E, Seidl K, Brachmann J, IRIS Investigators as Joint Study of the German University Hospitals and German Society of Leading Cardiological Hospital Physicians [ALKK]. Immediate Risk-Stratification Improves Survival [IRIS]: study protocol. Europace. 2004;6:392-9).

impedance (Z). The total opposition presented to the flow of alternating current by an electrical circuit or device. Impedance includes the opposition to current caused by the physical characteristics of the material through which the current is flowing (resistance) and the opposition produced by capacitors and inductance coils (reactance). Impedance commonly is related to voltage (V) and current (I) by Ohm's law, Z=V/I. However, a true expression of impedance also includes the opposition to current produced by capacitance and inductance, that is, the reactance of the system. The impedance of a pacing system is a combination of the opposition to the flow of electrical current by the lead(s) electrode(s), the electrode-myocardial interface, and the body tissues. Impedance is expressed in ohms. See also *afterpotential, resistance*.

impedance mismatch. An important concept for cardiac wave propagation and the generation of arrhythmia in which a mismatch between the impedance associated with the source of current and the sink for the current flow will cause slowing of conduction and possible arrythmogenesis.

impedance plethysmography. A method by which changing tissue volumes can be determined from measurement of electrical impedance at the body surface. This technique has been used to optimize the atrioventricular interval by repetitively measuring cardiac output at various intervals and accepting the atrioventricular interval that yields the greatest cardiac output.

implantable cardioverter. A device that delivered an electrical shock, synchronized to a ventricular depolarization, to terminate malignant ventricular arrhythmias. The energy delivered by a cardioverter usually ranged from 0.025 to 5 J. Stand-alone implantable cardioverters are no longer manufactured. See also *cardioversion, defibrillation, implantable cardioverter-defibrillator, implantable defibrillator*.

implantable cardioverter-defibrillator (ICD). The generic term for permanent implantable devices designed to detect spontaneous ventricular tachycardia or ventricular fibrillation and to terminate these arrhythmias by the delivery of shocks. Contemporary implantable cardioverter-defibrillators have antitachycardia pacing functions and bradycardia pacing. Some devices also have antitachycardia pacing functions and cardioversion for the treatment of atrial tachy-dysrhythmias. See also *atrial defibrillator, cardioversion, defibrillation*.

implantable cardioverter-defibrillator analyzer. A noninvasive testing device that determines the functional status, including power supply, of an implantable defibrillator or cardioverter-defibrillator. A magnet within the analyzer triggers the release of charge from the defibrillator into a capacitor. When the capacitor is fully charged, it unloads to a special test resistor. A progressive increase in the amount of time it takes for the capacitor to fully charge, normally 10 seconds or less, indicates battery depletion. Implantable cardioverter-defibrillator analyzers are rarely used today, except in experimental circumstances or with older models of defibrillators.

implantable defibrillator. A device designed to deliver an electrical shock to defibrillate the heart. See also *implantable cardioverter-defibrillator*.

implantable hemodynamic monitor. A device that is permanently placed to measure specific hemodynamic variables. These devices are currently under investigation. Variables measured include right ventricular systolic and diastolic pressures, pulse pressure, estimated pulmonary artery diastolic pressure, heart rate and activity, right ventricular dP/dt (positive and negative), preejection interval, and systolic time interval.

implantable loop recorder (ILR). See *loop recorder*.

implantable pacemaker registration form. A form that is completed when a pacemaker is implanted to allow the pacemaker manufacturer to keep a record of the patient on file. The implantable pacemaker registration form is packaged with each pacemaker. When the form has been sent to the manufacturer to register the patient, an identification card, including the name of the manufacturer, the model and serial number of the pacemaker, and the date of implantation, is sent to the patient.

implantable pulse generator (IPG). An implantable arrhythmia-control device consisting of a battery and electronic components such as microprocessors, resistors, and capacitors. See also *implantable cardioverter-defibrillator, pacemaker, pulse generator*.

implantation. Any of the various surgical procedures by which an arrhythmia-control device is inserted into the body. Implantation of currently available devices requires placement of the electrode(s) in or on the heart and placement of the pulse generator in a pocket beneath the skin. The subcutaneous pocket for pacemakers usually is in an infraclavicular, prepectoral location. A device sometimes is placed in the abdominal region with epicardial pacing systems and sometimes in small children when transvenous pacing is not a viable option.

implant criteria. Guidelines established to justify implantation of a pacemaker, implantable cardioverter-defibrillator, or cardiac resynchronization therapy device. Implant criteria have been established by a task force of ACC/AHA/HRS and are updated intermittently. Medicare also has established guidelines, but these generally follow those established by the task force of the professional societies.

implant support device (ISD). A type of analyzer used during implantation of some cardioverter-defibrillator systems. An implant support device is capable of measuring sensing, pacing, and defibrillator lead characteristics. It also can be used to deliver test shocks for the measurement of defibrillation thresholds and to deliver tachycardia induction signals.

impulse. A wave of excitation in the myocardium. In pacing, impulse frequently refers to the electrical output delivered by a pacemaker.

impulse initiation. The initiating potential for automatic arrhythmias. 1. Focal atrial tachycardias and some ventricular tachycardias that occur in a normal heart have a discrete site of impulse initiation. 2. General term signifying the site of earliest activation, either in a paced rhythm or in an impulse as a result of inherent automaticity.

impulse propagation. From the point of impulse initiation, propagation of the electrical wave front through the myocardium. Impulse propagation may be normal in certain arrhythmias, such as automatic tachycardias occurring in a structurally normal heart, or abnormal as a result of prior infarction, cardiac surgery, or prior ablation.

I_{Na}. The fast inward sodium current responsible for the rapid upstroke (phase 0) present in atrial, Purkinje, and ventricular cells. I_{Na} is voltage-dependent and is activated when the cell depolarizes to threshold. It is blocked by class I antiarrhythmic agents.

I_{Na-B}. The background sodium current thought to be present in sinus nodal cells and to play a role in the spontaneous depolarization of phase 4.

I_{NaCa}. The sodium-calcium exchange current, which exchanges three sodium ions for each calcium ion across the cell membrane. I_{NaCa} is the primary mechanism for removal of calcium from the cell. It may contribute to delayed afterdepolarizations, because intracellular calcium overload leads to calcium release from the sarcoplasmic reticulum (calcium-induced calcium release), which in turn causes the sodium-calcium exchanger to generate an inward current as calcium is extruded from the cell.

inactivated state. According to the modulated receptor hypothesis, ion channels exist in three states: activated, inactivated, and resting. After being activated, channels pass into the inactivated state, during which time the channel is closed and cannot conduct ions. The channel must then return to the resting state before it can be activated again. See also *modulated receptor hypothesis*.

I_{NaK}. The sodium-potassium pump, which moves three sodium ions outward across the cell membrane for every two potassium ions that move inward. The sodium-potassium pump requires adenosine triphosphate and is blocked by digitalis glycosides.

inappropriate shocks. When implantable cardioverter-defibrillator therapies (shocks) occur for supraventricular arrhythmias or the detected noise, inappropriately sensed as ventricular tachycardia or fibrillation, the resulting shocks are termed inappropriate. Common causes for inappropriate shocks include sinus tachycardia, atrial fibrillation with rapid ventricular rates, and atrioventricular node reentrant tachycardia.

inappropriate sinus tachycardia (IST). Sinus tachycardia is common in states of catecholamine excess such as exercise or emotion or in certain illnesses (e.g., accompanying fever). In certain patients, persistent or paroxysmal sinus tachycardia may occur without any obvious inciting factor. These patients have inappropriate sinus tachycardia. Three possible subsets of patients are 1) those with autonomic disorders, 2) those with high anxiety state, and 3) those with a history of high endurance physical training.

inappropriate therapy. See *inappropriate shocks*.

incessant tachycardia. An arrhythmia that is persistent and either is not terminable by any means or stops only for a brief time before spontaneously recurring. Incessant tachycardia sometimes occurs as a type of proarrhythmia in patients taking type IC antiarrhythmic agents, in patients with ventricular aneurysms, and in patients with the permanent form of junctional reciprocating tachycardia.

incomplete circuit. A pacing circuit that has been disrupted. An incomplete circuit is indicated by intermittent or complete loss of pacing or sensing. Causes of an incomplete pacing circuit include lead fracture, improper contact between the setscrew and the lead terminal pin, and air entrapment in the pacemaker of unipolar pacemakers. See also *open circuit*.

incremental pacing. See *decremental pacing*. See also *atrial decremental pacing, ventricular decremental pacing*.

indifferent clamp. A unipolar ground extension wire used to establish a temporary connection between a unipolar pacemaker and the patient before pacemaker implantation. Once the lead is connected to the pacemaker, the circuit extension from the pacemaker case to subcutaneous tissue completes the circuit, and thus immediate pacing is available. Indifferent clamps are not commonly used. They can provide continued pacing from the pacemaker while the subcutaneous pocket is being prepared.

indifferent electrode. 1. The pacemaker case in a unipolar pacing system. 2. An implantable subcutaneous reference electrode used to convert a bipolar pacemaker to a unipolar pacing system. The indifferent electrode can be inserted into one of the two apertures in the bipolar pacemaker neck to ground the terminal. The other aperture is used for the insertion of a unipolar lead or one terminal pin of a bifurcated bipolar lead for completion of the unipolar pacing system. See also *adaptor, anode*.

inducibility. The characteristic of a cardiac rhythm that allows it to be initiated with programmed stimulation.

infection. See *pacing system infection*.

inferior caval vein (ICV). See *IVC*.

inferior isthmus. 1. Synonymous with cavotricuspid isthmus, the arrhythmogenic substrate for typical atrial flutter. 2. Isthmus of myocardium that may be arrhythmogenic between an atriotomy scar and the inferior vena cava.

inflow tract. The inflow portion of the right ventricle from the tricuspid valve to the right ventricular apex and separated from the outflow tract by muscle bundles.

infra-His block. Conduction block to the ventricle during sinus rhythm, atrial pacing, or supraventricular tachycardia, occurring below the level of the His bundle. Retrograde infrahisian block may occur in ventricular tachycardia and ventricular pacing.

infrahisian conduction disease. Conduction slowing possibly with intermittent block occurring below the level of the His bundle. Manifestations of infrahisian conduction disease include antegrade and retrograde infrahisian block.

inframammary pacemaker placement. Implantation of a permanent pacemaker beneath the breast. Inframammary pacemaker placement can be used when there is concern that an effective cosmetic result cannot be obtained by placing the pacemaker in the usual infraclavicular position. Because of the small size of current pacemakers, they usually can be placed in the infraclavicular position without cosmetic compromise. See also *implantation*.

infranodal atrioventricular block. Atrioventricular conduction block occurring in the His bundle, bundle branches, or Purkinje network. During invasive electrophysiologic study, atrioventricular block during atrial pacing or supraventricular tachycardia occurs without a recorded His electrogram.

inhibited pacing. Pacing in which the pacemaker output pulse is suppressed when a spontaneous intrinsic cardiac event is sensed before the end of the escape interval. Inhibited pacing occurs when the rate of intrinsic events is faster than the programmed minimum rate of the pacemaker. See also *atrial-inhibited pacing mode (AAI), AV sequential dual-chamber inhibited pacing mode (DDI), AV sequential ventricular-inhibited pacing mode (DVI), ventricular-inhibited pacing mode (VVI)*.

inhibition. See *demand pacing*.

in-line bipolar lead. See *coaxial lead, in-line connector*.

in-line connector. The proximal end of a coaxial bipolar pacing lead. The in-line connector has two contact elements in series: a metal cathodal terminal pin and an anodal contact ring. The terminal pin completes the circuit between the pacemaker and the distal-tip electrode. The anodal contact ring, located a few millimeters from the cathodal pin, completes the circuit between the pacemaker and the proximal-ring electrode. The lead terminal pin and contact ring are inserted into the pacemaker neck aperture and secured in the connector block to form an electrical connection with the pacemaker circuitry. In-line connectors also are referred to as coaxial connectors. See also *bipolar lead, lead connector*.

in-line terminal pin. See *in-line connector*.

innocent bystander tracts. In the pathogenesis of reentrant arrhythmias, slow zones of conduction are responsible for the maintenance of reentrant circuits. Certain slow zones of conduction resulting from abnormal myocardium may not be directly responsible for the substrate for the clinical arrhythmia but instead represent a bystander site, anatomically related to the critical slow zone for the arrhythmia. These innocent bystander sites for one given arrhythmia may be arrhythmogenic for another not as yet clinically relevant arrhythmia. During entrainment mapping, pacing within an innocent bystander tract site may be mistaken for the critical slow zone. Typically, very long capture latencies are noted when pacing from an innocent bystander tract.

inositol triphosphate (IP$_3$). A second messenger that participates in the release of intracellular calcium from sarcoplasmic reticulum after stimulation of cell membrane receptors.

inotropic drugs. Pharmacologic agents that increase cardiac contractility and are used for severe systolic heart failure. Examples include digoxin, dobutamine, and milrinone.

inotropic therapy. Therapy for severe systolic heart failure with inotropic agents such as milrinone or dobutamine, meant to improve, usually temporarily, cardiac contractility.

input. The delivery or transfer of information to a circuit or a device. In pacing, input most often refers to the information selected by the user during programming of a pacemaker, that is, the variables to be changed and the chosen values.

insulation. A material that has a high electrical resistivity and prevents current flow. In pacing, insulation refers to the sheath that covers the lead conductor and prevents contact between the conductor and body tissue at any point other than the electrode-myocardial interface. Insulation materials used for pacing leads, such as polyurethane or silicone rubber, are biocompatible and are inert. See also *lead*.

insulation break. See *insulation failure*.

insulation failure. A crack or tear in the pacemaker lead insulation. An insulation failure may allow current leakage into the surrounding body tissue, thus reducing the impedance of the pacing system. Loss of sensing or capture may be an indication of insulation failure. See also *environmental stress cracking, metal ion oxidation*.

InSync ICD trial. See *Multicenter InSync ICD Randomized Clinical Evaluation*.

integrated circuit. A circuit in which multiple circuit elements are placed on a silicone wafer or chip and interconnected during manufacture. An integrated circuit does not necessitate the use of discrete elements, and thus the circuit size can be decreased and the reliability increased. Integrated circuits in pacemakers also have made possible an increase in the number and complexity of pacemaker functions, such as programming and telemetry, and a decrease in overall pacemaker size and power requirement. Microchips and silicone chips are integrated circuits.

integrated sensor. See *blended sensor*.

interatrial. From right to left atria or vice versa, as opposed to intra-atrial, which implies timing or some other aspect within a single chamber. Interatrial conduction occurs primarily through Bachmann's bundle and partially through the musculature of the coronary sinus and fossa ovalis.

interatrial conduction delay. Prolonged conduction from right to left atrium or vice versa.

Marked interatrial conduction delay may occur in very enlarged atria and after atrial surgery or ablation, promoting further atrial arrhythmia.

interatrial connections. Impulse propagation from the right atrium to the left atrium occurs through three principal routes: 1) Bachmann's bundle on the atrial roof, 2) the region of the fossa ovalis, and 3) the musculature of the coronary sinus.

intercalated disks. Structures that are located at cell-to-cell junctions and are partly responsible for the conduction characteristics of myocardial tissue.

intercostal muscle stimulation. Extracardiac stimulation of the intercostal muscles that may occur after device implantation. This does not cause any problems but can be very uncomfortable for the patient and may require reprogramming the device output or repositioning the responsible lead.

interfascicular reentry. Macroreentrant tachycardia involving both the anterior and the posterior fascicles of the left bundle branch. Two forms are recognized: antegrade anterior and antegrade posterior interfascicular reentry. Either the anterior or the posterior fascicle can be ablated to cure this arrhythmia.

interfascicular tachycardia. A type of reentrant tachycardia that usually, but not exclusively, occurs in dilated hearts. The reentrant circuit involves the left anterior and left posterior fascicles of the left bundle branch. Interfascicular tachycardia can be managed by ablating one of the left-sided fascicles.

interference. A block in the conduction of a normal impulse from one site of origin due to tissue refractoriness caused by activation from a different site of origin. In pacing, interference also may be caused by electromagnetic or electromyographic interference. See also *electromagnetic interference, electromyographic interference*.

interference mode. See *noise reversion mode*.

intermittent capture. Failure of a pacemaker output stimulus to consistently cause cardiac depolarization. See also *failure to capture*.

intermittent sensing. Failure of a pacemaker to consistently sense an intrinsic cardiac event. See also *failure to sense*.

internal cardioversion. Cardioversion performed with endovascular electrodes usually placed in the lateral right atrium and right ventricular outflow tract. With the advent of biphasic external cardioversion, internal cardioversion is rarely necessary for converting atrial fibrillation to sinus rhythm.

internal longitudinal resistance (r_i). The resistance to current flow within a cell. Internal longitudinal resistance is one of the passive properties that affects conduction and propagation. It is affected by many factors, including ischemia, intracellular pH, and extracellular potassium.

International Organization for Standardization (ISO). An organization founded in 1946 for the purpose of developing a common international set of manufacturing, trade, and communication standards. There are currently 91 member countries. The United States ISO representative organization is the American National Standards Institute.

international standard-1. See *IS-1*.

internodal conduction. The conduction of an impulse from the sinus node to the atrioventricular node. Complete internodal conduction from the sinus node to the atrioventricular node typically takes 30 to 70 milliseconds and is measured by the PA interval. See also *PA interval*.

interrogation. A telemetry process used to retrieve information from an implanted pacemaker or defibrillator. The information is transmitted, in a binary code, from the pulse generator to the external programming unit. Interrogation is used before and during programming to determine the programmed variables. It also may be used to initiate the transmission of stored data such as patient information, measured values, and intracardiac electrograms. See also *binary code, telemetry*.

interval. The time separating two events. In pacing, intervals are used to identify different segments of a surface electrocardiogram, intracardiac electrogram, and pacemaker timing cycle. Intervals commonly are measured in milliseconds.

interval irregularity. Spontaneous irregularity or variation in the cycle length of measured electrograms. Interval irregularity in sensed ventricular electrograms suggests either polymorphic ventricular tachycardia or rapidly conducted atrial fibrillation.

interval stability. Lack of variation in the cycle length of sensed electrograms in either the atrium or the ventricle. Interval stability suggests a reentrant tachycardia arising from the chamber where the electrograms have been sensed.

interventricular conduction delay (IVCD). Conduction delay occurring between the right and left ventricles or vice versa. Interventricular conduction delay is the result of either a cardiomyopathic process affecting the interventricular septum or significant His-Purkinje disease affecting the left ventricle more than the right ventricle.

interventricular dyssynchrony. Uncoordinated mechanical activation occurring because of delayed activation of the left ventricle during stimulation of the right ventricle or vice versa. Interventricular dyssynchrony typically occurs as a result of interventricular conduction delay and often occurs along with intraventricular dyssynchrony. See also *intraventricular dyssynchrony*.

intimal flap. During procedures in which dissection of either vascular endothelium or endocardium has occurred, the endocardium or intima is raised as a flap endocardial to the dissection plane. Intimal flaps are usually iatrogenic and occur during ablative and pacemaker procedures, particularly those involving the coronary sinus or pulmonary vein.

intra-atrial block (IAB). Disruption in the conduction of electrical impulses within the atria.

intra-atrial conduction. Electrical conduction occurring within the atria. Intra-atrial conduction is abnormal in patients with large atria, patients receiving antiarrhythmic drug therapy, particularly sodium channel blockers, and patients who have had previous atrial surgery or ablation. Intra-atrial conduction delay frequently manifests on the surface electrocardiogram with a long T-wave duration.

intra-atrial conduction interval. Interval that is a reflection of intra-atrial conduction from the time of impulse initiation to the completion of atrial activation. The intra-atrial conduction interval is sometimes measured in sinus rhythm during invasive electrophysiologic study from the onset of the P wave to the atrial electrogram on the distal coronary sinus catheter.

intra-atrial delay. Delay in conduction occurring in the atrial myocardium. Intra-atrial delay is proarrhythmic, that is, increased intra-atrial delay promotes the formation of atypical atrial flutter.

intra-atrial reentrant tachycardia (IART). When atrial electrical or myopathic processes are present, there can be prominent intra-atrial delay. Such delay promotes the formation of reentrant tachycardias (flutters); these are referred to as intra-atrial reentrant tachycardias. Intra-atrial reentrant tachycardias frequently occur in patients who have enlarged atria or have had previous surgical or ablation procedures performed in the atrium.

intra-atrial reentry. See *intra-atrial reentrant tachycardia*.

intra-atrial septal pacing. When the atrial pacing lead is placed on the intra-atrial septum, intra-atrial and interatrial conduction time are decreased. This decrease is a result of near simultaneous activation of the right atrium and left atrium. The P-wave duration typically shortens, and, hypothetically, pacing from this site may decrease both automatic and certain reentrant atrial tachycardias.

intracardiac echocardiography (ICE). 1. Linear phased-array echocardiography typically performed from the right atrium with visualization of all cardiac chambers and pulmonary veins. This form of intracardiac echocardiography can be used to obtain Doppler blood flow velocities and Doppler tissue velocities. 2. Circular array intravascular ultrasonography performed from either the right atrium or other cardiac chambers or within the pulmonary veins.

intracardiac electrogram (IEGM). See *electrogram*.

intracardiac mapping. Mapping performed endocardially. See also *mapping*.

intracardiac pacing catheters. Catheters placed endocardially to either the atrium or the ventricle for temporary pacing during electrophysiologic studies and ablation procedures.

intrafascicular reentry. Microreentrant circuits often involving the left posterior fascicle and surrounding Purkinje tissue may be responsible for ventricular tachycardia in structurally normal hearts. See also *interfascicular reentry*.

intra-His block. Atrioventricular block sometimes may occur within the His bundle itself. This is less common than compact atrioventricular nodal or infrahisian block. During invasive electrophysiologic study, intra-His block is recognized because of prominent delay between two components of the His bundle electrogram with loss of the second component when atrioventricular block occurs. Intrahisian block may occur rarely during supraventricular tachycardias or junctional tachycardia or in the retrograde direction during ventricular pacing or ventricular tachycardia.

intrahisian disease. Structural disease, or conduction delay, within the penetrating bundle of His. Intrahisian disease is fairly uncommon but may occur after certain surgical procedures or ablation procedures.

intramural scroll waves. Reentrant waves that either exclusively or predominantly involve the mid myocardial tissue.

intranodal conduction. The conduction of an impulse through the atrioventricular node. Complete intranodal conduction of an impulse across the length of the atrioventricular node typically takes 55 to 130 milliseconds and is measured by the AH interval. See also *AH interval, internodal conduction.*

intraventricular dyssynchrony. Mechanically uncoordinated ventricular contractions occurring within the same ventricular chamber. Intraventricular dyssynchrony may occur because of severe cardiomyopathy, multiple ventricular infarctions, or highly disordered intraventricular electrical conduction. See also *interventricular dyssynchrony.*

intrinsic activation. Creation of an action potential by spontaneous depolarization of cells within the specialized cardiac conduction system. A depolarization current passes across a cell membrane, alters the transmembrane potential, and results in an action potential.

intrinsic automaticity. The inherent property of individual myocardial conductive cells that allows them to depolarize spontaneously. The specialized conduction system of the heart

Intraoperative Evaluation			
Defect	Voltage threshold	Current threshold	Lead impedance
Wire fracture	High	High, normal, or low	High
Insulation break	High	High	Low
Lead dislodgement	High	High	Normal
Exit block	High	High	Normal

intraoperative evaluation. Specific measurements must be obtained at the time of device implantation to ensure that pacing and sensing thresholds are adequate. Measurements that should be taken as part of an intraoperative evaluation and expected values are shown in the table.

intrathoracic impedance. In implantable device systems, a measurement made between the right ventricular lead and the pulse generator which can be used to reflect intrathoracic fluid status or to determine minute ventilation as the basis for rate-adaptive pacing.

intraventricular asynchrony. Lack of synchrony that occurs within the ventricle. This is most commonly used to refer to left ventricular asynchrony or dyssynchrony between the septal and lateral wall, or, with more specific techniques, specific regions of the left ventricle may be noted to be asynchronous.

intraventricular conduction delay. Delays in electrical conduction within the left ventricle that result in intraventricular asynchrony. See also *intraventricular asynchrony.*

is organized in a function hierarchy such that cells with the fastest intrinsic rate impose their rhythm on cells with slower intrinsic rates. Thus, the sinus node, the cells of which have the fastest intrinsic rhythm, is the primary pacemaker of the heart, followed by the atrioventricular nodal cells, and, finally, the cells of the His-Purkinje system.

intrinsic conduction. Conduction through the normal electrical pathways.

intrinsic deflection (ID). The large, rapid peak-to-peak movement in atrial and ventricular electrograms. The intrinsic deflection correlates with local conduction, that is, the depolarization of cardiac cells adjacent to the electrode from which the signal is recorded. The respective conduction times of the atria and ventricles can be determined by the point at which the first large, rapid deflection crosses the baseline of the intracardiac recording. See also *intrinsicoid deflection.* •

intrinsic event. In cardiology, an inherent or spontaneous event within or originating from the heart; a native cardiac event.

intrinsic heart rate (IHR). The rate of spontaneous sinus node depolarization, independent
of the effects of the autonomic nervous system.
Intrinsic heart rate is determined by blocking
the parasympathetic and sympathetic nerves
with drugs such as atropine and propranolol,
respectively. The intrinsic heart rate is age-de-
pendent from approximately 15 to 70 years.
Sinus node dysfunction is indicated by intrinsic
heart rate values less than those expected for
a particular age. The regression of the intrinsic
heart rate with age is calculated by: IHR (beats
per minute) = (117.2) − (.53 × age in years).

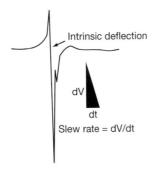

Intrinsic Deflection

Intrinsic deflection

dV

dt

Slew rate = dV/dt

*Modified from Kay GN. Basic aspects of cardiac pacing.
In: Ellenbogen KA, editor. Cardiac pacing. Boston: Blackwell Scientific Publications; 1992. p. 32-119. Used with
permission.*

intrinsicoid deflection. The surface electrocardiographic equivalent of the intrinsic deflection. Intrinsicoid deflection is the time at
which local ventricular activation has passed
under any given lead and is denoted by the
peak of the R wave in that lead. The intrinsicoid deflection may be delayed in the left precordial leads in the presence of left ventricular
hypertrophy.

intrinsic sympathomimetic activity (ISA). A
property of some β-adrenoreceptor blocking
drugs that causes mild agonist action while the
drug is occupying the β-receptor. This results in
slowing of the heart rate at rest but still allows
blunting of the heart rate response to exercise.
See also *β-adrenergic blocking drugs*.

introducer. See *lead introducer*.

investigational device exemption (IDE). The
term used by the U.S. Food and Drug Administration to indicate the status of a device that is
undergoing clinical investigation to determine
its safety and effectiveness before commercial
availability. The exemption requires safeguards
for humans who are subjects of investigators,
maintenance of sound ethical standards, and
procedures to ensure development of reliable
scientific data.

inward rectifier. The potassium current (I_{K1})
that plays a major role in maintaining the resting potential in atrial, Purkinje, and ventricular
cells.

ion channel. A pore in a cell membrane that selectively allows passage of one or more specific
ions into or out of the cell. Most ion channels
control the flow of ions and allow more ions to
pass at certain voltages.

IP₃. Abbreviation for *inositol triphosphate*.

IPG. Abbreviation for *implantable pulse generator*.

IRIS trial. See *Immediate Risk Stratification Improves Survival*.

IS-1. A designation for international standard-
1 lead connectors for low-voltage applications
such as pacing. They may be either unipolar,
designated by "IS-1 UNI," or bipolar, designated
by "IS-1 BI." The major portion of the lead connector is 3.2 mm in diameter. O-ring seals are
located on the lead connector. The IS-1 standard replaced a previously voluntary standard.
See also *VS-1*.

ISA. Abbreviation for *intrinsic sympathomimetic
activity*.

ischemia. In reference to the heart, the reduction
or cessation of blood flow into an area of the
myocardium due to narrowing or occlusion of a
coronary artery.

ischemic cardiomyopathy. Left ventricular
systolic dysfunction due to myocardial damage
from ischemic events.

ISD. Abbreviation for *implant support device*.

Ishikawa method. An echocardiographic method for optimization of the atrioventricular interval in which the optimal atrioventricular
delay is predicted by a simple method: slightly
prolonged atrioventicular delay minus the interval between the end of the atrial kick and
complete closure of the mitral valve (duration
of diastolic mitral regurgitation) at the atrioventricular delay setting (Ishikawa T, Sumita S,
Kimura K, Kikuchi M, Kosuge M, Kuji N, et al.
Prediction of optimal atrioventricular delay in
patients with implanted DDD pacemakers. Pacing Clin Electrophysiol. 1999;22:1365-71).

ISO. Trademark (Geneva, Switzerland). Abbreviation for *International Organization for Standardization*.

isochronic maps (isochronal maps). Activation maps in which either a line or a color code is given to all sites of similar timing relative to a reference electrogram or surface electrocardiogram. Isochronic mapping is a common form of mapping in electroanatomic and noncontact mapping systems.

isodiametric lead. An endocardial lead that has a constant diameter or dimension over its entire length. The diameter of the lead does not increase at the electrode and is designed to facilitate removal of an implanted lead.

isoelectrical. Electrically, neither negative nor positive. Isoelectrical signals produce no net current flow and thus, in electrocardiographic recordings, produce a straight line.

isoelectrical line. A period noted between two electrograms in which no discernible electrical activity is seen. Isoelectrical lines separate double potentials seen at sites of very slow conduction or conduction block.

isolated apical hypertrophy. Form of hypertrophic cardiomyopathy more common in the Japanese population in which the left ventricular apex is hypertrophied. Some debate persists as to whether indications for implantable cardioverter-defibrillators should be the same for this form of hypertrophic cardiomyopathy.

isometric exercise. A form of active exercise in which muscle tension is increased by applying pressure against stable resistance. In isometric exercises, there is no joint movement and the length of the muscle does not change. In pacing, isometric arm exercises, such as pressing the hands together or pulling one arm against the other, are used to assess pacemaker response to myopotentials.

isoproterenol. A short-acting, sympathomimetic, β-adrenoreceptor agonist that increases automaticity in the sinus node and subsidiary intrinsic pacemakers, increases conduction through the atrioventricular node and His-Purkinje system, augments contractility, and increases ventricular excitability. Isoproterenol is used to treat heart block and other bradycardias; however, in some patients, it may cause ventricular arrhythmias or chest pain. Isoproterenol may be useful for preventing torsades de pointes in acquired long QT syndrome. In electrophysiologic testing, isoproterenol is used to assist in the induction of tachycardias and in tilt testing. Isoproterenol causes an immediate increase in the pacing threshold, followed by a decrease in the pacing threshold.

isorhythmic atrioventricular dissociation. The independent depolarization of the atria and ventricles at identical, or nearly identical, rates. Isorhythmic atrioventricular dissociation may be caused by an interruption in atrioventricular conduction or by sinus bradycardia and a resultant atrioventricular nodal escape rhythm.

IST. Abbreviation for *inappropriate sinus tachycardia*.

isthmus. Any region of myocardium usually between two scars or anatomical boundaries such as a pulmonary vein or atrioventricular valve important in the sustenance of reentrant arrhythmia. Common isthmuses include the myocardium between the tricuspid valve and inferior vena cava and the region between an inferior myocardial infarction and the mitral valve.

isthmus-dependent atrial flutter. Common form of atrial flutter that uses the myocardium between the tricuspid valve and the inferior vena cava as its slow zone for reentrant arrhythmia sustenance. See also *atrial flutter, cavotricuspid isthmus*.

I_{TO}. Transient outward current across cell membranes that is carried by potassium and is responsible for phase 1 of the action potential in epicardial cells. Its absence from endocardial ventricular cells accounts for the different appearance of phase 1 in endocardium versus epicardium. $I_{TO,1}$ is blocked by quinidine and 4-aminopyridine.

$I_{TO,F}$. Fast form of repolarizing current. See also I_{TO}.

$I_{TO,S}$. Slow form of early repolarizing current. See also I_{TO}.

IVC. Abbreviation used primarily for *inferior vena cava* but also used for *isovolumic contraction*. See *inferior caval vein*.

IVCD. Abbreviation for *interventricular conduction delay*.

IVD. Abbreviation for *interventricular delay*.

j

J. Abbreviation for *joule*.

Jackson-Pratt drain. A drain that can be used at an operative site for collection of fluid. The drain has a one-way valve that prevents fluids from returning to the site. Such a drain may rarely be of benefit in the surgical management of an infected pulse generator pocket.

James fibers. See *atriohisian fibers*.

J box. See *junction box*.

Jervell and Lange-Nielsen syndrome. Congenital long QT syndrome associated with deafness. Jervell and Lange-Nielsen syndrome has autosomal recessive inheritance.

JET. Abbreviation for *junctional ectopic tachycardia*.

J lead. See *atrial J lead*.

joule (J). The international unit of measurement for energy or work. One joule of work occurs when one coulomb of current flows across a potential of 1 volt for 1 second. In pacing, microjoules are used to quantify the amount of energy delivered by a pacemaker output pulse to the electrode-myocardial interface. In cardioversion-defibrillation, joules are used to quantify the energy of defibrillation shocks. See also *energy, watt*.

J retention wire. Part of the atrial J-shaped lead design used in the Accufix and Encor (Telectronics, Inc., Englewood, Colorado) series of pacing leads. Over time, the retention wire could break and migrate and penetrate the lead, and a major vessel or cardiac structure could be lacerated.

J-shaped electrode. An atrial lead that has a preformed shape that resembles a J. This shape was designed to facilitate placement in the atrium and, more importantly, to minimize atrial lead dislodgement at a time when passive fixation atrial leads were more commonly used. When a stylet is placed in the lead, the lead is straight (i.e., the J shape is not appreciated). When the lead is in the atrial cavity and the stylet is withdrawn, the lead assumes the J shape.

J-shaped retention wires. See *J retention wire*.

jugular vein. Central venous route that was once used for permanent lead placement and commonly used for temporary lead placement.

J Retention Wire

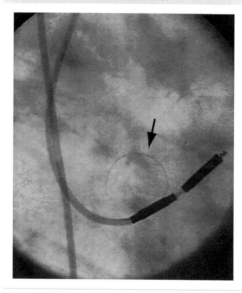

The jugular route is undesirable for permanent lead placement because the lead must be tunneled either over or under the clavicle and there is a greater chance of both erosion and conductor fracture.

junctional arrhythmia. Any arrhythmia originating in the atrioventricular junctional tissue.

junctional ectopic tachycardia (JET). Form of tachycardia resulting from abnormal automaticity affecting the compact atrioventricular node. This tachycardia may occur in fetal life or in children and also after cardiac surgery, typically valvular surgery. Junctional tachycardia also may arise from the His bundle. Junctional tachycardia may present as a narrow complex supraventricular tachycardia, as an atrial tachycardia-atrial fibrillation when the junctional focus has exit block to the ventricle, as a ventricular arrhythmia with atrioventricular dissociation when the focus has exit block to the atrium, and rarely as complete heart block when the rapidly firing junctional focus has exit block to both the atrium and the ventricle and sinus beats are not able to propagate through the refractory nodal structures to the ventricle.

junctional escape beat. An escape beat that originates from any site in the atrioventricular junctional tissue, including the compact atrioventricular node and His bundle. Junctional escape beats may become apparent in cases of sinus bradycardia or atrioventricular block. See also *escape beat, junctional escape rhythm*.

junctional escape rhythm. An arrhythmia defined by the occurrence of consecutive junctional escape beats. Junctional escape rhythms usually occur at a rate of 40 to 60 beats per minute. See also *junctional escape beat*.

junctional rhythm. 1. A rhythm that originates in the vicinity of the atrioventricular junctional tissue. On the surface electrocardiogram the P wave may be inverted in the inferior electrocardiographic leads (because it is retrogradely conducted), absent, or hidden or partially hidden in the QRS complex. 2. Automatic or reentrant rhythms that originate either in the compact atrioventricular node, His bundle, or related tissue.

junctional tachycardia. A tachycardia in or near the atrioventricular junction. Junctional tachycardia sometimes is used to describe a rapid arrhythmia that occurs primarily in infants. This arrhythmia may present as tachycardia-induced cardiomyopathy and is thought to be due to abnormal automaticity. See also *AV nodal reentrant tachycardia, nonparoxysmal junctional tachycardia, permanent form of junctional reciprocating tachycardia*.

junctional tissue. The tissue of the cardiac conducting system that surrounds the atrioventricular node, including the atrioventricular node and the His bundle. In normal hearts, this is the only electrical connection between the atria and the ventricles.

junction box. A protective enclosure into which wires or cables of an electrical system are fed and connected. In electrophysiologic testing, a junction box is used for the selection of specific electrode pairs for stimulation of the myocardium or recording of cardiac events. Switches on the face of the junction box correspond to the stimulating and recording electrodes and allow the operator to change functions during testing. The junction box also provides an isolated ground during the stimulation and recording of cardiac activity. A junction box also is referred to as a J box.

J wave. A low-amplitude, low-frequency wave at the terminal portion of the QRS on the surface electrocardiogram. J waves are frequent in hypothermia and rare in hypercalcemia. J waves also are known as Osborne waves.

k

K. The symbol for potassium. See I_K, I_{Kl}, and so on, for potassium currents.

KB-R 7943. New sodium-calcium exchange inhibitor, possibly selectively inhibiting calcium entry (reverse mode); potential activity on the sinus node and atrial myocardium promotes inotropic effects on the ventricular myocardium.

KChAB. A member of the family of molecular chaperones. This specific molecule is a chaperone for several potassium channels, including Kv1.3 and Kv4.3 (which produces the transient outward current Ito). See also *chaperone*.

KChIPs. Proteins that bind calcium (ejection fraction and containing calcium ions). Important in the regulation of Kv for potassium channels and thus the transient outward current (I_{TO}).

KChIP 2. A functional modifier of Kv4.3 potassium channel, acting as a chaperone and altering channel kinetics and resulting in the amplification of fast transient outward current (I_{TO}). KChIP 2 is a calcium-binding protein capable of binding three or four calcium ions at distinct sites.

KCNE1. Membrane protein that associates with *KCNQ1* α subunits to form channels that are responsible for the I_{Ks} currents that determine the duration of action potential in cardiac muscle. Mutations in the genes coding for these subunits cause long QT syndrome type 1 and the Jervell and Lange-Nielsen syndrome.

KCNE potassium channel subunits. Membrane glycoproteins made up of one transmembrane domain. Subunits of this family of potassium channels modulate the characteristics of voltage-dependent potassium channels. The *KCNE* subunits are divided into five subfamilies: *KCNE1, KCNE2, KCNE3, KCNE4,* and *KCNE1L.*

KCNH2. Potassium voltage-gated channel, subfamily H (ether-a-go-go–related), member 2. *KCNH2* gene belongs to the family of genes that code for potassium channels. *KCNH2* and *KCNE2* genes interact to form a functional potassium channel. Mutations in the *KCNH2* gene are one of the causes of Romano-Ward

syndrome. Other mutations have been associated with the short QT syndrome.

KCNQ1. A gene located on human chromosome 11p15.5. This gene codes for a voltage-gated potassium channel important in cardiac repolarization. It associates with *KCNE1* to form the I_{Ks} cardiac potassium current. Mutations in this gene have been associated with long QT 1 syndrome and familial atrial fibrillation.

KCNQ1/KCNE1. See *KCNQ1.*

KCNQ2. Gene coding for a voltage-gated potassium channel, KQT-like, member 2. Abnormalities in this gene affect neurogenic M channel currents and result in some forms of epilepsy.

Kearns-Sayre syndrome. A rare mitochondrial encephalomyopathy consisting of the following triad: age at onset younger than 20 years, chronic progressive external ophthalmoplegia, and pigmentary degeneration of the retina. Additional clinical features of the disease include cardiac conduction defects and cerebellar ataxia. Conduction abnormalities can occur at multiple levels of the conduction system. Atrioventricular block or infrahisian block can occur suddenly.

Kent bundle. See *Kent fiber.*

Kent fiber. A muscular bundle within the heart that provides an accessory atrioventricular connection. A Kent fiber can transmit impulses that ordinarily would travel from the atria to the ventricles via the normal conduction system. An active Kent fiber can provide the substrate for atrioventricular reentrant tachycardias and is associated with syndromes such as Wolff-Parkinson-White syndrome and concealed accessory pathways. See also *accessory pathway, atrioventricular fibers.*

Kent potentials. Electrical potentials that arise from electrically active tissue that bridges the atrium and ventricle and bypass the atrioventricular node. This tissue is associated with ventricular preexcitation and reentrant tachyarrhythmias (also called Jackman potentials). These signals are found via unipolar or bipolar mapping catheters placed in proximity to an accessory pathway and represent electrical conduction through the accessory pathway. Kent potentials may be antegrade or retrograde.

Kir channels. Inward rectifier potassium channels with a primary role of maintenance of membrane potentials. The Kir channels are subdivided into seven families (Kir1-Kir7).

Koch's triangle. See *triangle of Koch*.

Kv channels. Voltage-dependent channels important for cardiac repolarization. They are composed of four α subunits that form the pore of the channel. Nine Kv channels have been identified (Kv1-Kv9).

Kv1. Potassium channel gene, a member of the Kv family with a distinguishing data subunit. Also called Shaker family 1 potassium channel. See also *Kv channels*.

Kv1.4. Member of the Kv voltage-dependent Shaker family of potassium channels. Responsible in part for the transient outward current (I_{TO}). The *KCNA4* gene codes for the Kv1.4 potassium channel. See also *Kv channels*.

Kv1.5. Potassium channel, member of the voltage-gated Kv channel family. Also referred to as HK2 and responsible in part for the delayed-rectifier potassium current I_{Kur}. The *KCNA5* gene codes for this potassium channel.

Kv4.1. Member of the voltage-gated potassium channel (Shaker) family. Kv4.1 is responsible in part for the transient outward repolarizing current (I_{TO}) and is coded by the *KCND3* gene. See also *Kv channels*.

Kv4.2. Member of the voltage-gated potassium channel (Shaker) family. Kv4.2 is partly responsible for the transient outward (I_{TO}) current and is coded by the *KCND2* gene. See also *Kv channels*.

Kv4.3. Member of the voltage-gated potassium (Shaker) family of channels. The Kv4.3 channel is partly responsible for the transient outward current (I_{TO}) and is coded by the *KCND3* gene.

KvLQT. Voltage-dependent potassium channel of the Shaker family. Mutation responsible for long QT syndrome.

KvLQT1. Voltage-gated potassium channel, also referred to as Kv7.1. KvLQT1 is a major subunit of the I_{Ks} channel. Activation of this channel begins shortly after depolarization, in contrast to Ikr channel, which is more prominent at the end of the plateau phase of the action potential. See also *HERG, I_{Kr}, I_{Ks}*.

labeling. From a regulatory standpoint, labeling any printed material that relates to a product. It may include the technical manual, labels, and markings on the package or box.

labetalol. A nonselective, β-adrenergic blocking agent with α-adrenergic blocking activity. For side effects, see β-*adrenergic blocking drugs*.

ladder diagram. A representation of the propagation of cardiac impulses in space and time. Ladder diagrams are useful for conceptualizing the mechanism of arrhythmias. In pacing, they sometimes are used to describe pacer timing cycles graphically.

lamin A/C. One of the extracellular matrix proteins, a group that also includes fibronectin. Lamin is bound to the intracellular actin microfilaments via the dystrophin glycoprotein complex. This framework allows a communication between intracellular actin microfilaments and the extracellular matrix.

LA-PV conduction. Electrical conduction that occurs between the left atrium (LA) and the pulmonary vein (PV) via the ostium of the pulmonary vein. In sinus rhythm, a manifestation of this conduction is the pulmonary vein potential recorded when catheters are placed in the pulmonary vein. The object of pulmonary vein isolation done for paroxysmal atrial fibrillation is to modify or completely abolish LA-PV conduction.

large-tip catheter. Ablation catheters with electrodes larger than 5 mm. These include 8-mm and 10-mm catheters. The large tip allows for greater power delivery at sites of either thick myocardium or poor surrounding blood flow.

LAS. Abbreviation for *low-amplitude signal*.

laser. Acronym for light amplification by stimulated emission of radiation. The term commonly is used to describe a device in which crystal, gas, or other suitable atoms are stimulated by focused light waves. In pacing, lasers are used to weld the edges of a titanium pacer case together to create a hermetic seal. Lasers also are used in the manufacture of some porous-surfaced electrodes. See also *ablation*.

laser ablation. The removal or destruction of tissue by the use of laser. Laser ablation sometimes is used to eliminate the site of origin of an arrhythmia or to interrupt the circuit through which it travels. See also *ablation*.

laser lead extraction. Removal of a permanent pacemaker, implantable cardioverter-defibrillator, or coronary sinus lead with the aid of a laser. The laser used for lead extraction is an excimer laser system. It generally is easier and thought to be safer than mechanical methods for breaking through dense, fibrous tissue.

LASF. Abbreviation for *left anterior superior fascicle*.

lasso catheter. Circumferential multielectrode mapping catheter typically placed at the ostium of a pulmonary vein during ablation for atrial fibrillation. The pulmonary vein electrograms are recorded on the lasso catheter during ablation until entrance block is obtained.

latency. The interval between the introduction of and the response to a stimulus. In pacing, latency is the interval between a pacemaker output pulse and the subsequent depolarization (a P wave or a QRS complex). Latency may occur to such a degree that the output pulse artifact appears separate from the depolarization on an electrocardiographic recording. The difference in the time required for depolarization after a pacemaker output pulse may be due to the patient's condition, the type of leads implanted, and the position of the lead. In electrophysiology, latency is said to occur when the S_2 to A_2 interval exceeds the S_1 to A_1 interval. See also *AV interval latency*.

latency interval. The difference between the time required to depolarize a cardiac chamber after an output pulse and the time required to depolarize the cardiac chamber during an intrinsic event. The latency interval is expressed in milliseconds. See also *AV interval latency*.

late perforation. See *perforation*.

late potentials. High-frequency, low-amplitude signals detected at the terminal portion of the signal-averaged QRS. Late potentials may represent electrical activity from regions of slow conduction. See also *signal-averaged electrocardiography*.

late potentials in ventricular tachycardia. In the catheter ablation procedures for automatic arrhythmias, potentials that occur earliest in reference to the surface QRS morphology (in the case of ventricular tachycardia) are targeted for ablation. On the contrary, in patients with reentrant ventricular tachycardias, such as those associated with prior myocardial infarction, electrical potentials may be found that correspond to all stages of the cardiac cycle (i.e., early, mid, and late). Very late potentials (i.e., occurring after the surface QRS) may be considered sites that are also extremely early, occurring before the next QRS complex. These late potentials in ventricular tachycardia have to be assessed for their arrhythmogenicity and whether or not they represent sites critical to the ventricular tachycardia using entrainment maneuvers. See also *entrainment*.

lateral cardiac veins. Tributaries of the coronary sinus used for left ventricular lead implantation. The lateral wall of the left ventricle is drained by many venous structures. These include a lateral cardiac vein, a posterolateral vein, and often an anterolateral vein and their tributaries. These veins together constitute the lateral veins.

lateral left atrial isthmus. Myocardial tissue located between the mitral valve and the left inferior pulmonary vein. Particularly after isolation of the left inferior pulmonary vein, the lateral left atrial isthmus may form an important conducting structure in the genesis of left atrial flutter and may be targeted for catheter ablation.

LBB. Abbreviation for *left bundle branch*.

LBBB. Abbreviation for *left bundle branch block*.

LBBB-type conduction delay. Left bundle branch block-type conduction delay. Some patients may not have a typical left bundle branch block pattern on the surface electrocardiogram but rather have a wide QRS with a predominant S wave in lead V_1 and an R wave in leads V_5 and V_6, suggestive of left bundle branch block. These patients probably have significant conduction disease involving both the right and the left bundle branches but preferentially affecting the left bundle branch to a greater degree. See also *left bundle branch block*.

lead. An insulated wire used to conduct pacemaker output pulses from the pacemaker or implantable cardioverter-defibrillator to the heart or to transmit depolarization potentials from the myocardium to the sensing circuit of the pacemaker or implantable cardioverter-defibrillator. The proximal end of the lead connects with the pacemaker, that is, the terminal pin fits into the pacemaker neck aperture. The distal end of the lead is an electrode that interfaces with the myocardium. The body of the lead is composed of conductive wires, ribbons, or coils surrounded by insulation. Leads are classified as atrial or ventricular, endocardial (transvenous) or epicardial (myocardial), unipolar or bipolar, and active or passive fixation. See also *active fixation lead, atrial J lead, atrial lead, bipolar lead, endocardial lead, epicardial lead, passive fixation lead, permanent lead, screw-in lead, temporary lead, unipolar lead, ventricular lead*.

lead adaptor. See *adaptor*.

lead body. The conductor coil and the surrounding insulation material.

lead chatter. Electromechanical artifacts that can occur between the cathodal ring electrode and the lead tip or between a functioning lead and an abandoned lead. These artifacts, or chatter, can be sensed and result in output inhibition in the ventricle. Theoretically, chatter on the atrial lead in a dual-chamber pacemaker could result in inappropriate tracking and an increased ventricular pacing rate.

lead clippers. Instrument used to separate connector from pacemaker or defibrillator lead wire. Cleanly cuts the lead so that the inner coil is exposed.

lead conductor fracture. See *conductor fracture*.

lead configuration. 1. The form or shape of a pacing lead, for example, an atrial J lead. 2. The polarity configuration in a pacing system (unipolar or bipolar). Polarity configuration is more appropriately referred to as lead polarity configuration. See also *bipolar lead, unipolar lead*.

lead connector. 1. The proximal end of a pacing lead that is inserted into the pacemaker connector block. The lead connector creates an electrical connection with the pacemaker circuitry and seals out body fluids. 2. The hardware used for splicing a lead. Lead connector also sometimes is used incorrectly as a synonym for lead adaptor or lead extender. See also *adaptor, IS-1, lead extender, lead splice, terminal pin, VS-1*.

Lead Connectors

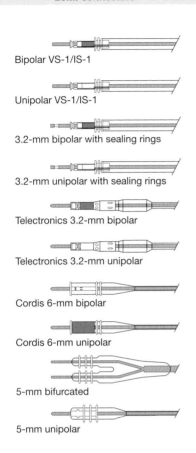

Bipolar VS-1/IS-1

Unipolar VS-1/IS-1

3.2-mm bipolar with sealing rings

3.2-mm unipolar with sealing rings

Telectronics 3.2-mm bipolar

Telectronics 3.2-mm unipolar

Cordis 6-mm bipolar

Cordis 6-mm unipolar

5-mm bifurcated

5-mm unipolar

lead dislodgement. See *dislodgement.*

lead extender. An additional length of pacing lead that can be used to extend the lead. The need for a lead extender is uncommon, but an extender may be used, for example, if a pacing lead is placed via the subclavian or cephalic vein and the pulse generator is implanted in the abdomen or flank.

lead extraction. Removal of a chronically implanted pacing lead. Several extraction techniques have been described, including manual extraction, Dotter retriever extraction, and Byrd extraction. See also *Byrd extraction technique, Cook Lead Extraction device, Dotter retriever.*

lead extraction kit. A collection of tools used for lead extraction for the superior approach through the vein entry site. It includes the extraction sheaths, a locking stylet designed to pass to the tip of the lead, and accessory tools, including stylets, gauge pins, equipment to cut

the lead and to dilate the conductor coil, and a soft grip for holding the lead.

lead fracture. See *conductor fracture.*

lead impedance. The opposition to current by the components of the pacing lead system (lead terminal pins, conductors, and electrodes). Lead impedance is a portion of the total pacing system impedance. See also *impedance.*

leading-circle reentry. A subtype of the reentrant mechanism whereby an impulse travels around a central region of functional block. The central zone around which the impulse circles is perpetuated by inward activation from the traveling wave front. There is no excitable gap in this type of arrhythmia, and the cycle length equals the refractory period of the tissue.

leading edge. The voltage upslope of a depolarization as recorded on an intracardiac electrogram or electrocardiogram.

lead integrity. The physical and functional status of a pacing lead. The presence of lead integrity indicates that the lead is intact and functioning properly.

lead introducer. A thin tube sheath through which a catheter or endocardial lead is inserted into a vein for passage into the heart. The lead introducer may be inserted percutaneously or with direct visualization and provides entry into the vessel over a previously inserted guidewire. A pacing lead is inserted into a vein through the lumen of the lead introducer, and the lead introducer is withdrawn and removed. Lead introducers are available in prepackaged procedure kits consisting of a needle, guidewire, syringe, dilator, and removable sheath. See also *peel-away sheath, split-sheath lead introducer.* •

lead maturation. See *threshold maturation.*

lead perforation. See *perforation.*

lead pin. See *lead terminal pin.*

lead pin cap. See *lead terminal cap.*

lead polarity configuration. The designation of a lead as either unipolar or bipolar. See also *bipolar lead, unipolar lead.*

lead redundancy. The capability of a multifilar lead conductor to provide continued stimulation and sensing if one of the wires breaks. In a bipolar pacing system, lead redundancy also refers to the ability to use the pacing system in a unipolar configuration if one of the conductors of the lead fractures. Lead redundancy also may refer to positioning of the intracardiac portion of the lead with excess slack. This may be desirable in a pediatric patient to allow for patient growth.

lead ring. The nonactive electrode in bipolar leads, usually located a few millimeters proximal to the tip electrode.

Lead Introducer

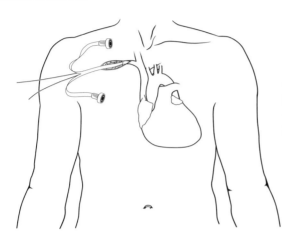

Modified from Furman S, Hayes DL, Holmes DR Jr. A practice of cardiac pacing. Mount Kisco (NY): Futura Publishing Company Inc./Blackwell; 1986. Used with permission.

Lead Introducer, Peel-Away

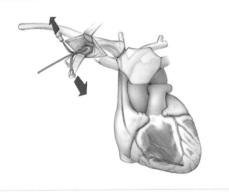

lead splice. A connecting unit used to reconnect fractured leads or to extend leads. A lead splice is a metal conductor surrounded by an insulator with an appropriate receiving port on each end for lead insertion. After a lead is inserted, two setscrews are tightened, or the connector is crimped, to anchor the lead within the splice. It is difficult, if not impossible, to splice many of the leads used currently, and the procedure should be undertaken only by someone experienced in the technique.

lead terminal cap. A plastic cap designed to fit over the lead connector. A lead terminal cap may be used on a lead that is no longer useful for the current pacing system and is abandoned rather than explanted. A lead terminal cap also may be used on a lead that has been inserted prophylactically during open heart surgery in case permanent cardiac pacing might be required in the future. Lead terminal caps also may be used to reverse the polarity of a bifurcated bipolar lead from bipolar to unipolar. See also *adaptor*.

lead terminal pin. The proximal end of a lead connector. The lead terminal pin is inserted into the connector block and the pin is secured by setscrews, or some other securing mechanism, to complete the circuit between the electrode and the pacemaker circuitry. See also *connector block, lead connector, pacemaker header*.

lead-tip configuration. The form or shape of the distal tip of a pacing lead, for example, finned, flanged, tined, or pronged. Lead-tip configuration usually is related to the method of lead fixation. See also *active fixation, passive fixation*.

lead wire. See *conductor*.

leakage current. A trivial amount of current that escapes throughout the pacing cycle and is not part of the output pulse.

LED. Abbreviation for *light-emitting diode*.

left anterior fascicle. A portion of the specialized conduction system of the ventricle. The left anterior fascicle arises from the main left bundle branch. Isolated block in the left anterior fascicle is not uncommon and creates a characteristic pattern on the surface electrocardiogram with a frontal plane axis of −60°.

left anterior fascicular block. Blockage of the

fascicle of the left bundle that innervates the superior and anterior aspects of the left ventricle. Electrocardiographically, this results in slight QRS widening with a leftward axis (i.e., directed superiorly and to the left, the resultant axis is –30° or more negative). Also called left anterior hemiblock.

left anterior fascicular ventricular tachycardia. Form of ventricular tachycardia typically occurring in normal hearts but also may occur in association with dilated cardiomyopathy. In one manifestation of this arrhythmia, a focal site of origin in the left anterior fascicle, representing either localized microreentry or an automatic focus, is responsible for the tachycardia. In another manifestation, a reentrant tachycardia involving the left anterior fascicle, portions of the ventricular myocardium and the left posterior fascicle are responsible for the tachycardia (interfascicular tachycardia).

left anterior superior fascicle (LASF). The left bundle branch generally divides into two fascicles, the left anterior fascicle and the left posterior fascicle. Sometimes there is a third fascicle, occurring either directly from the left bundle or as a branch of the left anterior fascicle and located in the vicinity of the ventricular outflow tract, and it is called the left anterior superior fascicle. This fascicle is an embryonic remnant present in some adults (Lancisi fiber).

left atrial-esophageal fistula. Important complication associated with ablation procedures for atrial fibrillation. A fistulous tract develops between the posterior wall of the left atrium or posterior wall of the proximal pulmonary veins and the anterior aspect of the esophagus. This potentially lethal complication manifests as, for example, endocarditis, air embolization, dysphagia, or hematemesis. Emergency surgical correction is required once this condition is recognized. Lower power ablation and monitoring for esophageal injury may limit the prevalence of this complication.

left atrial posterior wall. Portion of the left atrium located posteriorly between and in the region of the pulmonary veins. An important posterior relationship to the posterior left atrium is the esophagus.

left atrial reverse remodeling. A return to a more normal left atrial size. This has been reported after initiation of cardiac resynchronization therapy.

left bundle branch (LBB). A portion of the specialized ventricular conducting system. The left bundle branch arises from the His bundle as it splits at the summit of the ventricular septum. The left bundle branch activates the left ventricle and is responsible for the initial depolarization of the ventricle (depolarization of the septum from left to right). The left bundle branch divides into the left anterior fascicle and the left posterior fascicle.

left bundle branch block (LBBB). A disruption or delay in conduction through the left bundle branch. On an electrocardiographic recording, ventricular depolarization that occurs during left bundle branch block shows a notched or slurred, widened monophasic R wave in surface lead I and a QS or rS pattern in lead V_1. The QRS interval is prolonged to at least 120 milliseconds.

left cervicothoracic sympathetic ganglionectomy. Rarely performed surgical procedure for patients with long QT syndrome.

left fascicles. Branches of the left bundle branch of the infrahisian conduction system. See also *left anterior fascicle, left anterior superior fascicle, left posterior fascicle, left posterior inferior fascicle*.

left hemiblock. Conduction block occurring in one of the branches of the left bundle, either the left anterior fascicle or the left posterior fascicle.

left inferior pulmonary vein (LIPV). Left-sided pulmonary vein that drains the lower lobe of the left lung. The left inferior vein has an important anatomic relationship with the descending aorta. The left inferior and left superior veins may arise from a common ostium or be separated by a margin of tissue called the carina. See also *pulmonary vein*.

left intraventricular conduction delay. See *intraventricular conduction delay*.

left midseptal (LMS) region. Region on the mitral anulus anterior to the course of the coronary sinus and inferior to the aortic mitral continuity. The left midseptal region may be a site of accessory pathways. When these pathways conduct in a retrograde direction, the His bundle catheter and the mid coronary sinus may show nearly simultaneous atrial electrograms during orthodromic tachycardia or ventricular pacing.

left posterior fascicle. A portion of the specialized conduction system of the ventricle. The left posterior fascicle arises from the main left bundle branch and is a fanlike structure that activates the posterolateral left ventricle. Isolated block in the left posterior fascicle is rare. Left posterior fascicular block creates a characteristic pattern on the surface electrocardiogram with a frontal plane axis of +120°.

left posterior fascicular ventricular tachycardia. Type of ventricular tachycardia that usually occurs in normal hearts. Either localized microreentry or an automatic focus may be located in the left posterior fascicle (Belhassen's tachycardia). This tachycardia manifests with a wide QRS complex, right bundle branch block pattern, and a superior access. This tachycardia may be treated with calcium channel blockers or β-blockers and is particularly amenable to catheter ablation.

left posterior inferior fascicle. Posterior branch of the left bundle branch system of the infrahisian conduction system.

left superior pulmonary vein (LSPV). Pulmonary vein entraining the upper lobe of the left lung. It has a tributary that usually drains the lingula of the left lung. The left superior pulmonary vein has an important relationship with the left atrial appendage, which is located anterior to this vein. The left superior pulmonary vein and the left inferior pulmonary vein may arise from a common vein or may have a small rim of tissue separating them called the carina. See also *pulmonary vein.*

left superior vena cava. A congenital anomaly in which the left superior vena cava persists. A persistent left superior vena cava usually connects to the coronary sinus and usually can be negotiated for placement of permanent atrial or ventricular pacing leads.

left ventricular Capture Management. Trademark for an algorithm for cardiac resynchronization therapy (Medtronic, Inc., Minneapolis, Minnesota) that automatically monitors left ventricular capture thresholds and, if programmed to "Adaptive," adjusts left ventricular amplitude to ensure capture. This algorithm is based on timing a right ventricular sense (or lack thereof) after a left ventricular pace. The algorithm determines when a right ventricular sense occurs due to left ventricular-right ventricular conduction (capture) rather than due to atrioventricular conduction (loss of capture).

left ventricular ejection fraction (LVEF). The percentage of left ventricular blood volume that is ejected through the aortic valve during systole. The normal left ventricular ejection fraction varies by the method used for the measurement and by laboratory, but it is usually 55% to 60%.

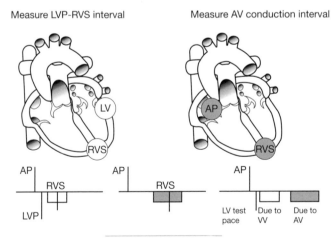

Left Ventricular Capture Management

Measure LVP-RVS interval   Measure AV conduction interval

AP, atrial paced event; LVP, left ventricular paced event; RVS, right ventricular sensed event. Modified from Medtronic, Inc [homepage on the Internet]. Minneapolis: Medtronic, Inc; c2007 [cited 2007 Jan 12]. Introducing Left Ventricular Capture Management to Ensure Cardiac Resynchronization Therapy. Available from: http://www.medtronic.com/physician/hf /concerto_lvcm.html. Used with permission.

left ventricular lead. Nonspecific term for a lead used to stimulate the left ventricle. It could be a lead placed in the coronary venous circulation, on the left ventricular epicardial surface, or, rarely, on the endocardial surface of the left ventricle.

left ventricular noncompaction. Relatively newly recognized syndrome with embryonal-type noncompact myocardium is found particularly at the left ventricular apical region. Left ventricular noncompaction may be associated with ventricular arrhythmia, preexcitation syndromes, and sudden cardiac death. The exact cause and best treatment for this condition are not known.

left ventricular outflow tract (LVOT). Left ventricular myocardium at or near the level of the aortic valve. The left ventricular outflow tract may be the source of ventricular tachycardia in otherwise normal hearts.

left ventricular outflow tract ventricular tachycardia. Form of ventricular tachycardia that may arise in structurally normal hearts. The ventricular myocardium below, at, or sometimes just above the aortic valve exhibits either triggered automaticity or abnormal automatic rhythms. The portion of the left ventricular outflow tract in the region of the mitral anulus (aortic mitral continuity) is also a site of origin of this type of tachycardia.

left ventricular protection period (LVPP). The period after a left ventricular event, either paced or sensed, when the device will not pace the left ventricle. It is designed to prevent the device from pacing into the left ventricle vulnerable period.

left ventricular stimulation thresholds. Threshold of stimulation when pacing the left ventricle. See also *pacing threshold*.

left ventricular systolic dysfunction. Abnormal myocardial contraction (systole). There are many causes, the most common being myocardial damage due to ischemic disease or idiopathic cardiomyopathic changes.

Lenègre's disease. Idiopathic fibrosis of the cardiac conduction system that diffusely affects the bundle branches. See also *Lev's disease*.

length constant. The distance over which the propagating electrical potential declines to 37% of its initial value. The length constant usually is represented by the Greek letter λ. See also *time constant*. The time constant represented

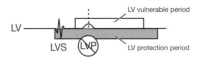

Left Ventricular Protection Period

LVP, left ventricular paced event; LVS, left ventricular sensed event. Modified from Guidant Corporation [homepage on the Internet]. Natick (MA): Boston Scientific Corporation; c2007 [updated 2004 Jun; cited 2007 Jan 12]. CONTAK RENEWAL TR: Cardiac Resynchronization Therapy Pacemaker. Available from: http://www.guidant.com/products /ProductTemplates/CRM/Contak_Renewal_TR.shtml. Used with permission.

by the Greek letter τ is the time taken for the electrical potential to decrease to 67% of its original value.

leucine isoleucine zippers. Repeating pattern or motif of four or five consecutive leucine or isoleucine residues in a primary sequence. The leucines can join to form a stable bond. This and other types of structural motifs allow for the ability of transcription factors to select a specific gene and regulate its expression.

level detector. In pacing, a component of the pacemaker sensing circuitry that receives and processes signals by amplitude and slew rate. The signal, evaluated as its leading edge passes through the level detector, is distinguished as an intrinsic depolarization even if the signal has an appropriately high amplitude and a rapid slew rate.

Lev's disease. Idiopathic degeneration of the cardiac conduction system with a predilection for the proximal portions of the bundle branches. Loss of fibers occurs and leaves "ghost" structures. See also *Lenègre's disease*.

Lewis diagram. A line drawing of an arrhythmia that is useful for explaining electrocardiographic phenomena. See also *ladder diagram*.

LGL. Abbreviation for *Lown-Ganong-Levine* (syndrome).

Li. Chemical symbol for *lithium*.

LiCuS. Chemical symbol for *lithium-cupric sulfide*.

lidocaine. A class IB antiarrhythmic agent that suppresses automaticity and afterdepolarizations in the His-Purkinje system and causes abnormal automaticity of the ventricles. Lidocaine has no appreciable effect on refractoriness in normal tissue, but it does increase refractoriness in tissue with an increased resting membrane potential. Lidocaine has efficacy in the treatment of ventricular arrhythmias, and it does not affect pacing thresholds.

ligament of Marshall. A vestigial fold of the pericardium that contains small blood vessels, fibrous bands, and nervous filaments surrounded by fat. The ligament courses obliquely above the left atrial appendage and lateral to the left superior pulmonary vein. The oblique vein of Marshall is contained within the ligament and drains into the coronary sinus.

light-emitting diode (LED). An electronic component that emits a characteristic light when energized, typically red or green but also infrared or yellow. Light-emitting diodes are used as indicator lamps and on other electronic displays, such as numerical readouts.

LiI. Chemical symbol for *lithium-iodide*.

limbus. Area surrounding the fossa ovalis on its right atrial aspect. The superior portion of the limbus is sometimes specifically referred to as the superior limbus, consisting of myocardium arranged in a circular manner around the fossa ovalis. The inferior portion of the limbus, also called the inferior limbus, is continuous with the muscle fibers that constitute the posterior portion of the eustachian ridge. See also *eustachian ridge, fossa ovalis*.

linear ablation. Type of ablation usually performed for treatment of macroreentrant tachycardias and fibrillation. Energy may be delivered in a sequential point-to-point manner or continuously while dragging the ablation catheter.

linear bipolar lead. See *coaxial lead, in-line connector*.

linear connector. See *in-line connector*.

linear left atrial ablation. Linear catheter ablation may be performed in the left atrium as part of catheter ablation for atrial fibrillation or left atrial flutter. Common sites for linear left atrial ablation include the myocardium between the mitral anulus and the left lower pulmonary vein, the roof of the left atrium between the right upper and left upper pulmonary veins, the posterior left atrium between the left-sided pulmonary veins and the right-sided pulmonary veins, and between the mitral anulus and the right lower pulmonary vein.

linear lesion. Ablative lesion produced by linear ablation performed either by "dragging" the catheter after a preset amount of time or with

serial point-to-point ablations in the myocardium connecting two otherwise electrically inert sites.

line of block. 1. During catheter ablation, particularly linear ablation, connecting two electrically inert structures (e.g., the anulus, myocardial scar). Electrical conduction after a successful line is created cannot cross the line in either direction. This is referred to as line of block. Sometimes unidirectional conduction may be possible across the line. When conduction is blocked bidirectionally, line of block is present. 2. In some patients, particularly with diseased myocardium or in certain anatomic locations where there is poor conduction (e.g., crista terminalis, eustachian ridge, site of prior myotomy), a line of block may be present even before catheter ablation.

linking. The phenomenon whereby a wave front tends to follow the pathway of previous excitation preferentially because of the residual electrophysiologic effects of the last depolarization. An example of linking is perpetuation of bundle branch block by repetitive transseptal concealed conduction of the previous beat in the retrograde direction into the contralateral bundle branch.

lipid rafts. Specialized membrane domains rich in certain lipids, cholesterol, and proteins. There are three types of lipid rafts: caveolae, glycosphingolipid-enriched membranes, and polyphosphoinositol-rich rafts.

LIPV. Abbreviation for *left inferior pulmonary vein*. Also called left lower pulmonary vein.

LITE protocol. Acronym for low-intensity treadmill exercise, a protocol that was designed to optimize rate-adaptive pacing variables in patients with minute ventilation rate-adaptive pacemakers (Lewalter T, MacCarter D, Jung W, Bauer T, Schimpf R, Manz M, et al. The "low intensity treadmill exercise" protocol for appropriate rate adaptive programming of minute ventilation controlled pacemakers. Pacing Clin Electrophysiol. 1995;18:1374-87).

lithium (Li). A chemical element that may be used as a battery anode. Lithium chemistry is energy-efficient. It has high voltage and energy density but relatively high cell impedance, which limits its use in low-current pacing applications. The reliability and longevity of lithium contribute to its use as the anode in almost all pacemaker batteries.

lithium-cupric sulfide (LiCuS). A battery chemistry in which the anode is lithium and the cathode is cupric sulfide. Lithium-cupric sulfide batteries provide 2.1 V of potential per battery cell. The internal impedance of a lithium-cupric sulfide battery changes little during its lifespan and decreases only after approximately 90% of battery life has been expended. In pacing, the decrease in impedance also causes reduction of the voltage and indicates the elective replacement time of a pacemaker. End of life, that is, the time for mandatory pacemaker replacement, is indicated by a second-level voltage reduction to 1.7 V.

lithium-iodide (LiI). A battery chemistry in which the anode is lithium and the cathode is iodide. Lithium-iodide batteries provide 2.8 V of potential per battery cell. The internal impedance increases during the life span of the cell, causing a linear decay in voltage output. A voltage output of 2.4 V indicates that 85% to 90% of battery life has been expended, and a rapid decrease in voltage occurs beyond this point. In pacing, the decrease in voltage output indicates that the pacemaker is approaching end of life, and this usually is observable as a decrease in the magnet rate.

lithium-iodine batteries. Batteries used in contemporary pacemakers. See also *lithium-iodide*.

lithium-silver-vanadium-oxide batteries. Power source for contemporary implantable cardioverter-defibrillators.

lithium-vanadium cell. See *lithium-vanadium-silver-pentoxide battery*.

lithium-vanadium-pentoxide (LiVO₅). Power source for early implantable cardioverter-defibrillators.

lithium-vanadium-silver-pentoxide battery. Battery used in contemporary implantable cardioverter-defibrillators. The lithium serves as the anode and the vanadium as the cathode.

lithotripsy. A technique that uses shock waves to break up stones in the kidney, ureter, urinary bladder, and gallbladder. This definition is germane to device therapy because the lithotripter can cause clinically significant device interference. In certain patients the device needs to be reprogrammed before the procedure.

Littleford introducer. See *lead introducer*.

LiVO₅. Chemical symbol for *lithium-vanadium-pentoxide*.

L-loop transposition. During embryonic development of the heart, the prospective apex of the ventricle bends initially to the right and then swings through an arc of about 120°. This is normal, or d-loop, rotation and results in a normally situated heart with the apex pointing to the left. In some instances an abnormal looping of the bulboventricular apparatus occurs, referred to as L-loop rotation. In this case, the tubular heart initially bends to the left and then swings through an opposite arc. This configuration results in the apex of the four-chambered heart pointing to the right and may produce simple dextrocardia or situs inversus. L-loop transposition typically occurs with the combination of situs solitus and L-loop rotation. The aorta is located anteriorly (ventral) to the pulmonary artery and arises from the right ventricle.

LMS. Abbreviation for *left midseptal*.

load. A device or circuit operated by the energy output of another device or circuit. In pacing, load usually refers to the components of the pacing system that drain battery energy. See also *external load*.

loading doses. When it is necessary to achieve a target plasma level of drug rapidly, a loading dose is used. The magnitude of the loading dose is dependent on the volume of distribution of the drug. A larger volume of distribution requires a larger loading dose. The loading dose is independent of the clearance of the drug.

local activation time. Timing of activation at the site of electrode contact on the myocardium relative to a control site, usually the QRS complex (or P wave in the case of the atrium). Local activation time measurements in comparison with neighboring local activation times constitutes the basis for activation mapping of tachycardia circuits and tachycardia origin sites.

LocaLisa. Trademark for a type of three-dimensional visualization system for electrophysiologic procedures (Medtronic, Inc., Minneapolis, Minnesota). Three pairs of electrodes are placed on the chest and measure currents and current flow in three dimensions, enabling real-time visualization of catheter movement and position.

locking stylet. A stylet designed to be placed in the lumen of a pacing or implantable cardioverter-defibrillator lead at its proximal end after the terminal pin(s) has been transsected. When introduced into the lumen, the stylet locks into a position at the distal end of the lead and creates traction forces. The mechanism is that of a hook that engages the lead coils when activated.

lockout. A pacemaker programming feature that prevents selection of pacing variables that are in conflict with the pacemaker's logic, are potentially hazardous, or are otherwise undesirable singly or in combination. During lockout, programming of the pacemaker is prohibited until the proper combination of pacing variables is established.

logic circuit. A circuit used in electronic equipment to perform operations for the appraisal of input signals. In pacing, logic circuits are used for functions such as noise sampling, controlled delivery of pacemaker output pulses, multipro-

longevity estimate. Feature in some pacemakers that estimates the time to elective replacement of the pulse generator. See also *elective replacement indicator.*

long PR interval. See *first-degree AV block.*

long QT syndrome. A group of disorders of repolarization associated with ventricular arrhythmias, especially polymorphic ventricular tachycardia (torsades de pointes). Long QT syndrome may be congenital or acquired. There are many acquired causes, including antiarrhythmic agents that affect repolarization, some phenothiazines, and hypokalemia. The mechanism underlying the arrhythmias associated with the long QT syndrome is thought to be either afterdepolarization or dispersion of repolarization.

Long QT Syndrome

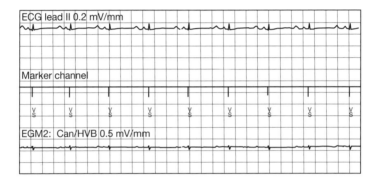

grammability, and telemetry. The logic circuit consists of digital hardware and is hardwired rather than programmed.

lone atrial fibrillation. Atrial fibrillation without evidence of underlying heart disease after careful evaluation. There is wide variation in the literature, suggesting that lone atrial fibrillation may represent 10% to 50% of cases of atrial fibrillation.

longevity. The amount of time a pacemaker will function properly, with its full capabilities, under normal operating conditions. Theoretically, pacemaker longevity is determined from battery capacity and average circuit current drain. The nominal values typically selected for the calculation of pacemaker longevity are based on 100% pacing at 70 pulses per minute with a nominal output and pulse duration and a resistance of 500 ohms.

long RP tachycardia. Classification of supraventricular tachycardia in which a visualized P wave occurs closer to the subsequent QRS complex rather than the preceding QRS complex. The interval from the R wave to the P wave is longer than that from the P wave to the subsequent R wave. Causes of long RP tachycardia include atrioventricular tachycardia with decrementally conducting retrograde pathways, atrioventricular node reentrant tachycardia, atrial tachycardia, and sinus tachycardia.

loop recorder. A monitoring and recording device used to capture paroxysmal arrhythmias or to correlate the electrocardiogram with nonspecific spells. The device is continuously monitoring but a segment is saved for review only if the patient triggers the device to do so. The device usually can be programmed to save a specific length of the recording. There are also implantable loop recorders that may automatically store events based on preprogrammed criteria.

loss of capture. In pacing, failure of the myocardium to depolarize in response to a pacemaker output stimulus of a given voltage amplitude and pulse duration that previously had resulted in depolarization. Causes include insufficient stimulus strength, separation of the electrode from the myocardium, and placement of the stimulating electrode in contact with a nonresponsive portion of the myocardium such as scar tissue. See also *capture*.

loss of sensing. In pacing, failure of the pacemaker sensing circuit to detect intrinsic cardiac signal. Causes include poor contact between the sensing electrode and the myocardium, loss of lead integrity, and decreased battery output.

low-amplitude signal (LAS). High-frequency activity detected at the terminal end of the QRS complex by signal-averaged electrocardiography. Low-amplitude signals generally are thought to be abnormal if they last longer than 38 milliseconds. Low-amplitude signals may represent slow conduction in patients prone to ventricular arrhythmias. See also *signal-averaged electrocardiography*.

low atrial septal pacing. Pacing when placing the atrial catheter in the vicinity of the coronary sinus ostium rather than in the usual high right atrial or right atrial appendage location. Low right atrial pacing sometimes is used to minimize the occurrences of atrial fibrillation. The P-wave morphology with low atrial septal pacing is with a negative P wave in leads 2, 3 and aVF with a somewhat shortened P-wave duration. Low atrial septal pacing may be combined with atrial appendage pacing and is then referred to as dual-site atrial pacing.

lower rate. The preset or programmed rate at which a pacemaker emits an output pulse in the absence of intrinsic cardiac activity. See also *minimum rate*.

lower rate interval (LRI). See *ventricular escape interval*.

lower rate limit (LRL). See *minimum rate, ventricular escape interval*.

lower rate programming. Setting the floor of the pacing rate. Typically programmed at 40 to 60 beats per minute for pacemakers implanted in adults. Some clinical situations benefit by programming to a very low lower rate in an effort to avoid pacing, and some clinical situations benefit from programming to a significantly higher rate.

Lown-Ganong-Levine (LGL) syndrome. The term used to describe the association of supraventricular tachycardias, short PR intervals, and an absence of delta waves on the surface electrocardiogram. This syndrome is thought to be caused by atriohisian fibers. However, the existence of a specific Lown-Ganong-Levine syndrome has been questioned.

low-pass filter. An electronic filter that allows the passage of frequencies below a given cutoff. A low-pass filter acts mathematically as a differentiator, that is, it emphasizes low slew rates in the input signal.

low-threshold lead. A lead that incorporates some design feature intended to lower chronic pacing thresholds. Although many leads can be classified as low-threshold leads, steroid-eluting leads are the classic example.

LQT1. Long QT 1 syndrome. Important cause of resulting substrate for sudden cardiac death caused by an abnormality in the IkKs channel. Abnormal gene is *KCNQ1*, and the mutated protein is KvLQT1.

LQT2. Long QT 2 syndrome. Caused by an abnormality in the I_{Kr} channel. Abnormal gene is *KCNH2*, and the mutated protein is HERG.

LQT3. Long QT 3 syndrome. Type of long QT syndrome caused by an abnormality in the sodium channel (I_{Na}). Abnormal gene is *SCN5A*, and the mutated protein is hH1 (Nav 1.5). A similar mutated protein and gene are responsible for Brugada's syndrome and Lenègre's syndrome.

LQT4. Long QT 4 syndrome. Type of long QT syndrome. The abnormal structure is ankyrin. The abnormal gene is *ANK2*, and the mutated protein is ankyrin.

LQT5. Long QT 5 syndrome. Caused also by an abnormality in I_{Ks} channel, like long QT 1 syndrome. The mutated protein is minK.

LQTS. Long QT syndrome. An important set of disorders that may result in sudden cardiac death. Mutations in the cardiac channels, mostly related to potassium currents but also may be related to sodium currents, are responsible for this syndrome. Examples include a loss of function mutation in HERG (responsible for I_{Kr}) causes long QT 2 syndrome, a loss of function mutation in the regulatory protein (MiRP1) causes long QT 6 syndrome (LQT6), and a loss of function mutation in KvLQT1 (responsible for I_{Ks}) causes long QT 1 syndrome (LQT1).

LRI. Abbreviation for *lower rate interval*.

LRL. Abbreviation for *lower rate limit*.

LSPV. Abbreviation for *left superior pulmonary vein*.

L-type calcium channels. Type of membrane ion channel for calcium, labeled L type for long-lasting. L-type calcium channels are found in many excitable tissues, including neural, myocardial, and nodal tissue. L-type calcium channels are made up of five subunits. The α_1 subunit is the site of action for calcium channel blockers.

lubricity. The property of a material that reduces friction and thereby facilitates the motion of materials in contact with one another. In pacing, the lubricity of materials used as lead insulators facilitates simultaneous insertion of two leads through the same venous pathway to the heart. As an example, lead insulators made of polyurethane are lubricious and allow simultaneous insertion of leads. See also *polyurethane*.

lumenless lead. A lead delivered via a sheath, in contrast to the standard pacing lead that is positioned with a stylet placed in the lumen of the lead. The lumenless design allows for smaller French size and theoretically allows more specific selection of pacing site.

Luo-Rudy dynamic model. Mathematically based model for cellular electrophysiology developed by Luo-Rudy, later revised to incorporate more plasma membrane and sarcoplasmic membrane currents.

LVEF. Abbreviation for *left ventricular ejection fraction*.

LVOT. Abbreviation for *left ventricular outflow tract*.

LVPP. Abbreviation for *left ventricular protection period*.

Lyme disease. A spirochetal infection, usually tick-borne, caused by the organism *Borrelia burgdorferi*. The acute systemic infection may manifest characteristic skin eruptions, myalgias, arthritis, fever, and carditis. A manifestation of the carditis may be conduction system abnormalities, which occasionally require temporary pacing. With treatment of the underlying infection, the carditis resolves and permanent pacing is neither needed nor indicated.

ьe cured by ablation of a critical portion of the circuit. See also *microreentrant circuit, reentry.*

macroreentrant tachycardia. See *macroreentrant circuit.*

macroreentry. An important mechanism for arrythmogenesis involving a zone of slow conduction and two limbs within the atrium or ventricle. Macroreentry is characterized by the ability to entrain the arrhythmia by pacing from the chamber in which the arrhythmia is noted.

MADIT. See *Multicenter Automatic Defibrillator Implantation Trial.*

MADIT-II. See *Multicenter Automatic Defibrillator Implantation Trial II.*

MADIT-CRT. See *Multicenter Automatic Defibrillator Implantation With Cardiac Resynchronization Trial.*

magnesium. A divalent cation with electrophysiologic effects. Hypomagnesemia may cause torsades de pointes. Administered intravenously, magnesium can be effective for treating the polymorphic ventricular tachycardia

s in acquired long QT syndrome, even ┐ting of a normal serum magnesium эerimentally, magnesium has been suppress drug-induced early afterde- ns and their resultant arrhythmias.

ıavior. In relation to implantable ⸱ices, the response of a permanent ⸱ to magnet application is general- ⸱nous pacing, and the behavior of ⸱ıble cardioverter-defibrillator varies ⸱ufacturers and possibly among mod- ⸱ıtions of a specific manufacturer. •

ectroanatomic map (MEAM). ıapping arrhythmias that combines ⸱mic mapping techniques and mag- ⸱tion. A three-dimensional electro- ⸱ıp is created of the arrhythmia in or chambers of interest. The point- ⸱ping is done with the aid of mag- ⸱ion.

rference. In pacing, the disrup- al pacemaker function by a mag- ∩ҽtıc or electrostatic field. Such a field can result in intermittent interference with the activity of the pacemaker reed switch. See also *electromagnetic interference.*

magnetic navigation. Method of manipulating catheters for mapping arrhythmias with the use of large magnets. By remote manipulation of the magnetic field, point-to-point mapping with a mapping catheter can be performed. Magnetic navigation has the potential advantage of allowing mapping of complex anatomic structures such as the pectinate muscles or pulmonary veins with a possibly lower risk of cardiac perforation.

magnetic resonance imaging (MRI). A noninvasive diagnostic test in which a fluctuating magnetic field is used to produce thin, high-resolution tomographic slices through various body structures. The magnetic field created by magnetic resonance imaging causes asynchronous function in any pacemaker in which the magnet function is "on." Some animals with certain types of pacemakers, when exposed to

Magnet Application: Implantable Cardioverter-Defibrillator Response	
Manufacturer	**Response**
Medtronic, Inc.*	Pacing mode, pacing rate, and interval as programmed. Ventricular fibrillation and ventricular tachycardia detection is suspended. "Patient alert" audible tones will occur if applicable and enabled
Boston Scientific[†]	If "enable magnet use" is "on" (nominal), device will emit beeping synchronous tones on the R wave. If after 30 seconds the beep does not change to a continuous tone, the magnet must be taped over the device to temporarily inhibit therapy. If beeping changes to a continuous tone after 30 seconds, tachy mode has gone to "off" and magnet can be removed. To turn device back to "monitor and therapy," magnet should be placed back over device for 30 seconds until R-wave synchronous tones are heard If "enable magnet use" is programmed to "off" (nominally "on"), then a magnet will *not* inhibit therapy. No tones will be emitted, and a programmer is needed to turn device off
St. Jude Medical[†]	Two programmable options for magnet response: "normal" (nominal) or "ignore." In "normal" response, when magnet is placed over the device, it blinds detection and delivery of therapy. In current devices, no tone is emitted from the device, but future devices will have a "vibrate" mode. Bradycardia pacing is not affected by a magnet placed over the device and must be reprogrammed if asynchronous pacing is needed If "ignore" is programmed, the blinding is null and void
ELA Medical, Inc.[‡]	When magnet is applied, it disables tachy therapy and arrhythmia detection. Brady function is to pace in VVI or DDD mode, depending on the programmed mode at the magnet rate (corresponding to battery voltage), pacing outputs are set to maximum, rate hysteresis and atrioventricular extension are set to zero, and atrioventricular delay is set to the programmed atrioventricular delay at rest
Biotronik[§]	When a magnet is positioned over device, tachyarrhythmia therapy and detection are suspended. Pacing function remains as programmed

* Minneapolis, Minnesota.
† Natick, Massachusetts.
‡ Arvada, Colorado.
§ Berlin, Germany.

magnetic resonance imaging, have unpredictable rapid pacing. It is also possible to obtain angiographic images with magnetic resonance imaging.

magnet-initiated tests. Tests initiated by the placement of a magnet over an implanted pacemaker. Magnet-initiated tests are used to assess certain pacemaker functions, such as elective replacement time, safety margins, and autothresholds. See also *autothreshold test, elective replacement inidicator, end of life, safety margin test.*

magnet mode. A pacing mode activated automatically in most pacemakers by placement of a magnet over the pacemaker. The magnet mode usually is fixed-rate pacing that continues as long as the magnet is held over the pacemaker. The magnet mode often is used to assess battery status. A change in the pacing rate or pulse duration indicates that the battery has reached the elective replacement time or end of life. The magnet mode response differs among devices and manufacturers. See also *magnet rate.*

magnetocardiography. Measurement of magnetic fields emitted by electrically active myocardial cells. It has been promoted as providing information that may be complementary to that of electrocardiography. This technique has been advocated for predicting arrhythmic events, mortality, and conduction system disease.

magnet rate. The rate at which a pacemaker emits an output pulse when a magnet is placed over the pacemaker. The magnet rate varies among different pacemakers, but often it is used as an indication of battery status, that is, elective replacement time or end of life. See also *elective replacement indicator, end of life.*

magnet reversion. Response of some pacemakers at the time elective replacement indicators occur.

Mahaim bypass tract. See *Mahaim fiber.*

Mahaim fiber. A specific type of accessory pathway that has the following properties: 1) decremental antegrade conduction, 2) absence of retrograde conduction (ventricle to atrium), and 3) the ventricular insertion of the pathway is either into ventricular tissue (often distant from the anulus) or into the bundle branch system (often to the distal right bundle branch). Mahaim fibers are responsible for antidromic tachycardia in some patients. Orthodromic tachycardia does not occur with Mahaim fibers. Mahaim fibers are almost exclusively located on the right side. The electrocardiogram in patients with Mahaim fibers typically shows minimal preexcitation, consistent with a right-sided accessory pathway that is decremental and slowly conducting. Other unusual pathways include nodoventricular, nodofascicular, or fasciculoventricular pathways. Nodoventricular pathways connect the atrioventricular node to the ventricles, nodofascicular pathways connect the atrioventricular node to the His-bundle branch system, and fasciculoventricular pathways connect the His-bundle branch system to the ventricles. Electrophysiologically, the term also includes atriofascicular accessory pathways with atrioventricular nodal-like properties. Atriofascicular, nodoventricular, and nodofascicular accessory pathways all may participate in reentrant tachycardias. Fasciculoventricular fibers are not known to cause tachycardias and merely cause a small delta wave on the surface electrocardiogram that remains unchanged with atrial premature ventricular complexes or changes in rate. See also *accessory pathway, atriofascicular fibers, fasciculoventricular fiber, nodofascicular fiber, nodoventricular fiber.*

Mahaim physiology. Accessory bypass tracts that have decremental conduction in the antegrade direction and have no retrograde conduction are said to exhibit Mahaim physiology.

Mahaim potential. An accessory pathway potential seen during antegrade conduction via a Mahaim fiber. Compared with pathway potentials with other accessory bypass tracts, Mahaim potentials are particularly important because they usually are easy to see given the long conduction time from atrium to ventricle and represent the primary target for successful ablation.

main timing event. In an implantable cardioverter-defibrillator, a signal that indicates the presence of tachycardia or the occurrence of an event such as intrinsic sensing, a pacemaker output pulse, shock delivery, the beginning of charging, or an internal charge dump. The main timing event may be telemetered to a programmer in real time or stored within the implantable cardioverter-defibrillator as part of the episode log.

make-and-break potentials. Electrical potentials that are generated by an intermittent fracture of the conductor coil of a pacing or implantable cardioverter-defibrillator lead as contact is "made" and "broken" by the fractured ends of the wires. These potentials manifest as artifacts on the electrogram.

malignant vasovagal syncope. Vasovagal syncope in which the patient has little or no prodrome before the syncopal event. The term also may be used to describe syncope that has no recognized precipitating stimulus.

malignant ventricular arrhythmias. Potentially life-threatening ventricular arrhythmias such as ventricular fibrillation or rapid ventricular tachycardias may be referred to as malignant.

Managed Ventricular Pacing (MVP). See *ventricular pacing avoidance algorithm.*

MAP. Abbreviation for *monophasic action potential.*

mapping. A generic term for methods to elucidate the mechanism, site of origin, and target for ablation of cardiac arrhythmias. Mapping may entail point-to-point mapping in which a catheter is moved sequentially from one location to another, multielectrode mapping, electroanatomic mapping, or noncontact mapping.

mapping catheter. Catheter used in the mapping process to define the mechanism or site of origin of a cardiac arrhythmia. See also *mapping*.

mapping of organized atrial arrhythmias. Specifically refers to methods of mapping atrial arrhythmias that may have initially presented as atrial fibrillation. During the electrophysiologic study, the arrhythmias may organize to either macroreentrant flutter circuits or point source tachycardia. Mapping of these organized arrhythmias is sometimes performed to target these circuits or sources of focal tachycardia for ablation.

MAR. Abbreviation for *mean atrial rate*.

Marey's reflex. An automatically mediated reflex in which baroreceptor fibers located in the arch of the aorta and at the bifurcation of the carotid arteries can sense increased pressure in these vessels and signal the cardiovascular regulatory center to slow the heart rate. See also *Bainbridge reflex, parasympathetic nervous system*.

marker channel. A term often used in a generic sense to indicate an event marker. See also *event marker*.

marker pulse. A spike on an electrocardiographic recording that precisely indicates the sensing and pacing activity of a pacemaker. The amount of energy delivered by marker pulses differs from that of normal triggered output pulses. Marker pulses provide enough energy to cause a deflection of the marker channel but not enough to depolarize the heart.

Marshall's vein. Remnant of the left superior vena cava that courses between the left-sided pulmonary veins and the left atrial appendage. Marshall's vein is rich in autonomic innervations and may be the source of atrial fibrillation in some patients.

MAS. Abbreviation for *measured average sensor*.

maturation. See *threshold maturation*.

maximum available battery capacity. The reduced amount of useful anodal or cathodal material in a battery as a result of internal chemical reactions. The maximum available battery capacity always is less than the theoretical battery capacity. See also *battery capacity, theoretical battery capacity*.

maximum diastolic potential. Largest-amplitude diastolic potential sometimes targeted for catheter ablation of macroreentrant ventricular tachycardia.

maximum pacing interval. The greatest amount of time that a pacemaker will wait before emitting a pacemaker output pulse in the absence of a sensed event. The maximum pacing interval usually is expressed in milliseconds. See also *escape interval, lower rate, minimum rate interval*.

maximum rate interval (MRI). The shortest amount of time between two consecutive output pulses from the same channel of the pacemaker circuitry. The maximum rate interval determines the maximum rate at which output pulses can be delivered.

maximum sensor-driven rate. See *maximum sensor rate*.

maximum sensor rate (MSR). The fastest sensor-driven pacing rate that can be achieved in a rate-adaptive pacing system. In a single-chamber demand pacemaker with rate-adaptive capability (SSIR), the maximum sensor rate is the same as the programmed upper rate limit. In a dual-chamber rate-adaptive pacemaker (DDDR), the maximum sensor rate is not necessarily equal to the maximum tracking rate.

maximum tracking interval (MTI). Maximum tracking rate expressed in milliseconds.

maximum tracking rate (MTR). The fastest atrial rate at which consecutively paced ventricular complexes maintain 1:1 synchrony with sensed atrial events. The maximum tracking rate is a function of dual-chamber pacing modes and can be defined as a preset or programmable value. The maximum tracking rate is limited to the total atrial refractory period (TARP). For example, if the TARP = 500 milliseconds, the maximum tracking rate is limited to 120 beats per minute (60,000 ÷ 500 ms). The maximum tracking rate also is known as the upper rate limit. See also *total atrial refractory period, upper rate response*.

maximum tracking rate interval (MTRI). The maximum tracking rate expressed in milliseconds. For example, a maximum tracking rate of 120 beats per minute is equal to a maximum tracking rate interval of 500 milliseconds.

max track. See *maximum tracking rate*.

maze procedure. A surgical procedure used to treat patients with atrial fibrillation. The atria are cut in multiple regions and sewn back together to create many dead-end pathways. The right atrial appendage (RAA) and left atrial appendage (LAA) are excised, and the pulmonary veins (PV) are isolated. Thus, no region of the

Maze Procedure

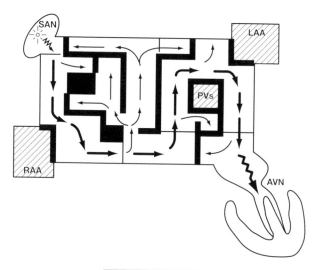

AVN, atrioventricular node; SAN, sinus node. From Cox JL, Schuessler RB, D'Agostino HJ Jr, Stone CM, Chang B-C, Cain ME, et al. The surgical treatment of atrial fibrillation. III. Development of a definitive surgical procedure. J Thorac Cardiovasc Surg. 1991;101:569-83. Used with permission.

atrium by itself is sufficient to support the re-entrant circuits of atrial fibrillation; however, the sinus impulse can still activate all portions of both atria to provide atrial contraction.

maze III procedure. Surgical procedure for the treatment of atrial fibrillation. The maze III procedure is a modification of the original maze procedure and involves either surgical incisions or ablative lesions placed as a box around the pulmonary veins and linear ablation connecting this box to the mitral anulus. May be combined with a right-sided maze procedure, atrial flutter ablation, or cryoablation in the coronary sinus.

M cells. Midmyocardial ventricular cells. These myocardial cells have a distinct action potential that differs from that of endocardial and epicardial cells. The differences in these action potential forms and durations are responsible for the ST-segment characteristics.

McNemar's test. Statistical test for checking whether two sets of variables occur in a similar proportion.

MCV. Abbreviation for *middle cardiac vein.*

MEA. Abbreviation for *multielectrode array.*

MEAM. Abbreviation for *magnetic electroanatomic map.*

mean atrial rate (MAR). Atrial rate index, continuously calculated by the pulse generator, to determine when it should respond to faster or slower atrial rates, specifically with mode switching or rate-adaptive atrioventricular operations.

measured average sensor (MAS). A term specific to devices by St. Jude Medical (St. Paul, Minnesota) to indicate a nonprogrammable value that the pulse generator determines based on the average sensor level during the preceding 18 hours. The measured value can be used to select the threshold value. If the sensor is programmed to function automatically, the measurement can be used to report the functioning value of the sensor.

measured data. Telemetered data obtained from the pulse generator, generally including details of the lead and battery status and intrinsic and sensor-driven heart rates.

mechanical dyssynchrony. Dyssynchronous myocardial contraction, usually referring to ventricular myocardium. Mechanical dyssynchrony may make symptoms of congestive heart failure worse for a given overall ventricular function. Mechanical dyssynchrony may result from electrical dyssynchrony (bundle branch block), electromechanical dyssynchrony, ischemia, or prior myocardial infarction. Dyssynchrony may be interventricular, in which one ventricle contracts earlier than another, or intraventricular, in which specific regions of the myocardium, usually the free wall and septum of the left ventricle, do not contract at the same time in a given ventricular chamber.

mechanically induced electrical artifact. Artifacts in pacemakers, defibrillators, or other electrical recording systems caused by motion, make-or-break fractures in leads, or mechanical interaction between two cavitary structures, such as redundant pacemaker leads.

mechanical sensing. The determination of mechanical changes within the body by the use of sensors that measure movement resulting from respiration or body motion. In pacing, mechanical sensing may be used to adjust pacing rate. See also *activity sensor, motion sensing*.

mechanical synchrony. Near simultaneous, synchronous activation of the ventricular myocardium. Typically, the free wall and septum of a given ventricular chamber contract nearly simultaneously and the right and left ventricles contract nearly simultaneously in the presence of a normal conduction system.

mechanoelectrical feedback. Feedback system used in certain programmable devices in which mechanical changes such as contraction or translational movement are transduced to electrical signals.

mechanoelectrical transducers. Transducers that can translate motion or contraction into electrical signals that then may be displayed.

mechanoelectrical transduction. See *mechanoelectrical feedback*.

medical advisory. See *recall*.

medical device notification. See *safety alert*.

Medicare guidelines for pacemaker implantation. In the United States, guidelines determined by Medicare to justify implantation of a permanent pacemaker. If the indication for pacing does not meet Medicare guidelines, reimbursement may be denied. At one time, permission for pacemaker implantation had to be obtained before the procedure. For the most part, this requirement has been abandoned, but the indication still must be well documented and must meet Medicare criteria.

Medtronic. Corporation that manufactures and markets pacemakers, implantable cardioverter-defibrillators, biventricular devices, and other implantable devices and catheters.

membrane depolarization. Process by which the natural negative polarity of myocardial cells is lost due to an electrical activation wave front reaching the cell. Membrane depolarization is mostly the result of the rapid influx of extracellular sodium into the cell.

membrane potential. The voltage difference across a cell membrane at rest. Cardiac cells are negative intracellularly relative to the extracellular fluid. Membrane potential is expressed in millivolts.

membrane pumps. Structures in the myocardial cell membrane responsible for the maintenance of normal cellular polarity. Membrane pumps may be exchange pumps in which one ion is exchanged for another.

memory affect and ventricular pacing. During ventricular pacing, abnormal depolarization occurs, manifested by a wide QRS complex. This abnormal depolarization, in turn, causes repolarization abnormality, usually with ST- and T-wave changes occurring opposite an axis to the QRS axis. This abnormal repolarization may persist even on cessation of pacing and with normalization of the QRS. This is referred to as cardiac memory associated with ventricular pacing. Clinically, the relevance of this finding is that P-wave inversions or ST changes may occur after cessation of pacing, mimicking the effects of ischemia.

memory chip. An integrated component of microcomputer circuits in which information is stored. In pacing circuitry, memory chips store the operational requirements of the pacemaker. Memory chips also are used in programmers, which can be updated with new memory chips to include new functions. See also *erasable programmable read-only memory, random-access memory, read-only memory*.

memory loop. 1. In pacing, a metal coil used in some leads to retain lead shape and maintain flexibility. For example, memory loops often are used in atrial J leads. 2. A type of event-recording device.

memory value. In electrophysiologic testing, a representation of the timing of the last pacing train that successfully reverted a tachycardia. The memory value is used as a starting point for scanning in subsequent delivery of pacing trains.

mercury-zinc. See *zinc-mercuric oxide*.

MERFS. See *Multicentre European Radiofrequency Survey*.

MERIT-HF. See *Metoprolol CR/XL Randomized Intervention Trial in Heart Failure*.

METAFER. See *Use of Metoprolol CR/XL to Maintain Sinus Rhythm After Conversion From Persistent Atrial Fibrillation*.

meta-iodobenzylguanidine (MIBG). A guanethidine analogue that is actively taken up into sympathetic nerve terminals by the uptake-1 mechanism. When labeled with iodine 123, meta-iodobenzylguanidine can provide a scintigraphic image of cardiac sympathetic innervation.

metal-induced oxidation (MIO). Synonym for metal ion oxidation. See also *metal ion oxidation*.

metal ion oxidation (MIO). A process thought to be responsible for deterioration of some polyurethane pacing leads in which certain corrosion products of metal parts within the lead act as catalysts for auto-oxidation of the polyurethane.

metal-oxide semiconductor field-effect transistor (MOSFET). A type of transistor used in high-voltage switching, as in implantable cardioverter-defibrillators.

metoprolol. A β_1-selective, β-adrenergic blocking agent without intrinsic sympathomimetic activity. Because it is β_1-selective, metoprolol may cause less bronchospasm than some other β-adrenergic blocking agents. For side effects, see *β-adrenergic blocking drugs*.

Metoprolol CR/XL Randomized Intervention Trial in Heart Failure (MERIT-HF). This was a prospective study to determine whether metoprolol controlled release/extended release (CR/XL) once daily, in addition to standard therapy, would lower mortality in patients with impaired systolic function and clinical heart failure. Patients were randomized to various doses. Metoprolol CR/XL once daily in addition to optimum standard therapy improved survival and the drug was well tolerated. Outcome data from this trial, specifically modes of death in heart failure by New York Heart Association functional class, are frequently quoted (Effect of metoprolol CR/XL in chronic heart failure: Metoprolol CR/XL Randomised Intervention Trial in Congestive Heart Failure [MERIT-HF]. Lancet. 1999;353:2001-7).

metoprolol succinate. Commonly used β-blocker for the treatment of hypertension and heart failure. This drug also is used in the treatment of atrioventricular nodal dependent arrhythmias, such as atrioventricular node

reentrant tachycardia or atrioventricular reentrant tachycardia.

mexiletine. A class IB antiarrhythmic agent that has little effect on refractoriness or conduction in normal atrial or ventricular tissue. Mexiletine is a lidocaine congener and has efficacy in the treatment of ventricular arrhythmias. It is metabolized by the liver. Its plasma half-life has been reported to be 10 hours in normal individuals and 17 hours in patients who have had myocardial infarction. Side effects of mexiletine include gastrointestinal and central nervous system effects, and these effects appear to be dose-related.

MIBG. Abbreviation for *meta-iodobenzylguanidine*.

μA. Abbreviation for *microampere*.

microampere (μA). One millionth of an ampere. Microamperes are the units of measurement for very small amounts of electrical current flow. In pacing, microamperes frequently are used to measure direct current drain in the pacemaker circuitry. Typically, pacemakers continuously draw 10 to 30 microamperes of current from the battery. See also *ampere, current*.

microchip. See *integrated circuit*.

μC. Abbreviation for *microcoulomb*.

microcoulomb (μC). One millionth of a coulomb. Microcoulombs are the units of measurement for very small amounts of charge. See also *charge, coulomb*.

microdislodgement. In pacing, the displacement of a permanent pacemaker lead that is not apparent radiographically. Microdislodgement is a diagnosis made by exclusion, that is, other explanations of the clinical problem must be found. For example, to diagnose microdislodgement, inadequate intrinsic cardiac signals or loss of lead integrity must be excluded.

microinstability. Fluctuations in sensing and pacing thresholds when the lead position appears grossly normal or unchanged radiographically (i.e., microdislodgement).

μJ. Abbreviation for *microjoule*.

microjoule (μJ). One millionth of a joule. Microjoules are used to measure very small amounts of electrical energy. In pacing, microjoules describe the work performed by a pacemaker with each output pulse and may be defined as the product of the pulse duration in milliseconds, the voltage in volts, and the current in milliamperes. Typically, the output of an implanted pacemaker ranges from 1 to 50 microjoules. See also *energy, joule.*

microprocessor. An integrated circuit that is one of the principal components of a microcomputer. It allows processing according to various programs stored in memory. The elements of a microprocessor are contained in a single silicone chip. The use of microprocessors in pacemaker and implantable cardioverter-defibrillator circuitry has made possible an increase in the number and complexity of device functions such as programmability, telemetry, data storage, and decreased size of pulse generators.

microreentrant circuit. A reentrant pathway of tachycardia in which impulse conduction occurs through relatively small areas of the myocardium or specialized conduction tissue. Many ventricular tachycardias probably are due to microreentrant circuits. See also *macroreentrant circuit, reentry.*

microreentry. Mechanism for the genesis of arrhythmia in which the reentrant circuit is highly localized. Unlike macroreentrant tachycardias, which have a large, excitable gap and typically involve large areas of atrial or ventricular myocardium, microreentrant circuits are localized and difficult to entrain. Microreentrant arrhythmias do not have features of automaticity, such as warm-up phenomenon or overdrive suppression.

microscopic heterogeneities. Fibrosis, anisotropy, tissue inflammation, or ischemia that occurs at a microscopic level. Microscopic heterogeneities occur in some forms of dilated cardiomyopathy and may be responsible for the multiple reentrant circuits and other ventricular arrhythmias found in this disorder.

microvolt T-wave alternans. Alternation in the microvoltage T-wave amplitude. It may be complete or relative and is a marker for arrhythmogenicity. Microvolt T-wave analysis may be useful to predict risk of sudden death or malignant ventricular arrhythmia in certain inherited disorders of repolarization and ischemic heart disease.

microwave (MW). Form of energy that can be used for myocardial ablation. Microwave ablation can be used in the treatment of ventricular or atrial disorders. Prior pacemakers had problems with microwave interference from home microwave ovens.

microwave ablation. Destruction of arrhythmogenic tissue with energy of a higher frequency than that used in radiofrequency ablation. Lesions are caused by heating the nearby tissue by means of induction of an electrical field rather than by flow of electrical current as with radiofrequency ablation. See also *ablation.*

mid-diastolic potential. Electrical activity recorded during endocardial catheter mapping of ventricular tachycardia. This mid-diastolic activity may arise from the zone of slow conduction and is one criterion used in determining the site for attempted ablation.

middle cardiac vein (MCV). The most proximal tributary of the coronary sinus, which drains blood from the posterior cardiac surface. Occasionally, the middle cardiac vein arises from a separate ostium in the right atrium. The middle cardiac vein or one of its lateral tributaries may be used for biventricular pacing. Accessory pathways may involve the musculature of the middle cardiac vein. See also *accessory pathway.*

midmyocardial cells (M cells). See *M cells.*

midodrine. An α-adrenergic agonist/vasopressor used to treat orthostatic hypotension. May be used in the therapeutic approach to vasodepressor syncope.

midseptal accessory pathways. Accessory pathways located on the anulus on the atrioventricular septum. Mid-septal pathways often lie in the closest anatomic proximity to the compact atrioventricular node. Ablation of mid-septal accessory pathways is associated with an increased risk of creating atrioventricular block. These pathways may be either right midseptal or left midseptal.

migration. The displacement of a pulse generator or lead from its original implantation site. Downward migration of a pulse generator may cause retraction of the endocardial electrode and thus result in failure to pace or sense. Migration can be prevented by anchoring the pulse generator to the underlying muscle fascia with sutures threaded through the suture hold in the pacemaker header. This also was prevented by encasing the pacemaker in a woven mesh pouch before implantation, but this approach is now rarely used. See also *pouch.*

MILIS. See *Multicenter Investigation of Limitation of Infarct Size.*

milliampere (mA). One thousandth of an ampere. Milliamperes are the units of measurement for low levels of electrical current flow. In pacing, milliamperes frequently are used to measure pacemaker output pulses. See also *ampere, current*.

millisecond (ms). One thousandth of a second. Milliseconds commonly are used to measure intracardiac conduction events, pacemaker timing functions, and other pacing intervals.

millivolt (mV). One thousandth of a volt. Millivolts are used to measure low levels of voltage. In cardiology and pacing, millivolts commonly are used to measure the amplitude of intrinsic P waves or R waves, cellular membrane potentials, and pacemaker sensitivity levels. See also *volt, voltage*.

minimum pacing interval. See *minimum rate interval*.

minimum rate. The maximum time the pacemaker timing circuitry will wait for intrinsic activity to occur before initiating a pacemaker output pulse. The minimum rate is a preset or programmable function and is measured in pulses per minute. The minimum rate is measured most accurately between two consecutive paced complexes. See also *minimum rate interval*.

minimum rate interval. The maximum time between two consecutive output pulses from the same channel of the pacemaker circuitry. The minimum rate interval can be determined by dividing 60,000 by the preset or programmed minimum rate of the pacemaker. The minimum rate interval is expressed in milliseconds. The minimum rate interval also is referred to as the minimum pacing interval. See also *minimum rate*.

minK. Cardiac cell channel protein important for the I_{Ks} component of the delayed rectifier current. The function of this protein may underlie responses to activated protein kinase C.

minute ventilation (MV). In respiratory physiology, the total volume of air breathed per minute. In rate-adaptive pacing, minute ventilation is one of the variables that is monitored and is used to adjust the paced heart rate proportionately. Minute ventilation (MV) is the product of tidal volume (TV, the total amount of air inhaled and exhaled during each breath cycle) and respiratory rate (RR), MV = TV × RR. See also *minute volume sensing*.

minute ventilation sensor. See *minute ventilation, minute volume sensing*.

minute volume. See *minute ventilation*.

minute volume sensing. A sensor system used in rate-adaptive pacing to effect proportionate changes in paced heart rate. Because of the high correlation between changes in transthoracic impedance and tidal volume, changes in transthoracic impedance are used in rate-adaptive pacing to estimate tidal volume and calculate minute ventilation. Respiratory rate and transthoracic impedance are measured directly. Minute ventilation (MV) is then calculated as the product of tidal volume (TV) and respiratory rate (RR), MV = TV × RR.

MIO. Abbreviation for *metal-induced oxidation, metal ion oxidation*.

MIRACLE. See *Multicenter InSync Randomized Clinical Evaluation*.

MIRACLE ICD. See *Multicenter InSync ICD Randomized Clinical Evaluation*.

MIRACLE ICD II. See *Multicenter InSync ICD Randomized Clinical Evaluation II*.

misprogramming. The response of a pacemaker, different from the intended response, after programming of the pacemaker with an external programmer. See also *dysprogramming, phantom programming*.

mitochondrial disorders. Form of inherited disorders typically passed on from mother to son. Unlike other genetically transmitted disorders that involve the nuclear DNA, the mitochondrial nucleic acids are the origin for transmission of these disorders. Examples include mitochondrial cardiomyopathy and certain hypercoagulable disorders. Kearns-Sayre syndrome is also a mitochondrial disorder. See also *Kearns-Sayre syndrome*.

mitral isthmus. 1. Atrial myocardium located between the mitral anulus and either the left lower pulmonary vein or the right lower pulmonary vein. It may be the arrhythmogenic substrate (slow zone) for left atrial flutter. Incision or ablation of the mitral isthmus is part of the endocardial or epicardial maze procedure. 2. Region of ventricular myocardium between the mitral valve and an inferior or inferolateral myocardial infarction. It may be the arrhythmogenic substrate for a common form of ventricular tachycardia (mitral isthmus ventricular tachycardia).

mitral isthmus ablation. Cardiac ablation involving the atrial mitral isthmus for left atrial flutter or the ventricular myocardial isthmus for a common form of ventricular tachycardias. See also *mitral isthmus*.

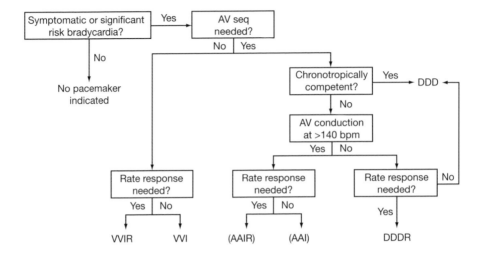

Mode Selection Algorithm

Complex selection algorithm

Simple selection algorithm

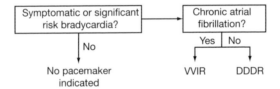

mixed venous oxygen saturation sensors. A sensor that utilizes a light-emitting diode and photoelectric cell to detect mixed venous oxygen saturation. For rate-adaptive pacing, the sensor is incorporated in the lead body, and fluctuations in oxygen saturation are used to adapt the paced rate.

M-mode echocardiogram. See *M-mode echocardiography.*

M-mode echocardiography. Form of echocardiographic imaging in which a single dimensional "slice" of ultrasound interrogation occurs. M-mode echocardiography is associated with high-resolution (high frame rate) imaging but does not display two- or three-dimensional structures. Doppler imaging, including color Doppler, can be performed in association with M-mode echocardiography.

M-mode imaging. See *M-mode echocardiography.*

Mobitz type I second-degree AV block. A partial disruption of atrioventricular conduction

in which progressive lengthening of the PR interval occurs until one atrial impulse is blocked. Following the nonconducted impulse, the first subsequent PR interval is normal. Mobitz type I is an electrocardiographic diagnosis and may occur due to delay and block occurring in either the atrioventricular node or the His-Purkinje system. Mobitz type I second-degree atrioventricular block is also known as Wenckebach block. See also *first-degree AV block, Mobitz type II second-degree AV block, second-degree AV block, third-degree AV block.*

Mobitz type II second-degree AV block. A partial disruption of atrioventricular conduction characterized by intermittent conduction of atrial impulses (P waves) through the atrioventricular node with no lengthening of the PR interval before blocked beats. Mobitz type II is an electrocardiographic diagnosis and may result from block in either the atrioventricular node or the His-Purkinje system. See also *first-degree*

AV block, Mobitz type I second-degree AV block, second-degree AV block, third-degree AV block.

mode. The preset or programmed response (paced or sensed, and inhibited or triggered) from a pacemaker in the presence or absence of intrinsic cardiac events. See also *NBG code, pacing mode.*

mode selection algorithm. A systematic approach that considers underlying conduction system abnormality and other variables to determine the best pacing mode.

Mode Selection Trial in Sinus Node Dysfunction (MOST). This was a prospective study in which patients with sinus node dysfunction were randomized to dual-chamber pacing or ventricular pacing and followed to a primary end point of death from any cause or nonfatal stroke. Secondary end points included the composite of death, stroke, or hospitalization for heart failure, atrial fibrillation, heart failure score, the pacemaker syndrome, and quality of life. Dual-chamber pacing, compared with ventricular pacing, did not improve stroke-free survival. However, dual-chamber pacing reduced the risk of atrial fibrillation, reduced signs and symptoms of heart failure, and slightly improved the quality of life (Lamas GA, Lee KL, Sweeney MO, Silverman R, Leon A, Yee R, et al, Mode Selection Trial in Sinus-Node Dysfunction. Ventricular pacing or dual-chamber pacing for sinus-node dysfunction. N Engl J Med. 2002;346:1854-62). Subsequent data analysis provided valuable insights into the potential adverse effects of ventricular pacing.

mode switching. The capability of a pacemaker that senses and tracks atrial activity to switch modes automatically to a non-tracking mode in the presence of intrinsic signals that the pacemaker determines to be a pathologic atrial rhythm disturbance. For example, if, in a patient with a DDDR pacemaker, atrial fibrillation with rapid ventricular pacing develops in response to the sensed atrial fibrillation, the pacemaker automatically reprograms to a nontracking mode, such as the VVIR or DDIR mode, until the pacemaker recognizes reestablishment of a physiologic atrial rhythm.

mode switch log. A record of mode-switch episodes that is stored within the pulse generator until the data are cleared. Data collected in the log may include the timing and duration of the event, shortest interval, and, in some devices, an electrogram of the event.

modified atrial-based timing system. An atrial-based timing system of a pacemaker that deviates from the basic rules of an atrial-based timing system. The deviation usually is device-specific. See also *atrial-based timing system.*

modified ventricular-based timing system. A ventricular-based timing system of a pacemaker that deviates from the basic rules of a ventricular-based timing system. The deviation usually is device-specific. See also *ventricular-based timing system.*

modulated parasystole. Variation in cycle length observed in a rhythm arising from a protected focus. Complexes from areas other than the parasystolic focus delay the next parasystolic beat when they occur in the first half of the parasystolic cycle, and they accelerate firing of the parasystolic focus when they occur in the latter half of the cycle. Although "protected," the parasystolic focus is affected by electronic conduction from impulses coming from elsewhere.

modulated receptor hypothesis. The theory that ion channels exist in three states (activated, inactivated, and resting) and that ion-channel blocking drugs have different effects because they interact with the channel in one or more of the different states. Channels may conduct ions

Mode Switching

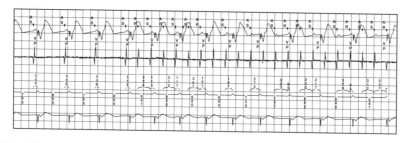

while in the activated state but then become inactivated by changes in voltage. These channels must then return to the resting state before they can be activated again. Most clinically useful antiarrhythmic drugs are activated-state blockers.

modulated-receptor model. See *modulated receptor hypothesis.*

modulation. Alteration of a carrier signal by superimposition of a specific coded electrical signal. The combination of the two signals causes a change of the carrier signal that is apparent by a change in the amplitude (voltage) or the signal frequency. Modulation of the carrier signal normally is used to transmit data, and the alteration caused by the superimposed signal is representative of specific information to be transmitted. In pacing, modulation is used to implement the communication between a programmer or telemetry. For example, the carrier signal emitted from the external programmer or pacemaker is modulated with a pattern of signals to indicate information to be transmitted. The altered carrier signal then is decoded by the programmer or pacemaker. The transmitted information either is displayed to the user by the programmer or is implemented by the pacemaker. See also *amplitude modulation.*

modulator circuit. The circuit that superimposes a coded electrical signal on a carrier signal, causing a change in the amplitude or frequency of the carrier signal. In pacing, a modulator circuit is used, for example, during programming or telemetry. The modulator circuit of the implanted pacemaker appropriately alters the carrier signal to represent information to be transmitted from the pacemaker to the programmer. See also *modulation.*

monitor mode. A programmable mode in implantable cardioverter-defibrillators in which the rhythm is monitored but tachy therapies are not enabled, a mode allowing the caregiver to monitor a given tachycardia. This mode may be used in patients undergoing a procedure or when there is concern that the implantable cardioverter-defibrillator could deliver inappropriate therapies because of detection of electromagnetic interference. During a monitor-only time, the patient should be continuously monitored externally and emergency resuscitation equipment and capable personnel should be available.

monitor zone. In implantable cardioverter-defibrillators, a detection zone for ventricular tachycardia may be programmed "on" without any programmed therapies. This feature is used when assessing medical or ablative therapy for symptomatic but hemodynamically tolerated tachycardias.

monomorphic. Usually refers to the P wave or QRS morphology during atrial or ventricular tachycardia, respectively. When the morphology of the P wave or QRS is uniform, monomorphic tachycardia results. Monomorphic tachycardias are generally more amenable to ablation than multimorphic or polymorphic tachycardias.

monomorphic ventricular tachycardia. Ventricular tachycardia that shows uniform morphology on the surface electrocardiogram. The induction of monomorphic ventricular tachycardia during an electrophysiologic study usually is a specific response. See also *polymorphic ventricular tachycardia.*

monophasic. Description of energy delivery or measured current that is either positive or negative in its entirety. See also *biphasic.*

monophasic action potential (MAP). A representation of a transmembrane action potential recorded extracellularly by a monophasic action potential catheter. In electrophysiologic studies, monophasic action potential recordings may be used to assess action potential duration and to search for delayed or early afterdepolarizations in vivo. See also *monophasic action potential (MAP) catheter.*

monophasic action potential (MAP) catheter. An electrode used for recording monophasic action potentials in vivo. Previously, these catheters were suction catheters. Currently, monophasic action potential catheters are contact electrodes.

monophasic waveform. A waveform whose excursions from a zero-potential baseline are either positive or negative, but not both. In cardiac pacing, negative (cathodal) monophasic waveforms typically are presented to the stimulating electrode, whereas positive (anodal) waveforms appear at the indifferent electrode or the anode in a widely spaced bipolar configuration. Currently, defibrillator shocks typically are monophasic, but biphasic defibrillator shocks may become the standard.

moricizine. An antiarrhythmic drug whose class is debated. Moricizine has been described as a combination of a class IA drug and a class IB drug. It also has been described as a class IC drug because its predominant effect is to slow conduction without affecting refractoriness. Moricizine has efficacy in the treatment of supraventricular and ventricular arrhythmias. Side effects include central nervous system effects and proarrhythmia. In the Cardiac Arrhythmia Suppression Trial (CAST), moricizine was associated with increased mortality compared with placebo treatment during the prerandomization phase. Moricizine also is known as ethmozine.

morphology discrimination. Variable used in certain defibrillators to distinguish ventricular from supraventricular arrhythmia. The morphology of the measured electrogram by the ventricular lead is compared between that measured during a detected tachycardia and that measured during normal rhythm.

MOSFET. Abbreviation for *metal-oxide semiconductor field-effect transistor*.

MOST. See *Mode Selection Trial in Sinus Node Dysfunction*.

motion sensing. The use of a specially designed sensor system that detects body motion or vibration and causes proportionate changes in the paced heart rate. Motion sensing is used in some rate-adaptive pacing systems. Motion detection usually is accomplished via a piezoelectric crystal or an accelerometer. See also *activity sensing, in rate-adaptive pacing*.

M-PATHY. See *Multicenter Study of Pacing Therapy for Hypertrophic Cardiomyopathy*.

MPI. Abbreviation for *myocardial performance index*.

MP35N. A hypoallergenic, biocompatible, and corrosion-resistant cobalt-nickel alloy. In pacing, MP35N has been widely used as the conductor coil of the pacing lead(s). See also *alloy*.

MRI. Abbreviation for *magnetic resonance imaging, maximum rate interval*.

ms. Abbreviation for *millisecond*.

MSR. Abbreviation for *maximum sensor rate*.

MTI. Abbreviation for *maximum tracking interval*.

MTR. Abbreviation for *maximum tracking rate*.

MTRI. Abbreviation for *maximum tracking rate interval*.

multiblock. Cardiac conduction disease, usually severe, manifests sometimes as conduction block occurring at more than one level, for example, atrioventricular conduction block occurring at both the compact atrioventricular node and infrahisian conduction system.

Multicenter Automatic Defibrillator Implantation Trial (MADIT). This was a study in which patients with coronary disease who had prior myocardial infarction, nonsustained ventricular tachycardia, and an ejection fraction less than 35% had improved survival with an implantable cardioverter-defibrillator compared with conventional drug therapy, primarily amiodarone. Therapy with an implantable cardioverter-defibrillator reduced mortality by 54% (Moss AJ, Hall WJ, Cannom DS, Daubert JP, Higgins SL, Klein H, et al, Multicenter Automatic Defibrillator Implantation Trial Investigators. Improved survival with an implanted defibrillator in patients with coronary disease at high risk for ventricular arrhythmia. N Engl J Med. 1996;335:1933-40).

Multicenter Automatic Defibrillator Implantation Trial II (MADIT-II). This was a prospective trial of patients with a prior myocardial infarction and a left ventricular ejection fraction of 30% or less randomized to receive an implantable cardioverter-defibrillator or conventional medical therapy. The primary end point was death from any cause. The mortality rate was 14.2% in the device group and 19.8% in the conventional therapy group (Moss AJ, Zareba W, Hall WJ, Klein H, Wilber DJ, Cannom DS, et al, Multicenter Automatic Defibrillator Implantation Trial II Investigators. Prophylactic implantation of a defibrillator in patients with myocardial infarction and reduced ejection fraction. N Engl J Med. 2002 Mar 21;346:877-83. Epub 2002 Mar 19).

Multicenter Automatic Defibrillator Implantation With Cardiac Resynchronization Trial (MADIT-CR). This is a prospective, randomized trial under way to determine whether combined therapy with cardiac resynchronization and an implantable cardioverter-defibrillator will reduce the combined end point of all-cause mortality or heart failure events compared with an implantable cardioverter-defibrillator only in patients in New York Heart Association (NYHA) functional class II with nonischemic or ischemic cardiomyopathy and patients in NYHA functional class I with ischemic cardiomyopathy, left ventricular dysfunction (ejection fraction ≤30%), and prolonged intraventricular conduction (QRS duration ≥130 milliseconds).

Multicenter InSync ICD Randomized Clinical Evaluation (MIRACLE ICD). This was a prospective, multicenter, randomized, double-blind, parallel-controlled clinical trial designed very similar to the MIRACLE trial. It was intended to assess the safety and clinical efficacy of a combined implantable cardioverter-defibrillator and cardiac resynchronization system in patients with dilated cardiomyopathy, New York Heart Association functional class III or IV heart failure (a cohort of patients with class II was also enrolled), interventricular conduction delay (QRS >130 milliseconds), and an indication for an implantable cardioverter-defibrillator. The trial showed significant improvements in quality of life, functional class, cardiopulmonary exercise capacity, and the composite clinical response in the active cardiac resynchronization group compared with control subjects. The magnitude of improvement was comparable to that in the MIRACLE trial, a finding suggesting that patients with heart failure who have an indication for an implantable cardioverter-defibrillator benefit as much from cardiac resynchronization therapy as those patients without an indication for an implantable cardioverter-defibrillator (Young JB, Abraham WT, Smith AL, Leon AR, Lieberman R, Wilkoff B, et al, Multicenter InSync ICD Randomized Clinical Evaluation [MIRACLE ICD] Trial Investigators. Combined cardiac resynchronization and implantable cardioversion defibrillation in advanced chronic heart failure: the MIRACLE ICD Trial. JAMA. 2003;289:2685-94).

Multicenter InSync ICD Randomized Clinical Evaluation II (MIRACLE ICD II). This was a prospective trial of patients with New York Heart Association functional class II clinical status and an indication for cardiac resynchronization therapy (CRT). They were randomized to parallel arms of CRT-on and CRT-off (control). Functional improvement at 6 months was not significant in the CRT arm, but the composite response of clinical variables that combined mortality, serious morbidity, and symptoms was improved significantly and compatible with less disease progression (Abraham WT, Young JB, Leon AR, Adler S, Bank AJ, Hall SA, et al, Multicenter InSync ICD II Study Group. Effects of cardiac resynchronization on disease progression in patients with left ventricular systolic dysfunction, an indication for an implantable cardioverter-defibrillator, and mildly symptomatic chronic heart failure. Circulation. 2004 Nov 2;110:2864-8. Epub 2004 Oct 25).

Multicenter InSync Randomized Clinical Evaluation (MIRACLE). This was the first prospective, randomized, double-blind, parallel-controlled clinical trial designed to validate the results from previous cardiac resynchronization therapy studies and evaluate the therapeutic efficacy and mechanisms of potential benefit of this therapy. Primary end points were New York Heart Association functional class, quality-of-life score, and 6-minute hall walk distance. Patients with moderate to severe symptoms of heart failure associated with a left ventricular ejection less than 35% and a QRS duration more than 130 milliseconds were randomized to cardiac resynchronization therapy or a control group for 6 months while conventional therapy for heart failure was maintained. Compared with the control group, patients randomized to cardiac resynchronization therapy had a significant improvement in quality-of-life score, 6-minute walk distance, functional class ranking, treadmill exercise time, peak oxygen consumption, and left ventricular ejection fraction. Patients randomized to cardiac resynchronization therapy had a highly significant improvement in a composite clinical heart failure response end point, fewer hospitalizations, and fewer intravenous medications for the treatment of worsening heart failure (Abraham WT, Fisher WG, Smith AL, Delurgio DB, Leon AR, Loh E, et al, MIRACLE Study Group. Cardiac resynchronization in chronic heart failure. N Engl J Med. 2002;346:1845-53).

Multicenter Investigation of Limitation of Infarct Size (MILIS). This study was a broad-based study assessing multiple aspects of myocardial infarction, including prognosis after cardiac arrest due to ventricular tachycardia or ventricular fibrillation associated with acute myocardial infarction (Tofler GH, Stone PH, Muller JE, Rutherford JD, Willich SN, Gustafson NF, et al. Prognosis after cardiac arrest due to ventricular tachycardia or ventricular fibrillation associated with acute myocardial infarction [the MILIS Study]. Multicenter Investigation of the Limitation of Infarct Size. Am J Cardiol. 1987;60:755-61).

Multicenter Study of Pacing Therapy for Hypertrophic Cardiomyopathy (M-PATHY). This was a prospective, multicenter trial that assessed pacing therapy in symptomatic patients with hypertrophic cardiomyopathy, a resting gradient of 50 mm Hg or more, and symptoms refractory to drug therapy. No significant differences were evident between pacing and no pacing for subjective or objective measures of symptoms or exercise capacity. After 6 additional months of pacing (unblinded), functional class and quality-of-life score were improved compared with baseline, but peak oxygen consumption was unchanged. The study concluded that pacing cannot be regarded as a primary treatment for obstructive hypertrophic cardiomyopathy (Maron BJ, Nishimura RA, McKenna WJ, Rakowski H, Josephson ME, Kieval RS. Assessment of permanent dual-chamber pacing as a treatment for drug-refractory symptomatic patients with obstructive hypertrophic cardiomyopathy: a randomized, double-blind, crossover study [M-PATHY]. Circulation. 1999;99:2927-33).

Multicenter Unsustained Tachycardia Trial (MUSTT). This was a prospective trial in which patients without inducible sustained ventricular tachycardia followed in a registry and patients with inducible sustained ventricular tachycardia were randomized to no antiarrhythmic therapy or to electrophysiology-guided therapy (i.e., sequential rounds of antiarrhythmic drug [AA Rx] therapy and drug nonresponders received an implantable cardioverter-defibrillator). The primary end point was arrhythmic death or cardiac arrest, and the secondary end point was overall mortality, and cardiac mortality. The risk of arrhythmic death or cardiac arrest at 5 years was reduced 27% for patients receiving electrophysiology-guided therapy (AA Rx or implantable cardioverter-defibrillator) (Buxton AE, Fisher JD, Josephson ME, Lee KL, Pryor DB, Prystowsky EN, et al. Prevention of sudden death in patients with coronary artery disease: the Multicenter Unsustained Tachycardia Trial [MUSTT]. Prog Cardiovasc Dis. 1993;36:215-26).

Multicentre European Radiofrequency Survey (MERFS). This study, conducted by the Working Group on Arrhythmias of the European Society of Cardiology, was a voluntary retrospective survey designed to assess the number of radiofrequency catheter ablation procedures performed in specific European institutions and the incidence of procedure-related complications with respect to the different types of ablative procedures (Hindricks G, The Multicentre European Radiofrequency Survey [MERFS] investigators of the Working Group on Arrhythmias of the European Society of Cardiology. The Multicentre European Radiofrequency Survey [MERFS]: complications of radiofrequency catheter ablation of arrhythmias. Eur Heart J. 1993;14:1644-53).

multielectrode array (MEA). Type of basket electrode specifically used with a noncontact mapping system. Multiple laser-etched electrodes are arranged on a central spine and placed in the cardiac chamber to be mapped. The electrodes do not make contact with the myocardium. Using an inverse solution principle, virtual electrograms (calculated electrograms based on constructed geometry) are visualized and aid in the mapping and ablation of cardiac arrhythmias.

multifilar lead. A pacing lead whose conductor is composed of two or more small-diameter wires connected or wound in parallel. Multifilar leads are flexible, durable, and redundant and allow a reduction of the lead diameter with an increase in the functional performance of the lead. Multifilar leads distribute stresses caused by flexion throughout the wires and thereby reduce the likelihood of lead or conductor fracture. Redundancy ensures that fracture of a single wire of the conductor coil will not cause conduction failure through the lead. See also *unifilar lead*.

multifocal. Originating from multiple sites. In electrophysiology, multifocal is used to describe an arrhythmia that originates from two or more foci.

multifocal atrial tachycardia. A chaotic atrial arrhythmia that has three or more different P-wave morphologies and a rate more than 100 beats per minute. Multifocal atrial tachycardia often is associated with severe illness, especially chronic pulmonary disease. Multifocal atrial tachycardia sometimes responds to verapamil, a result suggesting triggered activity as the underlying mechanism.

multifocal rhythm. Generic term indicating that the cardiac rhythm arises from multiple foci (e.g., multifocal atrial rhythm, multifocal ventricular rhythm).

multiform. Having multiple morphologies during a tachycardia. Multiform ventricular tachycardia may be a forerunner of ventricular fibrillation. Multiform ventricular arrhythmias are not as amenable to radiofrequency ablation as monomorphic arrhythmias.

multiform tachycardia. See *polymorphic ventricular tachycardia*.

multinodal. A characteristic of all programmable pacemakers in which the pacemaker has the capability of operating in more than one pacing mode. The desired mode of operation is chosen by the physician and the pacemaker is programmed to that mode.

multiple electrode mapping. Method of mapping cardiac arrhythmias by placing multiple electrode tip catheters in the heart. Multielectrode mapping is commonly used for the mapping of complex atrial and ventricular arrhythmias. Frequently a multielectrode catheter is placed in the coronary sinus to aid multielectrode mapping of both the left atrium and the left ventricle.

multiple wavelet hypothesis. The hypothesis that fibrillation consists of numerous separate wave fronts that course simultaneously throughout the myocardium between islands of refractory tissue. The wave fronts follow ever changing paths and vary in size.

multiplex transmission. A method by which two or more signals are combined for simultaneous transmission and reception over a single communications link. In pacing, multiplex transmission is the basis for transtelephonic electrocardiographic monitoring.

multipolar basket catheter. Type of mapping catheter in the shape of a basket (spindles around a central spine) placed in a cardiac chamber. Each spindle has several electrodes. Multielectrode basket catheters are designed such that the electrodes make contact with the myocardium to generate the electrogram. Multielectrode basket mapping has the advantage that often an activation sequence can be calculated from a single or a few beats of tachycardia.

multiprogrammability. The capability to noninvasively adjust three or more pacemaker variables with an external programmer. Multiprogrammability makes it possible to optimize or customize pacemaker function to meet the specific needs of the patient. In contemporary pacemakers programmable variables are extensive. See also *programmability*.

multiprogrammable pacemaker. An implantable pacemaker in which three or more pacing variables can be altered by external, noninvasive programming. See also *multiprogrammability*.

multisite pacing. Generic term for pacing from more than one site within the atria or ventricles. For example, multisite ventricular pacing could indicate multiple sites within the right ventricle, pacing right and left ventricles, or pacing multiple sites of the left ventricle.

Multisite Stimulation in Cardiomyopathies. This study was a single-blind, randomized, crossover evaluation of cardiac resynchronization therapy with two arms: one arm enrolled patients who were in normal sinus rhythm and had standard criteria for cardiac resynchronization (MUSTIC-SR) and the other arm enrolled patients with chronic atrial fibrillation and otherwise standard criteria for cardiac resynchronization (MUSTIC-AF). In the MUSTIC-SR group, significant improvement was found in the primary end point of 6-minute walk and in secondary end points, including change in quality of life, New York Heart Association class, peak oxygen consumption, hospital admissions, worsening heart failure, total mortality, and patient preference for pacing mode. The MUSTIC-AF group had significant improvements in the following primary and secondary end points: 6-minute hall walk, peak oxygen consumption, and hospitalizations. Although there was a trend toward improvement in quality of life with biventricular pacing, statistical significance was not met (Cazeau S, Leclercq C, Lavergne T, Walker S, Varma C, Linde C, et al, Multisite Stimulation in Cardiomyopathies [MUSTIC] Study Investigators. Effects of multisite biventricular pacing in patients with heart failure and intraventricular conduction delay. N Engl J Med. 2001;344:873-80).

muscarinic receptors. Postganglionic parasympathetic binding sites. Muscarinic receptors are stimulated by acetylcholine and blocked by atropine.

muscarinic-receptor stimulation. Stimulation of muscarinic receptors, which is one of the methods for stimulating the autonomic nervous system.

muscle potential oversensing. See *myopotential triggering*.

muscle stimulation. See *diaphragmatic stimulation.*

muscular dystrophy. A group of genetic, degenerative diseases primarily affecting voluntary muscles. The disease also may involve the cardiac conduction system and lead to sudden cardiac death.

musculoskeletal interference. See *myopotential.*

Mustard procedure. Surgical procedure performed for congenital transposition of the great vessels in which right atrial blood is circuited (baffled) to the left ventricle and thus to the pulmonary artery and lung. The pulmonary venous flow is similarly baffled to the right ventricle, which in turn is connected to the aorta.

MUSTIC. See *Multisite Stimulation in Cardiomyopathies.*

MUSTIC-AF. See *Multisite Stimulation in Cardiomyopathies.*

MUSTIC-SR. See *Multisite Stimulation in Cardiomyopathies.*

MUSTT. See *Multicenter Unsustained Tachycardia Trial.*

mV. Abbreviation for *millivolt.*

MV. Abbreviation for *minute ventilation.*

MVP. Abbreviation for *Managed Ventricular Pacing.* See *ventricular pacing avoidance algorithm.*

MW. Abbreviation for *microwave.*

myocardial ablation. Catheter ablation for cardiac arrhythmias targeting atrial or ventricular myocardium.

myocardial anisotropy. Architecture of the myocardial cells in which the tissues are not arranged in parallel. Marked changes in direction of cell arrangement results in slowing of conduction and the potential to generate reentrant cardiac arrhythmias.

myocardial lead. See *epicardial screw-in lead.*

myocardial pacing. See *epicardial pacing.*

myocardial performance index (MPI). Also known as the Tei index, the myocardial performance index is a Doppler-derived variable of cardiac function used in the serial evaluation and risk stratification of patients with left ventricular systolic and diastolic dysfunction of various causes. The myocardial performance index has been used to assess selection of patients for and response to cardiac resynchronization.

myocardial sutureless lead. See *epicardial screw-in lead.*

myocardial synchrony. Simultaneous and orderly activation of the myocardium, usually referring to ventricular myocardium that optimizes mechanical function.

myocardium. The thick, contractile middle layer of the heart wall, composed of cardiac muscle. In the normal heart, the atrial myocardium and the ventricular myocardium contract sequentially in response to spontaneous intrinsic electrical impulses from the sinus node. The myocardium also contracts in response to electrical impulses delivered via an extrinsic source of electrical energy such as a pacemaker or implantable cardioverter-defibrillator. See also *endocardium, epicardium.*

myopotential. An electrical signal originating in muscle as a result of voluntary or involuntary movement. Skeletal muscle myopotentials may be sensed by a pacemaker implanted near the muscles involved and interpreted incorrectly as cardiac depolarizations. Myopotentials often result in an irregular baseline on electrocardiographic recordings. See also *noise.*

myopotential inhibition. The inhibition of pacemaker output pulses by electrical signals that originate from skeletal muscle. The pacemaker senses the myopotential signals as intrinsic cardiac activity and inhibits the pacemaker output

Myopotential Inhibition

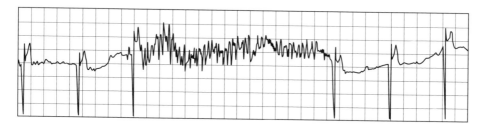

pulse. Myopotential inhibition occurs most often in unipolar pacing systems. See also *myopotential triggering*.

myopotential oversensing. See *myopotential triggering*.

myopotential triggering. The triggering of pacemaker output pulses by electrical signals that originate from skeletal muscle. For example, a DDD pacemaker could sense myopotential signals on the atrial sensing circuit as intrinsic cardiac activity and trigger a ventricular pacemaker output pulse. Myopotential triggering occurs most often in unipolar pacing systems. See also *myopotential, myopotential inhibition*.

myotomy-myectomy. Surgical treatment for hypertrophic obstructive cardiomyopathy. In a small percentage of patients undergoing myotomy-myectomy, the procedure is complicated by conduction system damage, most commonly atrioventricular block, requiring a subsequent pacemaker.

myotonic muscular dystrophy. One of multiple types of muscular dystrophy in which cardiac conduction system disease may develop.

n

Na. The chemical symbol for sodium.

Na+,Ca2+ exchanger. One of two primary mechanisms for removing calcium from the cytoplasm. Three sodium ions are exchanged for each calcium ion, thus making this exchanger electrogenic, generating an electrical potential across the plasma membrane. When the intracellular sodium concentration is increased, competition for calcium through this mechanism is enhanced, leading to an increase in intracellular calcium concentration. An important clinical example of this process occurs when the sodium-potassium adenosine triphosphate pump is diminished (with digoxin use), thus leading indirectly to increased intracellular calcium concentration and enhanced contractility.

Na+ channels. Also referred to as voltage-gated sodium channels. Voltage-dependent proteins located in the cell membranes of excitable tissues. Activation of sodium channels leads to cell depolarization. Currents traveling inward through the sodium channels of cardiac cell membranes are responsible for phase 0 of the cardiac action potential.

nadolol. A nonselective, β-adrenergic blocking agent without intrinsic sympathomimetic activity. Nadolol is excreted by the kidneys. Because it is hydrophilic, nadolol does not cross the blood-brain barrier and may cause fewer central nervous system side effects than some other β-adrenergic blocking agents. For side effects, see β-*adrenergic blocking drugs*.

Na+,H+ exchanger. Cell membrane protein that exchanges sodium and hydrogen ions. In effect, this protein ejects protons from cells and is critical in maintaining intracellular pH. Indirectly, this protein is also crucial for maintenance of cell volume.

Na+,K+ -adenosine triphosphatase. Enzyme located in the cell membrane, including the myocardial cell membrane that exchanges sodium for potassium ions. Activation of this protein is important for maintaining the cell membrane potential and normally low intracellular sodium concentration. Three sodium ions, along with adenosine triphosphate, attach to this enzyme intracellularly. When the adenosine triphosphate is hydrolized, a confirmational change in the protein occurs that causes the sodium to be released extracellularly and become attached to two potassium ions, in turn causing a confirmational change that directs the potassium ions intracellularly. Because one more sodium ion than potassium ion is exchanged, the pump is electrogenic, creating a negative intracellular environment.

Na+,K+-ATPase. See *Na+,K+-adenosine triphosphatase*.

Na+,K+-ATPase exchange pump. Na+,K+-adenosine triphosphatase.

NAPA. Abbreviation for N-*acetylprocainamide*.

narrow QRS complex ventricular tachycardia. Typically, ventricular tachycardias present with a wide QRS complex with a QRS complex duration of more than 120 milliseconds. Certain forms of ventricular tachycardia, including tachycardias that originate in the intraventricular septum or tachycardias involving the conduction system, may have a QRS duration less than 120 milliseconds, and they are referred to as narrow QRS complex ventricular tachycardias.

NASPE. Abbreviation for the *North American Society of Pacing and Electrophysiology*.

NASPE/BPEG code. See *NBG code*.

NASPE/BPEG defibrillator code. See *NBD code*.

NASPE/BPEG generic code. See *NBG code*.

natriuretic peptides. Peptides that cause the excretion of sodium in the urine (i.e., natriuresis). These peptides are produced by the heart and vasculature. A-type natriuretic peptide is secreted primarily by the atrial myocardium and occurs in response to dilatation of this chamber. B-type natriuretic peptide is produced largely by the ventricular myocardium and may be useful in the diagnosis of heart failure. C-type natriuretic peptide originates from endothelial cells lining blood vessels.

Naxos disease. A rare autosomal recessive syndrome characterized by arrhythmogenic right

NBD Code			
I	**II**	**III**	**IV**
Shock chamber	Antitachycardia-pacing chamber	Tachycardia detection	Antibradycardia pacing chamber
O = None	O = None	E = Electrogram	O = None
A = Atrium	A = Atrium	H = Hemodynamic	A = Atrium
V = Ventricle	V = Ventricle		V = Ventricle
D = Dual (A + V)	D = Dual (A + V)		D = Dual (A + V)

From Bernstein AD, Camm AJ, Fisher JD, Fletcher RD, Mead RH, Nathan AW, et al. North American Society of Pacing and Electrophysiology policy statement: The NASPE/BPEG defibrillator code. Pacing Clin Electrophysiol. 1993;16:1776-80. Used with permission.

ventricular dysplasia, woolly hair, and palmo-plantar keratoderma. It is identified on the Aegean island of Naxos at a frequency of 1:1,000.

NBD code. Abbreviation for the *NASPE/BPEG defibrillator code*. NASPE is the abbreviation for the *North American Society of Pacing and Electrophysiology*, and BPEG is the abbreviation for the *British Pacing and Electrophysiology Group*. A generic code of four letters created for implantable cardioverter-defibrillators. The first position designates the chamber that is shocked, the second position denotes the chamber in which antitachycardia pacing occurs, the third denotes the method of tachycardia detection, and the fourth is the chamber(s) in which bradycardia pacing occurs. Letters used include A for atrium, V for ventricle, D for dual, O for neither, E for electrogram, and H for hemodynamic (Bernstein AD, Camm AJ, Fisher JD, Fletcher RD, Mead RH, Nathan AW, et al. North American Society of Pacing and Electrophysiology policy

statement: The NASPE/BPEG defibrillator code. Pacing Clin Electrophysiol. 1993;16:1776-80).

NBG code. Abbreviation for the *NASPE/BPEG generic code*. NASPE is the abbreviation for the *North American Society of Pacing and Electrophysiology*, and BPEG is the abbreviation for the *British Pacing and Electrophysiology Group*. A generic pacemaker code for antibradycardias, rate-adaptive pacing, and antitachycardia devices. The NBG code is a five-position code.

NCAP. Abbreviation for *noncompetitive atrial pacing*.

near-field electrogram. On the atrial electrogram, the actual depolarization of the atrium is the near-field electrogram. This is in contrast to the ventricular electrogram, the far-field electrogram being sensed or seen on the atrial recording channel.

near-field signal. Electrograms recorded by intracardiac electrodes may have a complex signal. The signal arising from actual tissue-electrode

NBG Code			
Position	**I***	**II***	**III***
Category	Chamber(s) paced	Chamber(s) sensed	Response to sensing
	O = None	O = None	O = None
	A = Atrium	A = Atrium	T = Triggered
	V = Ventricle	V = Ventricle	I = Inhibited
	D = Dual (A + V)	D = Dual (A + V)	D = Dual (T + I)
Manufacturers' designation only	S = Single (A or V)	S = Single (A or V)	

* Positions I through III are used exclusively for antibradyarrhythmia functions.

contact is higher frequency and sharp and is referred to as a near-field signal. Signals picked up by the catheter, either without exact contact or from neighboring electrically active tissue, is more of a blunted low-frequency signal and is referred to as a far-field signal. See the figure *Far-field and near-field electrograms*.

near-syncope. The sensation of impending loss of consciousness without culmination in frank syncope.

needle's eye snare. A tool for use in the percutaneous retrieval of indwelling catheters, cardiac leads, fragments of catheter tubing or wire guides, and other foreign objects. This is a transfemoral grasping tool that forms a basket snare around the lead body.

negative AV interval hysteresis. Shortening of the AV interval after a spontaneous ventricular event is noted. The intent with negative AV interval hysteresis is to maintain ventricular pacing.

negative AV/PV delay. The measured AR (paced A to intrinsic R) conduction time minus the interval programmed for negative hysteresis delta value.

negative hysteresis. The shortening of the escape interval after spontaneous depolarizations, which results in shortening of the pacing interval. Negative hysteresis causes an increase in pacing rate and this, in turn, tends to suppress intrinsic activity such as ectopic beats and tachycardia.

neonatal lupus syndrome. A syndrome due to passage of maternal anti-Ro (SS-A) antibodies to the unborn fetus. Approximately half of infants with this syndrome have congenital complete heart block.

nesiritide. A natriuretic peptide used intravenously for the treatment of severe congestive heart failure.

neurally mediated syncope. See *neurocardiogenic syncope*.

neurocardiogenic syncope. Loss of consciousness due to hypotension with or without bradycardia. Neurocardiogenic syncope is caused by the Bezold-Jarisch reflex. The underlying mechanism is thought to be activation of afferent vagal nerves (C fibers), located predominantly on the inferior wall of the heart, with resultant reflex withdrawal of peripheral sympathetic outflow and an increase in efferent vagal activity to the heart. Neurocardiogenic syncope also is known as vasodepressor syncope and vagal syncope. See also *tilt-table testing*.

neurocardiogenic syndromes. Various syndromes that result from vasodepressor or vasovagal episodes. Syndromes include, but are not limited to, micturition syncope, defecation syncope, cough syncope, and swallow syncope.

neuropeptide Y. A peptide that is released from sympathetic nerve terminals. Once released, neuropeptide Y inhibits further release of norepinephrine by sympathetic nerves and causes vagal nerve terminals to reduce acetylcholine outflow.

New York Heart Association (NYHA) classification. A therapeutic and functional classification that denotes the level of physical activity of which a cardiac patient is capable.
- Class I: patients are not limited in terms of

NBG Code (continued)		
Position	IV	V
Category	Programmability and adaptive rate	Antitachyarrhythmia function(s)
	O = None	O = None
	P = Simply programmable	P = Pacing (Antitachyarrhythmia)
	M = Multiprogrammable	S = Shock
	C = Communicating	D = Dual (P + S)
Manufacturers' designation only	R = Rate modulation	

From Bernstein AD, Camm AJ, Fletcher RD, Gold RD, Rickards AF, Smyth NPD, et al. The NASPE/BPEG generic pacemaker code for antibradyarrhythmia and adaptive-rate pacing and antitachyarrhythmia devices. Pacing Clin Electrophysiol. 1987;10(4 Pt 1):794-9. Used with permission.

their activities; no symptoms occur with ordinary activities.

- Class II: patients have mild limitation of activity (i.e., they are comfortable with mild exertion and at rest).
- Class III: patients have marked limitation of activity and are comfortable only at rest.
- Class IV: patients are essentially confined to bed or chair; patients are symptomatic with any physical activity.

NiCd. The chemical symbol for *nickel-cadmium*.

nickel-cadmium (NiCd). A battery chemistry in which the anode is nickel and the cathode is cadmium. Nickel-cadmium is used in sealed storage batteries as primary cells that can be recharged. A nickel-cadmium battery has a high self-discharge rate and a battery capacity of less than 0.2 ampere-hours, and thus the battery cell must be charged regularly. Without recharging, the battery energy depletes in 6 to 8 weeks. In pacing, nickel-cadmium batteries were used as the power source for rechargeable pacemakers. These batteries had a low terminal impedance and only one cell was required to provide adequate output voltage for pacing. Rechargeable pacemakers are no longer available. See also *rechargeable battery*.

NIEPS. Abbreviation for *noninvasive electrophysiologic study*.

NIPS. Abbreviation for *noninvasive programmed stimulation*.

nitrous oxide (N₂O). See *N₂O*.

NMR imaging. Abbreviation for *nuclear magnetic resonance imaging*. See *magnetic resonance imaging*.

N₂O. Nitrous oxide. An anesthetic gas used in some ablation and complex pacemaker cases. Nitrous oxide, along with intravenous anesthetics, such as propofol, frequently is used for deep sedation in patients with automatic arrhythmias that are depressed by other anesthetic and analgesic agents.

nodofascicular bypass tract. Rarely occurring type of accessory pathway in which a direct connection is present between the atrioventricular node and either the distal portion of the His bundle or the bundle branches. Nodofasicular bypass tracts are distinguished from other atrioventricular bypass tracts by the absence of a direct electrical connection between the atrial myocardium and ventricular myocardium.

nodofascicular fiber. Myocardial tissue that directly connects the atrioventricular node and either the distal portion of the His bundle or bundle branch system. These fibers may rarely be responsible for reentrant tachycardias involving the atrioventricular node and bundle branch system.

nodoventricular accessory pathway. Type of accessory bypass tract in which a connection exists between the compact atrioventricular node and ventricular myocardium, bypassing the His bundle and proximal right bundle branch exit. These accessory pathways are rare and may be responsible for reentrant tachycardia. These types of accessory bypass tracts are distinguished from the more common type of accessory bypass tracts by the absence of a connection between the atrial myocardium to the ventricular myocardium.

nodoventricular bypass tract. See *nodoventricular accessory pathway*.

nodoventricular fiber. An accessory pathway that forms a connection between the atrioventricular node and the ventricle. These pathways are a type of Mahaim fiber and may participate in reentrant tachycardias.

noise. Current or voltage that can interfere with an electrical device or system. In pacing, noise refers to an extraneous spike, waveform, or signal from a noncardiac physiologic source or from the external environment. Noise may pass through the pacemaker sensing amplifier and interfere with pacemaker operation, usually by causing the pacemaker to respond in an inhibited or triggered mode. Examples of electrical noise include myopotentials, 60-Hz alternating current, electromagnetic interference, and radiofrequency signals. In pacing, noise also may result from improper electrode attachment to the conductor of the pacing lead. See also *electromagnetic interference*.

noise interference mode. See *noise reversion mode*.

noise mode operation. See *noise reversion mode*.

noise mode response. See *noise reversion mode*.

noise rate. A preset or programmed pacing rate, different from the original programmed pacing rate, that is initiated automatically in response to sensed noise interference. The noise rate varies in different pacemakers. In some pacemakers, noise detected during the noise window causes the pacemaker to become refractory and to function in the fixed-rate mode for one complete interval. In other pacemakers, the rate may change to continuously asynchronous fixed-rate pacing for some preset amount of time. See also *noise, noise reversion mode.*

noise response. The predetermined behavior of a pulse generator in the presence of interference. The response could include variations of, for example, rate, mode, and output.

noise reversion mode. A pacing mode automatically activated in some pacemakers when noise is sensed. The noise reversion mode usually consists of fixed-rate pacing for one complete paced interval. In some pacemaker models, the fixed-rate pacing may continue as long as noise is sensed, and normal pacemaker function resumes when noise is no longer sensed by the pacemaker. See also *noise, noise rate.*

noise sampling period. See *noise window, relative refractory period.*

noise window. The amount of time during the pacemaker refractory period when the pacemaker sensing amplifier is alert for noise signals. If noise is detected, the pacemaker changes to its noise reversion mode. Noise windows may occur in the atrial or ventricular channel, depending on the pacemaker model. See also *noise, noise rate, noise reversion mode.*

nominal (nominal settings, nominal values). The value of a setting at which a device will operate safely under normal conditions. In pacing, nominal values describe a set of pacing variables that will adequately pace the heart in most patients. Most pacemakers can be programmed relatively quickly and easily to a set of nominal variables, if necessary. See also *stat set, stat set values.*

noncapture. The presence of a pacemaker stimulus without depolarization in the chamber in which the stimulus was delivered. If the stimulus is delivered when the myocardial tissue is excitable, the noncapture represents true failure to capture. If the stimulus is delivered when the myocardial tissue is refractory, the noncapture represents one type of "functional" noncapture.

noncommitted DVI pacing. A type of atrioventricular sequential pacing. In noncommitted DVI pacing, if an intrinsic QRS complex is sensed before the end of the preset or programmed atrioventricular interval, the pacemaker will inhibit the ventricular output pulse.

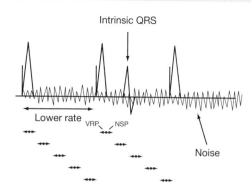

Noise Response

NSP, noise-sampling period; VRP, ventricular refractory period. Modified from Hayes DL, Strathmore NF. Electromagnetic interference with implantable devices. In: Ellenbogen KA, Kay GN, Wilkoff BL, editors. Clinical cardiac pacing and defibrillation. 2nd ed. Philadelphia: WB Saunders Company; 2000. p. 939-52. Used with permission.

Therefore, competition between the ventricular output pulse and an intrinsic ventricular event does not occur. See also *AV sequential ventricular-inhibited pacing mode (DVI), committed DVI pacing.*

noncommitted implantable cardioverter-defibrillator. See *noncommitted shocks.*

noncommitted shocks. Shocks that are delivered by an implantable cardioverter-defibrillator only if the tachycardia is reconfirmed after the capacitors have charged completely. If the tachycardia reverts spontaneously during capacitor charging, no shock will be delivered to the myocardium and the charge will be dumped. Noncommitted shock delivery is a programmable feature in some implantable cardioverter-defibrillators. See also *committed shocks.*

noncompetitive atrial pacing (NCAP). In some pulse generators, a feature that is designed to prevent competitive atrial pacing during the atrium's relative refractory period when competitive pacing could result in atrial arrhythmias. This feature delays atrial pacing when an atrial event is sensed during the postventricular atrial refractory period. •

noncontact mapping. Electrophysiologic mapping and navigation system used for ablation in both atria and ventricles. The unique feature of this system is the nonrequirement for catheter contact at a myocardial interface to obtain an electrogram. In this system, a far-field (virtual)

Noncompetitive Atrial Pacing

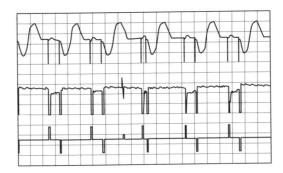

electrogram is obtained by the system and, with use of the inverse solution principle, the electrogram at the tissue site is calculated. Advantages of this system include the ability to map hemodynamically unstable tachycardias and poorly sustained tachycardias.

nonexcitatory stimulation. A stimulus that does not depolarize the cardiac chamber in which it was delivered. Any subthreshold stimulus could be considered nonexcitatory stimulation. However, this term is more likely to be used to describe the stimuli delivered with cardiac contractility modulation.

nonfluoroscopic navigation system. Methods used in an electrophysiology laboratory to minimize fluoroscopic exposure. These include noncontact mapping and electroanatomic mapping.

nonfluoroscopic three-dimensional mapping. Navigation systems and mapping systems allowing reconstruction of the cardiac chambers in three dimensions, used in addition to or in lieu of fluoroscopy. Currently used nonfluoroscopic three-dimensional mapping systems are noncontact mapping and electroanatomic mapping.

noninvasive electrophysiologic study. Electrophysiologic study done primarily to attempt induction of ventricular tachycardia, done via an implanted pacemaker or defibrillation, without use of intravenous elctrodes.

noninvasive emergency pacing. See *transcutaneous pacing.*

noninvasive programmed stimulation (NIPS). Arrhythmia induction performed via an implanted pacemaker or defibrillator such that the placement of catheters is not necessary.

noninvasive programming. See *programming.*

nonischemic cardiomyopathy. A cardiomyopathic process unrelated to underlying coronary artery disease and ischemic myocardial damage. The most common nonischemic cardiomyopathy is an idiopathic dilated cardiomyopathy.

nonlinear dynamics. See *chaos.*

nonparoxysmal junctional tachycardia (NPJT). An abnormal rhythm that arises from the atrioventricular junction. It is thought to be due to abnormal automaticity or triggered activity. It has gradual onset and termination, typically has a rate of 70 to 130 beats per minute, and often has concomitant atrioventricular dissociation. Nonparoxysmal junctional tachycardia most frequently is caused by digitalis toxicity, inferior myocardial infarction, myocarditis, or open-heart surgery.

nonpharmacologic therapy. Treatment of arrhythmias using means other than drugs. Nonpharmacologic therapy includes surgery, ablation, and the use of implanted arrhythmia-control devices.

nonphysiologic AV delay. A term sometimes used to describe the foreshortened atrioventricular interval of safety pacing.

nonphysiologic AV interval. See *safety pacing.*

nonprogrammable pacemaker. A pacemaker in which the pacing variables (e.g., rate, pulse width, sensitivity, voltage amplitude, refractory period) are preset during manufacture of the pacemaker and cannot be altered.

nonsustained tachycardia. An abnormally rapid heart rhythm, usually more than 100 beats per minute, that is not sustained. By convention, most investigators define a nonsustained tachycardia as one that persists for less than 30 seconds. See also *sustained tachycardia.*

nonsustained ventricular tachycardia (NSVT). A nonsustained tachycardia (see preceding entry) that originates from the ventricle.

nonthoracotomy lead. See *endocardial defibrillation lead, nonthoracotomy lead system.*

nonthoracotomy lead system. An implantable defibrillator lead system that is positioned without performing a thoracotomy. Nonthoracotomy lead systems are available in various configurations. The system may include endocardial leads positioned in the right ventricle, coronary sinus, or superior vena cava. In addition, a subcutaneous patch may be part of the system. A nonthoracotomy lead system is also known as a transvenous defibrillation lead system.

nonuniform conduction. When conduction velocities in three dimensions are distinctly different in either atrial or ventricular myocardium, nonuniform conduction of an impulse occurs. Nonuniform conduction may be associated with nonuniform refractoriness in diseased myocardium and promote the development of complex arrhythmias.

nonuniform recovery of excitability. See *dispersion of refractoriness.*

noradrenaline. See *norepinephrine.*

norepinephrine. The major catecholamine neurotransmitter of postganglionic sympathetic fibers. Norepinephrine is a potent stimulator of α_1, α_2, and β_1 receptors. Its effect on β_2 receptors is less pronounced.

normal sinus rhythm (NSR). Atrial activity that arises from the sinus node and drives the heart at a rate of 60 to 100 beats per minute.

North American Society of Pacing and Electrophysiology (NASPE). Founded in 1979, a professional organization whose goal is to disseminate information and education in the fields of implantable arrhythmia control devices, electrophysiology, and therapeutic approaches to cardiac arrhythmias.

North American Vasovagal Pacemaker Study I (VPS-I). In the North American Vasovagal Pacemaker Study, patients with a minimal number of syncopal episodes, syncope or presyncope induced with a tilt-table test, and a relative bradycardia were randomized to receive a dual-chamber pacemaker or no device. The study found a statistically significant reduction in syncopal episodes in the pacemaker group (Connolly SJ, Sheldon R, Roberts RS, Gent M, the Vasovagal Pacemaker Study Investigators. The North American Vasovagal Pacemaker Study [VPS]: a randomized trial of permanent cardiac pacing for the prevention of vasovagal syncope. J Am Coll Cardiol. 1999;33:16-20).

North American Vasovagal Pacemaker Study II (VPS-II). The North American Vasovagal Pacemaker Study II was a double-blind randomized trial to assess the efficacy of pacing therapy in vasovagal syncope. All patients received a pacemaker and were randomized to DDD pacing or no pacing (ODO). In contrast to the results of VPS-I, pacing therapy did not reduce the risk of recurrent syncope in patients with vasovagal syncope (Connolly SJ, Sheldon R, Thorpe KE, Roberts RS, Ellenbogen KA, Wilkoff BL, et al, VPS II Investigators. Pacemaker therapy for prevention of syncope in patients with recurrent severe vasovagal syncope: second Vasovagal Pacemaker Study [VPS II]: a randomized trial. JAMA. 2003;289:2224-9).

NPJT. Abbreviation for *nonparoxysmal junctional tachycardia.*

NSR. Abbreviation for *normal sinus rhythm.*

NSVT. Abbreviation for *nonsustained ventricular tachycardia.*

nuclear batteries. Batteries powered by a radioactive source. Plutonium 238 was used at one time as a pacemaker energy source.

nuclear magnetic resonance (NMR) imaging. See *magnetic resonance imaging.*

nuclear pacemakers. Pacemakers that use plutonium 238 as the energy source.

nuclear-powered pacemaker. A pacemaker powered by a radioisotopic material such as plutonium 238 or promethium 147. Heat produced in the battery by isotope decay is converted to electrical energy by a thermoelectric mechanism.

NYHA classification. See *New York Heart Association classification.*

O

O (none). Designation in the NBG and NBD codes for the lack of activity in a given chamber, be it sensing, pacing, or mode of response. See the figure *NBG code*.

OAO mode. A programmed mode in which there is atrial sensing but no pacing and no mode of response (i.e., the pulse generator does not react to any sensed atrial activity).

occlusive coronary sinus venography. Delineation of the coronary venous anatomy by injection of a contrast agent via a catheter with balloon occlusion of the proximal coronary sinus. The occluding balloon prevents retrograde reflux of the contrast dye and better pacification of the coronary sinus and tributaries. Occlusive coronary sinus venography often is performed before placement of left ventricular pacing leads or to visualize coronary sinus aneurysms or diverticula in epicardial accessory pathway ablation procedures.

ODO mode. A programmed mode in which there is atrial and ventricular sensing but no pacing and no mode of response (i.e., the pulse generator does not react to any sensed atrial or ventricular activity).

ohm (Ω). The basic unit of electrical resistance or impedance. When 1 ampere of current produces a voltage of 1 V across a conductor, the resistance or impedance is equal to 1 ohm.

Ohm's law. The mathematical expression of the relationship among voltage, current, and resistance. The current within a linear system is directly proportional to the voltage applied to the circuit. Ohm's law, in its most commonly used form, states that voltage (V) is the product of current (I) and resistance (R): V=IR.

one-dimensional reentry. Mechanism of arrythmogenesis in which the reentry circuit is confined to a one-dimensional layer of the myocardium (e.g., the endocardial layer or epicardial layer alone).

110-millisecond phenomenon. A term synonymous with ventricular safety pacing and nonphysiologic atrioventricular interval. In the first pacemakers to incorporate ventricular safety pacing, the shortened atrioventricular interval that occurred as a result of safety pacing was 110 milliseconds, and in most devices the nonphysiologic atrioventricular interval remains in the range of 100 to 110 milliseconds. See also *safety pacing*.

1:2 atrioventricular conduction. Sometimes a single atrial depolarization can result in two ventricular depolarizations. This phenomenon may occur in patients who have dual atrioventricular nodal physiology with sufficient differences in the conduction time through the fast pathway and the slow pathway and the absence of retrograde penetration via the fast pathway into the slow pathway. In sinus rhythm, a single P wave is associated with two QRS complexes. 1:2 Atrioventricular conduction also may rarely occur in patients with atrioventricular node conduction and accessory pathway conduction.

onset. A programmable function in some implantable cardioverter-defibrillators that modifies detection and allows the device to attempt to discriminate between sinus tachycardia and ventricular tachycardia. To diagnose ventricular tachycardia, the algorithm watches for an abrupt shortening in cycle length.

open circuit. An electrical circuit broken at one or more points. An open circuit does not have a complete path for current flow and thus cannot conduct current. In pacing, an open circuit occurs if the conductor of the pacing lead fractures or if the terminal pin is loose in the connector block. An open circuit is indicated by complete loss of pacing and sensing. See also *incomplete circuit*.

open-loop control system. Automatic modification of an adjustable variable (such as pacing rate) that is under the control of a variable (such as mechanical vibration) that is not itself affected by the adjustable variable. In pacing, open-loop control requires the use of sensors. The control systems are designed within the pacemaker circuitry to continually monitor and process information collected by the sensor(s). See also *closed-loop control system*.

open-loop rate-adaptive pacemaker system. See *open-loop control system.*

open-loop system. See *open-loop control system.*

OPSITE. See *Optimal Pacing SITE.*

OPT. Abbreviation for *optimized pharmacologic therapy.*

optical mapping. Use of optical dyes to visualize wave-front propagation in myocardial tissue. Optical mapping has been an important tool in understanding the three-dimensional aspects of wave-front propagation.

Optimal Pacing SITE (OPSITE). This trial was a prospective, randomized, single-blind, 3-month crossover trial that compared right ventricle- and left ventricle-only pacing and right ventricular and biventricular pacing. Pacing only the left ventricle and biventricular pacing provided modest or no additional favorable effect compared with right ventricular pacing (Brignole M, Gammage M, Puggioni E, Alboni P, Raviele A, Sutton R, et al, Optimal Pacing SITE [OPSITE] Study Investigators. Comparative assessment of right, left, and biventricular pacing in patients with permanent atrial fibrillation. Eur Heart J. 2005 Apr;26:712-22. Epub 2004 Dec 20).

optimized pharmacologic therapy (OPT). As the term relates to device therapy, one of the labeling criteria requirements of the U.S. Food and Drug Administration for cardiac resynchronization therapy. There is no specific definition, but the term generally implies that the patient is receiving optimal angiotensin-converting enzyme inhibitor or angiotensin II receptor blocker therapy, β-blockers, and diuretic therapy.

OptiVol. Trademark for a feature of a cardiac resynchronization system that automatically monitors intrathoracic fluid status (Medtronic, Inc., Minneapolis, Minnesota). The purpose is to assess a patient's fluid status by measuring, tracking, and reporting intrathoracic impedance. A change in intrathoracic impedance, and thus intrathoracic fluid status, may presage clinical deterioration and allow early treatment of cardiac compensation and prevent hospitalization for heart failure.

ORT. Abbreviation for *orthodromic reciprocating tachycardia.*

orthodromic atrioventricular reciprocating tachycardia. Common form of supraventricular tachycardia in which antegrade conduction of the reentrant circuit occurs via the atrioventricular node and the retrograde limb of the circuit is through an accessory pathway.

orthodromic atrioventricular reentrant tachycardia. See *orthodromic atrioventricular reciprocating tachycardia.*

orthodromic entrainment in ventricular tachycardia. Continuous resetting (entrainment) of the tachycardia which occurs with little change in the intraventricular activation sequence when pacing during ventricular tachycardia. Typically, entrainment performed from sites close to the exit or within the slow zone of the tachycardia circuit results in orthodromic entrainment. See also *entrainment.*

orthodromic pacemaker tachycardia. Form of pacemaker-mediated tachycardia in which the antegrade limb of the circuit is completed by the pacemaker. See also *pacemaker-mediated tachycardia.*

orthodromic paroxysmal supraventricular tachycardia. See *orthodromic atrioventricular reciprocating tachycardia.*

orthodromic propagation. Propagation in the usual direction of conduction. For example, in atrioventricular tachycardia in which an accessory pathway is present, when the tachycardia circuit involves antegrade conduction through the atrioventricular node (usual direction) orthodromic reciprocating tachycardia is said to result. See also *orthodromic atrioventricular reciprocating tachycardia.*

orthodromic reciprocating tachycardia (ORT). Atrioventricular reentrant tachycardia utilizing the atrioventricular node as the antegrade limb and an accessory pathway as the retrograde limb.

orthodromic tachycardia. See *orthodromic atrioventricular reciprocating tachycardia.*

orthogonal floating atrial lead. See *orthogonal sensing.*

orthogonal lead. A catheter with electrodes located circumferentially around the catheter such that it can record electrical activity with a vector perpendicular to the long axis of the catheter. Orthogonal leads are useful for recording accessory pathway activity from within the coronary sinus.

orthogonal sensing. In pacing, sensing that occurs at a right angle from the pacing lead. This term is used to describe atrial sensing in a single-lead VDD system in which P-synchronous pacing occurs in the ventricle and atrial activity is sensed from electrodes incorporated into the body of the lead, which is positioned in the atrial cavity.

orthorhythmic pacing. A type of burst stimulation in which the external stimuli are coupled to a sensed tachycardia at an interval that is related, by some proportion, to the tachycardia cycle length. In orthorhythmic pacing, the tachycardia termination window is not directly proportional to the tachycardia cycle length. Research to date demonstrates a higher degree of successful tachycardia termination with orthorhythmic pacing than with nonorthorhythmic pacing. See also *antitachycardia pacing, burst stimulation, coupled electrical stimulus.*

orthostatic hypotension. A decrease in blood pressure upon assuming an upright position. It has been more precisely defined as a sustained decrease in blood pressure more than 20 mm Hg systolic or 10 mm Hg diastolic that occurs within 3 minutes of head-up tilt. Orthostatic hypotension is thought to be a sign of autonomic dysfunction.

Osborne wave. A low-amplitude, low-frequency wave at the terminal portion of the QRS on the surface electrocardiogram. Osborne waves, also known as J waves, occur frequently in hypothermia and rarely in hypercalcemia.

oscillator. An electronic circuit that spontaneously generates a repetitive signal, such as a steady sine wave or a series of regular pulses. The frequency of the output may be constant or varied, depending on the circuit components and other factors such as programmable variables. In pacing, the oscillator circuit is composed of a resistance-capacitance network or a quartz crystal, which establishes the pulse interval. Examples of oscillator applications in pacing include pacemaker pulse generation, telemetry carrier signals, and microprocessor clocks. The oscillator circuit also may be referred to as the timing circuit. See also *quartz-crystal oscillator.*

ostial-atrial junction. Complex anatomic location between the pulmonary vein and left atrium. Also may refer to the junction of other venous structures and the atrium, such as the superior vena cava-right atrial junction. This complex region is highly arrhythmogenic and may represent an area of slowed and decremental conduction targeted during ablation procedures for atrial fibrillation.

ostial pulmonary vein. Portion of the pulmonary vein at a venous confluence or junction with the left atrium. The ostial pulmonary vein is often the site for placement of ablative lesions

in a circumferential manner for the treatment of atrial fibrillation.

ouabain. The common name for G-strophanthin. In higher concentrations (i.e., in vitro or intravenously), ouabain blocks Na+,K+-ATPase. Recently, the concept has developed that ouabain at low concentrations has the opposite effect (i.e., stimulation of Na+,K+-ATPase).

outflow tract. Anatomic region of the chest caudal to the great arteries. The right ventricular outflow tract is the ventricular myocardium just below the pulmonary valve, and the left ventricular outflow tract is the region of ventricular myocardium just below the aortic valve.

outflow tract ventricular tachycardia. Common form of ventricular tachycardia that typically arises in patients with structurally normal hearts. Right ventricular outflow tract tachycardia is more common than left ventricular outflow tract tachycardia. These tachycardias are characterized typically by being catecholamine-sensitive and can be treated with β-blockers or catheter ablation.

output. The current, voltage, energy, or power delivered by a circuit or device. In pacing, output refers to the electrical output generated by a pacemaker and delivered to the heart either to cause a depolarization or to mark a spontaneous depolarization in a triggered pacing mode such as AAT or VVT.

output (cardiac). See *cardiac output.*

output circuit. A portion of the pacemaker circuitry used for the delivery of appropriate electrical stimuli from the pacemaker to the heart. A capacitor within the output circuit is charged until a voltage-sensitive switch, controlled by the timing circuit, closes and results in the discharge of electrical stimuli through the pacing lead.

output (pacemaker). The electrical output delivered from a pulse generator. The output usually is defined in terms of pulse width (ms) and voltage (V).

output switching. An electrical switch that may be necessary to deliver required output. Different pathways require different configurations of switches. For example, in a biphasic shock the voltage on the capacitor is connected to the leads in one direction by two switches for the first phase and then reversed for the second phase by two other switches. The switches that are on in phase 1 are off in phase 2, and vice versa. A pacing pulse also has two pathways, one for the pace and a second for recharge. Extra switches are needed to achieve the necessary recharge.

oval fossa. Remnant of the fetal interatrial connection. The oval fossa is the site targeted for transseptal puncture and is bounded superiorly by the superior limbus and inferiorly by the inferior limbic continuation of the eustachian ridge. See also *eustachian ridge, fossa ovalis, superior limbus.*

overdrive pacing. Pacing at a rate faster than the intrinsic heart rate. Overdrive pacing gains electrical control of the heart by suppressing intrinsic activity or terminating a tachycardia. Overdrive pacing is especially useful for the termination of atrial flutter between 230 and 250 beats per minute. In some cases, it can be used for the termination of ventricular tachycardia. In torsades de pointes due to acquired long QT syndrome, overdrive pacing may be used to prevent tachycardias that usually are initiated by bradycardia or pauses. See also *external overdrive.*

overdriver. See *external overdrive.*

overdrive suppression. Inhibition of automaticity or conduction brought on by rapid pacing. Overdrive suppression usually is a transient phenomenon.

overpotential. See *overvoltage.*

oversensing. The sensing of events other than cardiac signals by the pacemaker circuitry or, less commonly, inadvertent multiple sensing of single cardiac pulses (double counting) by an implantable cardioverter-defibrillator. Events that are potentially oversensed include myopotentials, electromagnetic interference, T waves, P waves, and crosstalk between the atrial and ventricular channels. Depending on the pacing mode, oversensing may cause an inhibited or triggered mode of response from the pacemaker. In implantable cardioverter-defibrillators, oversensing may cause overdetection and inappropriate delivery of therapies. See also *undersensing.*

over-the-wire leads. Pacemaker leads used in cardiac resynchronization devices for left ventricular pacing. These leads have the advantage that once a wire has been negotiated into the selected left ventricular venous tributary of the coronary sinus the lead can be advanced over that wire.

overvoltage. A voltage greater than that at which a device or circuit is designed to operate. In pacing, overvoltage is supplied by the pacemaker output circuit to overcome the electrochemical polarization effects that take place at the electrode-myocardial interface. The overvoltage is greater than the voltage otherwise required for pacing at the stimulation threshold of the myocardium.

OVO mode. A programmed mode in which there is ventricular sensing but no pacing and no mode of response (i.e., the pulse generator does not react to any sensed ventricular activity).

oxygen consumption. The body's ability to take in oxygen, deliver it to working tissues (e.g., muscles), and use it to release cellular energy. Measurement of the body's highest rate of oxygen uptake ($\dot{V}O_2$max) is an important indicator of aerobic performance.

oxygen saturation sensing. Determination of the oxygen saturation level by the use of sensors that measure changes in the oxygen saturation of blood. Oxygen saturation reflects the utilization of oxygen from oxygenated hemoglobin and, therefore, reflects activity or exercise of the patient. Oxygen saturation sensors may be used in closed-loop rate-adaptive pacing systems to control pacing rate.

Oversensing

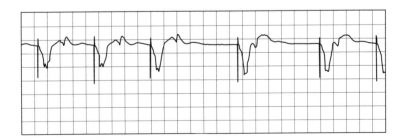

P

PAC. Abbreviation for *premature atrial complex, premature atrial contraction.*

paced activation sequence mapping. The activation sequence can be mapped using any of the available electroanatomic mapping systems. This maneuver is performed in the electrophysiology laboratory in two circumstances: 1) as part of a voltage mapping procedure used to define areas of slow conduction and scar—the paced activation sequence is mapped instead of the tachycardia when the tachycardia is associated with hemodynamic collapse or is not sufficiently sustained; 2) as an adjunct to entrainment mapping for reentrant tachycardias—after the tachycardia circuit has been mapped during continuous resetting when pacing (entrainment), another map is generated. If the maps thus generated are identical or nearly identical, concealed entrainment and overdrive suppression of a mistakenly diagnosed automatic arrhythmia are the diagnoses to consider. See also *electroanatomic mapping, scar-based ablation.*

paced AV interval. Programmed duration from the delivered atrial pacing stimulus to the ventricular pacing stimulus.

paced cycle length (PCL). The amount of time from the delivery of one programmed electrical stimulus to the next consecutive programmed electrical stimulus. Paced cycle length can be used to refer to the interval between pacemaker output pulses. However, it is used most frequently to refer to the interval between the stimuli of the drive train during programmed electrical testing. See also *drive cycle.*

paced depolarization integral (PDI). Integration of the paced R wave which yields the ventricular depolarization gradient. The ventricular depolarization gradient is dependent on activation sequence and the dispersion of activation. The ventricular depolarization gradient remains stable in a patient with a normal chronotropic response. Paced depolarization integral is a variable that has been used for rate-adaptive pacing.

pace limit. A mechanism of the pacemaker hardware or software designed to protect against extremely rapid stimulation of the myocardium by the pacemaker as a result of component malfunctions. Pace limit is a safety feature designed to prevent runaway pacemakers. Pacemakers typically are limited to a maximum rate of 180 pulses per minute. Pace limit also is referred to as rate limit. See also *runaway pacemaker.*

pacemaker (PM). 1. Physiologically, a small mass of specialized cells within the heart that periodically give rise to an electrical impulse that initiates a wave of depolarization and causes cardiac contraction. Normally, the sinus node is the primary pacemaker of the heart. However, in various arrhythmias or atrioventricular block, other myocardial cells such as the atrioventricular node or ectopic foci can assume the role of the dominant pacemaker. 2. A device that periodically delivers an electrical stimulus to the myocardium to initiate a wave of depolarization and cause cardiac contraction. Most pacemakers have the capacity to sense spontaneous intrinsic cardiac activity and to deliver output pulses through a lead to the endocardium or epicardium. The manner in which a pacemaker responds to sensed intrinsic activity and the manner in which it delivers output pulses depend on the preset or programmed mode. A pacemaker consists of the power source, the electronic circuitry, the pacemaker feed through(s), the lead connector(s), and the pacemaker header aperture(s) for connection of the pacing lead(s) to the pacemaker. A pacemaker may be an external system, connected to myocardial tissue by temporarily implanted pacing leads, or a fully implanted system, inclusive of the pacemaker and the lead(s). Used generically, the term pacemaker may refer to the full pacing system, that is, the power source, the electronic circuits, the encapsulation material, the lead(s), the connector(s), and the electrode(s). A pacemaker also is referred to as a pulse generator. See also *external pacemaker, permanent pacemaker, temporary pacemaker.*

179

pacemaker alternans. The alternate change in the morphology of QRS depolarization complexes initiated by ventricular pacemaker output pulses, as seen on an electrocardiographic recording. The alternate complexes occur at equally spaced intervals with a constant spike amplitude. Pacemaker alternans may be caused by pericardial effusion, respiratory phasic fluctuations, or unusual electrolyte or metabolic disturbances. Pacemaker alternans is not common.

pacemaker artifact. See *stimulus artifact*.

pacemaker can. See *pacemaker case*.

pacemaker case. The outer portion of the pacemaker that houses and protects the battery and electronic circuitry of the pacemaker. The pacemaker case usually is made of titanium and is sealed hermetically to protect the electronic components of the pacemaker from fluid invasion. Also referred to as the pulse generator can.

pacemaker circus-movement tachycardia (PCMT). See *pacemaker-mediated tachycardia*.

pacemaker click. An auscultatory finding in patients who have a pacemaker that describes an extra heart sound, which may be due to contact between the pacemaker lead and the tricuspid valve. In an asymptomatic patient, pacemaker click has no clinical significance.

pacemaker current. See I_f.

pacemaker dependent. There is no generally agreed on definition of pacemaker dependency. This lack of agreement confounds the clinician's efforts to categorize patients at greatest risk in the event of a sudden failure of the pacemaker system. Pacemaker dependence could be defined as being present when abrupt cessation of pacing results in bradycardia-related symptoms or signs that create an emergency or urgent clinical situation. Similarly, a history of symptoms or signs of an emergency or urgent situation in the absence of pacing, that is, before pacing, may constitute pacemaker dependency. From a practical standpoint, pacemaker dependency may be categorized in three classes. Class 1: abrupt cessation of pacing results in bradycardia-related symptoms or signs that create an emergency or urgent clinical situation, or there is a history of symptoms or signs of an emergency or urgent nature. Class 2: Patients are asymptomatic, have less than an urgent or emergency clinical situation when there is no intrinsic escape rate or rhythm at the lowest programmable rate setting of the implanted pacemaker, or remain asymptomatic if the escape rate is less than 30 beats per minute. Class 3: there is an escape rate more than 30 beats per minute and no history of an emergency or urgent clinical situation related to bradycardia. Patients in class 3 are not pacemaker-dependent.

pacemaker depolarization. Excitation of the myocardium as a result of pacemaker stimulus delivery.

pacemaker header. The superior portion of a pacemaker or implantable cardioverter-defibrillator that contains the connector block. The header houses the receptacles into which the lead connectors are inserted. Pacemaker headers usually are made of clear epoxy resin. See also *connector block, lead connector, lead terminal pin*.

pacemaker identification. See *radiopaque identification letters*.

pacemaker-induced arrhythmia (PIA). See *pacemaker-induced tachycardia*.

pacemaker-induced tachycardia. In a patient with a permanent pacemaker, any tachycardia that would not have occurred had the pacemaker not been present. There are multiple types of pacemaker-induced tachycardia. A tachycardia may be induced if competition occurs between pacing and intrinsic depolarization of a cardiac chamber. For example, if a pacemaker stimulus occurs in the vulnerable period of ventricular or atrial repolarization, the consequence could be ventricular or atrial tachycardia or fibrillation. Abnormally rapid rhythms caused by a runaway pacemaker are no longer a common occurrence but also constitute a form of pacemaker-induced tachycardia. See also *pacemaker runaway, runaway pacemaker*.

pacemaker-mediated tachycardia (PMT). A paced rhythm that can occur in patients with pacemakers capable of P-synchronous ventricular pacing. Pacemaker-mediated tachycardia begins with an event that allows atrioventricular dissociation and subsequent ventricular events to be conducted retrograde to the atria, resulting in atrial depolarization. The retrograde atrial depolarization is sensed and, after the appropriate atrioventricular interval, the pacemaker delivers a stimulus to the ventricle. Thus, the pacemaker provides the antegrade conduction pathway for the reentrant circuit, and the intrinsic conduction system of the heart provides the retrograde pathway. A repetitive cycle can

Pacemaker-Mediated Tachycardia

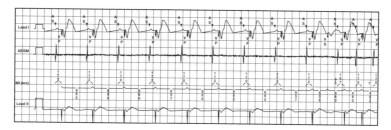

then be maintained. Pacemaker-mediated tachycardia also is called endless-loop tachycardia or pacemaker circus-movement tachycardia. Pacemaker-mediated tachycardia may be incessant or self-limited. Most dual-chamber pacemakers now have programmable features designed to prevent or terminate pacemaker-mediated tachycardia. See also *pacemaker-mediated tachycardia mechanism, pacemaker-mediated tachycardia protection, sensor-mediated tachycardia.*

pacemaker-mediated tachycardia mechanism. A process or event, intrinsic or pacemaker-related, that initiates a pacemaker-mediated tachycardia. Pacemaker-mediated tachycardia can be initiated by various mechanisms, including premature ventricular contractions, nonconducted premature atrial contractions, mode changes, loss of atrial capture, myopotentials, electromagnetic interference, echo beats, Wenckebach effect, and paroxysmal atrial tachycardia.

pacemaker-mediated tachycardia protection. A function of dual-chamber pacemakers that minimizes the initiation or continuation of a pacemaker-mediated tachycardia. Pacemaker-mediated tachycardia protection varies in different pacemakers and often is a programmable function. Examples of pacemaker-mediated tachycardia protection functions include lengthening of the programmed atrial refractory period, an automatic extension of the atrial refractory period after a sensed premature ventricular contraction, and a dropped ventricular output pulse after a predetermined number of beats at a specified rate or upper rate limit.

pacemaker monitor. A programmable function of some pacemakers that enables the pacemaker to monitor specific events occurring within the heart for a specific amount of time and to record and store this information for retrieval by telemetry. Examples of information available by use of the pacemaker monitor include the average pacing rate, the percentage of paced and sensed events, the number of premature ventricular contractions, and the data regarding sensor activation in pacemakers capable of rate adaption. See also *diagnostic data.*

pacemaker multiblock. During periods of intrinsic atrial rhythm or supraventricular tachycardia at rates that exceed the upper tracking rate (cycle length less than the total atrial refractory period), 2:1 or higher grade atrioventricular block results. See also *pseudo-Wenckebach response, total atrial refractory period.*

pacemaker neck. See *pacemaker header.*

pacemaker pocket. A surgically created cavity into which a pacemaker is placed at the time of implantation. The pacemaker pocket usually is subcutaneous and is located in the prepectoral region in adults. In most children, the pacemaker also is placed in the prepectoral position, but occasionally it is placed in the abdominal region. Implantable cardioverter-defibrillators and cardiac resynchronization devices are also usually placed in a prepectoral position.

pacemaker programming. See *programming.*

pacemaker radiography. Radiographic assessment of a temporary or permanent pacing system. Pacemaker radiography is used for visual identification of the pacing system and for visual inspection of pacing system components during troubleshooting of a pacing system malfunction. See also *radiographic identification, radiopaque identification letters.*

pacemaker reentry tachycardia. See *pacemaker-mediated tachycardia.*

pacemaker-related tachycardia. A tachycardia that is in any way related to the presence of the pacemaker. The tachycardia may be pacemaker-induced (atrial or ventricular tachycardia or fibrillation) or pacemaker-mediated (endless-loop tachycardia).

pacemaker runaway. With contemporary devices, a rare occurrence in which a malfunction of the central processing unit allows an acceleration of the pacing rate to extraordinarily fast rates, far above the upper rate limit, constituting life-threatening dysrhythmias. Known causes of pacemaker runaway include loss of the hermetic seal, allowing fluids into the circuitry and device exposure to therapeutic radiation.

Pacemaker Selection in the Elderly (PASE). This randomized trial assessed the effect of pacing mode on morbidity and mortality. The study found an improvement in quality of life with pacing compared with no pacing, but there was no significant difference between VVI and physiologic pacemakers in terms of mortality, cardiovascular events, or quality of life. A significant percentage of patients, 26%, who were intolerant of ventricular pacing had crossover to dual-chamber pacing (Lamas GA, Orav EJ, Stambler BS, Ellenbogen KA, Sgarbossa EB, Huang SK, et al, Pacemaker Selection in the Elderly Investigators. Quality of life and clinical outcomes in elderly patients treated with ventricular pacing as compared with dual-chamber pacing. N Engl J Med. 1998;338:1097-104).

pacemaker syndrome. An assortment of symptoms related to the adverse hemodynamic impact of the loss of atrioventricular synchrony. Pacemaker syndrome occurs most commonly in VVI pacing, with the atria contracting in any pacing mode if atrioventricular dissociation occurs. It may be associated with a significant decrease in blood pressure during pacing. Symptoms of pacemaker syndrome may include fatigue, dizziness, near-syncope or syncope, chest discomfort, dyspnea, cough, and neck pulsations.

pacemaker systems analyzer (PSA). An external testing device used to assess lead or pacemaker function by measuring various factors at the time of pacemaker or lead implantation or replacement. Measurements commonly include R-wave or P-wave amplitude (measured in millivolts), stimulation threshold (measured in volts and milliamperes), impedance (measured in ohms), and slew rate.

pacemaker Wenckebach. See *pseudo-Wenckebach response*.

pace mapping. An electrophysiologic testing technique used to identify the site of origin of a tachycardia, usually ventricular. Multiple sites are paced during sinus rhythm at the same cycle length as the tachycardia. The 12-lead electrocardiogram generated from pacing at each site is then compared with the electrocardiogram of the tachycardia to compare the morphology of the QRS (in ventricular tachycardia) or the morphology of the P wave (in atrial tachycardia). Pace mapping should not be confused with entrainment. See also *entrainment*.

pace per minute. Pacing rate. Although this term is sometimes used synonomously with beats per minute, it more correctly refers to an intrinsic rate.

pacing circuit. The electrical components of a pacemaker that provide the proper electrical stimuli (the pacemaker output pulses) and the properly timed delivery of the output pulses from the pacemaker to the myocardium in order to depolarize and capture the heart. See also *oscillator, output circuit*.

pacing configuration. Generic term referring to the polarity of the pacing system (i.e., unipolar vs. bipolar pacing).

pacing cycle length (PCL). The amount of time from the delivery of one programmed electrical stimulus to the next consecutive programmed electrical stimulus. Pacing cycle length can be used to refer to the interval between pacemaker output pulses. However, it is used most often to refer to the interval of the basic drive train during electrophysiologic testing.

Pacing Evaluation-Atrial Support in Cardiac Resynchronization Therapy (PEGASUS-CRT). This study is investigating the effect of a cardiac resynchronization therapy defibrillator programmed to DDD-70 or DDDR-40 to DDD-40. The primary end point is to assess the effect of atrial support pacing on a clinical composite score consisting of all-cause mortality, heart failure events, New York Heart Association class, and a global assessment tool. Secondary end points include quality of life, arrhythmia rates, and the effect of lead positions (ClinicalTrials.gov [homepage on the Internet]. Bethesda: U.S. Department of Health and Human Services National Institutes of Health [updated 2006 Nov 20; cited 2007 Feb 2]. PEGASUS CRT Study: Atrial Support Study in Cardiac Resynchronization Therapy. Available from: http://www.clinicaltrials.gov/ct/show/NCT00146848).

Pacing in Cardiomyopathy (PIC). This randomized clinical trial assessed the efficacy of pacemaker therapy in patients with hypertrophic cardiomyopathy and symptoms refractory to medical therapy. Although this trial suggested a potential therapeutic role for pacing in hypertrophic cardiomyopathy, a subsequent trial was less convincing and pacing is rarely used today for treatment of symptoms related to hypertrophic cardiomyopathy (Kappenberger LJ, Linde C, Jeanrenaud X, Daubert C, McKenna W, Meisel E, et al, Pacing in Cardiomyopathy [PIC] Study Group. Clinical progress after randomized on/off pacemaker treatment for hypertrophic obstructive cardiomyopathy. Europace. 1999;1:77-84).

pacing interval. The amount of time in a pacemaker timing cycle between two consecutive pacemaker output pulses. The pacing interval is a representation of the pacemaker rate and is either preset or programmable. The pacing interval is measured in milliseconds.

pacing mode. The manner in which a pacemaker provides rate and rhythm support. Pacing modes are described by the NBG code, a five-letter designation that indicates the chamber(s) paced, the chamber(s) sensed, the mode of response to sensed events (inhibited or triggered), programmability, and multisite pacing. Conventionally, only the first three positions (letters) of the NBG code are used to specify the pacing mode. See also *AAI, AAIR, AAT, AATR, AOO, DAD, DDD, DDDR, DDI, DDIR, DOO, DVI, DVIR, VAT, VDD, VDDR, VOO, VVI, VVIR, VVT.* •

pacing spikes. A term used synonymously for pacemaker stimuli or artifacts.

pacing system analyser (PSA). See *pacemaker systems analyzer*.

pacing system infection. Acute or chronic infection involving the pacemaker pocket, leads, or pulse generator. The most common warning signs of infection are local inflammation and abscess formation involving the pacemaker pocket and fever or systemic symptoms. Erosion of part of the pulse generator or lead(s) through the skin often is followed by secondary infection. Early postimplantation infections are caused most commonly by *Staphylococcus aureus* and often are associated with fever and systemic symptoms. Late infections are caused most commonly by *Staphylococcus epidermidis* and often are not associated with fever or systemic symptoms.

Pacing Therapies in Congestive Heart Failure I (PATH-CHF I). This single-blind, randomized, crossover, controlled trial was designed to evaluate the acute hemodynamic effects and to assess the long-term clinical benefit of right ventricular, left ventricular, and biventricular pacing in patients with moderate-to-severe chronic heart failure and interventricular conduction block. Acutely, biventricular and left ventricular pacing increased dP/dt and pulse pressure more than right ventricular pacing. There was a trend toward improvement of the primary end points: oxygen consumption at peak exercise and at anaerobic threshold during cardiopulmonary exercise testing and on 6-minute hall walk distance (Auricchio A, Stellbrink C, Sack S, Block M, Vogt J, Bakker P, et al, Pacing Therapies in Congestive Heart Failure [PATH-CHF] Study Group. Long-term clinical effect of hemodynamically optimized cardiac resynchronization therapy in patients with heart failure and ventricular conduction delay. J Am Coll Cardiol. 2002;39:2026-33).

Pacing Therapies in Congestive Heart Failure II (PATH-CHF II). This study was designed to assess the effect of cardiac resynchronization on echocardiographic variables; patients underwent hemodynamic testing before and after cardiac resynchronization. The study found that cardiac resynchronization may lead to a reduction in left ventricular volumes in patients with advanced heart failure and conduction disturbances (Auricchio A, Stellbrink C, Butter C, Sack S, Vogt J, Misier AR, et al, Pacing Therapies in Congestive Heart Failure [PATH-CHF] II Study Group; Guidant Heart Failure Research Group. Clinical efficacy of cardiac resynchronization therapy using left ventricular pacing in heart failure patients stratified by severity of ventricular conduction delay. J Am Coll Cardiol. 2003;42:2109-16).

pacing threshold. The minimum electrical stimulation (pacemaker output pulse) required to consistently initiate atrial or ventricular depolarization and cardiac contraction. The voltage required to obtain capture usually is greater than the value at which capture is lost. Pacing thresholds may change in response to physiologic changes such as exit block, maturation at the electrode-myocardial interface, and myocardial infarction and in response to changes brought about by external sources such as

Pacing Modes

VOO	Ventricular pacing; no sensing	DOO	Dual-chamber pacing; no sensing
VVI	Ventricular pacing; ventricular sensing and inhibition	DVI	Dual-chamber pacing; ventricular sensing and inhibition; no tracking of the atrium
VVT	Ventricular pacing; ventricular sensing and triggering	DVIR	Dual-chamber pacing; ventricular sensing and inhibition; no tracking of the atrium; AV sequential rate modulation
VVIR	Ventricular pacing; ventricular sensing with inhibition; rate-modulated pacing	DDI	Dual-chamber pacing; dual-chamber sensing and inhibition; no tracking of the atrium
VOOR	Ventricular pacing; no sensing; rate-modulated pacing	DDIR	Dual-chamber pacing; dual-chamber sensing and inhibition; no tracking of the atrium; AV sequential rate modulation
AOO	Atrial pacing; no sensing	VDD	Ventricular pacing; dual-chamber sensing; tracking of the atrium with ventricular inhibition
AAI	Atrial pacing; atrial sensing and inhibition	VDDR*	Ventricular pacing; dual-chamber sensing; tracking of atrium with ventricular inhibition and ventricular rate modulation
AAT	Atrial pacing; atrial sensing and triggering	DDD	Dual-chamber pacing; dual-chamber sensing and inhibition; tracking of the atrium
AAIR	Atrial pacing; atrial sensing with inhibition; rate-modulated pacing	DDDR	Dual-chamber pacing; dual-chamber sensing and inhibition; tracking of the atrium; AV sequential rate modulation
AOOR	Atrial pacing; no sensing; rate modulation	DOOR	Dual-chamber pacing; insensitive; AV sequential rate modulation
		OOO	Pacemaker is programmed "off" (allows assessment of underlying rhythm)

AV, atrioventricular.

*VDDR is a misnomer by the North American Society of Pacing and Electrophysiology/British Pacing and Electrophysiology Group code for pacing modes. The "R" in this context would generally indicate the capability of dual-chamber, sensor-driven pacing. However, VDD by definition excludes atrial pacing. The designation VDDR is being used by manufacturers for a device that operates in a P-synchronous mode except when sensor-driven, when pacing may be VVIR or DDDR, depending on the specific device.

From Hayes DL, Lloyd MA, Friedman PA. Cardiac pacing and defibrillation: a clinical approach. Armonk: Futura Publishing Company, Inc; 2000. p. 247-323. Copyrighted and used with permission of Mayo Foundation for Medical Education and Research.

pharmacologic therapy and defibrillation. Pacing thresholds may be measured invasively with a pacing systems analyzer or noninvasively via the programmer. Pacing thresholds usually are expressed in volts and milliamperes at a specified pulse duration. See also *acute pacing threshold, chronic pacing threshold, peak threshold, strength-duration curve, threshold maturation.*

pacing train. A series of pacing stimuli. A pacing train usually is delivered to induce or terminate a tachycardia.

PA interval. The amount of time that it takes for a wave of depolarization to travel from the sinus nodes to the atrioventricular node, that is, internodal conduction time. The PA interval is measured from the earliest onset of the P wave to the onset of atrial activation on the His-bundle electrogram. Typical values range from 10 to 45 milliseconds.

paired electrical stimuli. Two programmed electrical stimuli that are delivered in sequence at some preset or programmable interval. Paired electrical stimuli are used in electrophysiologic testing to initiate and terminate tachycardias and in antitachycardia pacemakers to terminate tachycardias by delivery of the stimuli at a critically timed interval.

palpitations. The sensation of rapid or irregular cardiac activity.

panel. See *advisory committee.*

paradoxical undersensing. Undersensing rarely may occur when the atrial sensitivity is programmed to a very sensitive setting (in which, typically, oversensing and not undersensing occurs). This is usually due to "ringing" or saturation of the atrial channel and results in virtual extension of an atrial blanking period, and thus rapid atrial events such as atrial fibrillation or atrial tachycardia are undersensed. When this occurs, failure to mode switch may result. Paradoxical undersensing is also more generally used to refer to situations in which undersensing of one chamber's events occurs because of oversensing of other electrical events (e.g., ventricular oversensing may give rise to extension of the postventricular atrial refractory period, and thus atrial events may be undersensed).

parahisian accessory pathways. Accessory pathways located close to the His bundle are referred to as parahisian pathways. These may be further subdivided into right anterior free wall pathways (in which risk of atrioventricular block with ablation is lower but catheter contact may be difficult), anteroseptal accessory pathways (higher risk of atrioventricular block with ablation but catheter contact obtained with ease), and midseptal accessory pathways (highest risk of atrioventricular block with ablation but usually no difficulty with obtaining catheter contact).

parahisian pacing. A maneuver used to distinguish retrograde atrial activation occurring over septal accessory pathway from that occurring over the normal ventriculoatrial conduction system. An electrode catheter is placed near the His bundle and pacing occurs at a constant cycle length with decreasing pulse amplitude, beginning at a high output. The His bundle is captured initially, but then His-bundle capture is

Parahisian Pacing

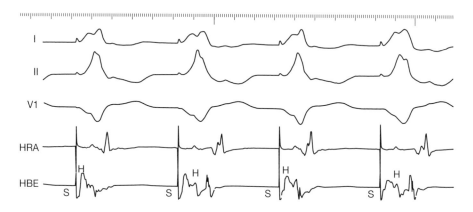

lost and ventricular capture occurs as the output is reduced. Changes in the ventriculo-His (VH) and ventriculoatrial (VA) intervals are assessed. In the presence of an accessory pathway, the VH interval lengthens and the VA interval remains constant as His-bundle capture is lost. However, with atrioventricular nodal conduction, both the VH and VA intervals prolong.

parameter. In pacing, a parameter is one of many elements that govern the function and behavior of a pacemaker. Many pacing parameters are programmable and may include, for example, pacing mode, pacing rate, pulse duration, atrioventricular interval, refractory periods, sensitivity, and voltage amplitude.

parasympathetic denervation. The interruption of vagal innervation. In the ventricles, the vagal fibers are located in the subendocardial region and thus can be damaged by transmural or subendocardial ischemia or infarction. Denervation supersensitivity to acetylcholine has been demonstrated in the sinus and atrioventricular nodes.

parasympathetic nervous system. The portion of the autonomic nervous system that is carried by the vagus nerve and its branches and activates muscarinic postganglionic receptors. Efferent parasympathetic activation causes sinus slowing, prolongation of conduction through the atrioventricular node, and shortening of refractoriness in both the atria and the ventricles. In the ventricles, the parasympathetic nerves course in a base-to-apex orientation within the subendocardium. See also *cardiovascular regulatory center, sympathetic nervous system.*

parasystole. A relatively regular rhythm originating in a protected focus. The focus can be modulated but cannot be reset by impulses from other sites in the heart. Parasystolic rhythms demonstrate variable coupling to the underlying cardiac rhythm and periodic fusion complexes. See also *modulated parasystole.*

paroxysmal atrial fibrillation. Atrial fibrillation that terminates spontaneously without the need for cardioversion. Episodes may be numerous and often arise from the pulmonary veins.

paroxysmal atrial tachycardia (PAT). An abrupt episode of tachycardia that emanates from an ectopic atrial focus. Paroxysmal atrial tachycardia may occur in normal hearts.

paroxysmal supraventricular tachycardia (PSVT). A term that usually refers to atrio-

ventricular nodal reentrant tachycardia or atrioventricular reentrant tachycardia involving an accessory pathway. However, paroxysmal supraventricular tachycardia also may be used to refer to all supraventricular tachycardias that begin abruptly.

paroxysmal tachycardia. A recurrent tachycardia that starts and stops suddenly and is characterized by sporadic periods of accelerated heart rate.

Parsonnet pouch. See *pouch.*

PASE. See *Pacemaker Selection in the Elderly.*

passive fixation. In pacing, positioning an endocardial pacing lead within a chamber of the heart such that the distal end of the lead is in contact with the endocardium but does not penetrate the myocardium. See also *passive fixation lead.*

passive fixation lead. A pacing lead with tines, fins, flanges, wedges, or some other mechanism constructed at or proximal to the distal-tip electrode to facilitate lodging of the lead within the trabeculae of the cardiac chamber in which the lead is placed. A passive fixation lead does not penetrate into the myocardium and no special action is required to achieve fixation. Contemporary passive fixation leads almost all use tines as the fixation mechanism. See also *fin, flange, low-threshold lead, porous electrode, porous-surface electrode, tine, totally porous electrode.*

passive properties. The aspects of cardiac cells that allow transmission of a signal without formation of an action potential. Generation of an action potential is an active property. Passive properties include membrane resistance, capacitance, and cable properties.

PAT. Abbreviation for *paroxysmal atrial tachycardia.*

patch clamp technique. A method for studying ion currents by fixing the transmembrane potential at different voltages. This is done on a small segment of membrane that has been removed with a micropipette.

patch electrode. A flexible epicardial electrode positioned surgically on the epicardial surface of the heart or on the pericardium for use with an implantable cardioverter-defibrillator. Patch electrodes are constructed of metal mesh or coils embedded in an insulating backing. The exterior face of the patch electrode is insulated to prevent current dissipation away from the heart upon shock delivery from the implantable cardioverter-defibrillator. A patch electrode may be used in combination with one or more additional patches, or with one or more intravascular defibrillation leads.

patch-patch configuration. An uncommonly used defibrillation electrode array consisting of two epicardial patch electrodes. Typically, one epicardial patch electrode is placed anteriorly and the other is placed over the posterolateral left ventricle. See also *patch electrode, springpatch*.

PATH-CHF. See *Pacing Therapies in Congestive Heart Failure I, Pacing Therapies in Congestive Heart Failure II.*

PATH-CHF I. See *Pacing Therapies in Congestive Heart Failure I.*

PATH-CHF II. See *Pacing Therapies in Congestive Heart Failure II.*

patient alert. A signal from the implanted pulse generator to make the patient aware of a warning or potential problem.

patient information storage. A function of most contemporary pulse generators whereby a portion of the memory is used to store information to supplement the patient record. Patient information storage may include the name, birth date, and sex of the patient; the date of pacemaker implantation; the type of pacing lead(s); the presence of retrograde conduction; pacing and sensing thresholds at the time of implantation; current drug therapy; and summarized history. See also *data storage*.

patient-triggered event record (PTER). A diagnostic feature of the pulse generator that the patient can initiate in an effort to correlate diagnostic information with symptoms. For example, the device may be triggered to save an event if the patient places a magnet over the device. The event stored may be in the form of sequential event markers or electrograms that are stored for a preset number of cycles both before and after the trigger.

PAVB. Abbreviation for *postatrial ventricular blanking.*

PAVE. See *Post AV Nodal Ablation Evaluation.*

PCL. Abbreviation for *pacing cycle length.*

PCMT. Abbreviation for *pacemaker circus-movement tachycardia.*

PC shock. Abbreviation for *programmer-commanded shock.*

PCV. Abbreviation for *percutaneous coronary venoplasty, posterior cardiac vein.*

PD. Abbreviation for *potential difference.*

PDF. Abbreviation for *probability density function.*

PDI. Abbreviation for *paced depolarization integral.*

peak amplitude. A term that is somewhat generic, referring to the greatest height or amplitude of a waveform as measured from baseline to the highest point.

peak endocardial acceleration sensor. A rate-adaptive sensor that measures mechanical vibrations generated by the myocardium during the isovolumetric contraction phase. This is accomplished by incorporating an accelerometer into the distal aspect of the pacing lead (i.e., near the lead-endocardial junction).

peak threshold. In pacing, the highest stimulation threshold that occurs after pacemaker and lead implantation. Peak threshold can also refer to sensing threshold, but generally it is used to refer to stimulation threshold. Peak threshold usually occurs 4 weeks or more after implantation and is attributed to the inflammatory tissue response caused by lead trauma and subsequent fibrotic tissue encapsulation of

---

Peak Endocardial Acceleration Sensor

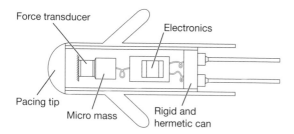

Force transducer
Electronics
Pacing tip
Micro mass
Rigid and hermetic can

From Hayes DL, Lloyd MA, Friedman PA. Cardiac pacing and defibrillation: a clinical approach. Armonk: Futura Publishing Company, Inc; 2000. p. 325-46. Copyrighted and used with permission of Mayo Foundation for Medical Education and Research.

the electrode tip. See also *acute pacing threshold, chronic pacing threshold, pacing threshold, sensing threshold, threshold, threshold maturation.*

pectinate muscles. Muscular bones that run in the right atrium. The terminal (or beginning, depending on perspective) portion of all the pectinate muscles come together at a vertical ridge called the crista terminalis. From the crista terminalis, the pectinate muscles run to various portions of the atrium, including the atrial appendage, and, at times, through the cavotricuspid isthmus up to and including the ostium of the coronary sinus. See also *crista terminalis.*

pectoral muscle stimulation. Inappropriate extracardiac stimulation from a pulse generator that results in electrical stimulation of a pectoral muscle. It manifests by an annoying episodic twitch or jerk of the pectoral muscle.

peel-away introducer. See *peel-away sheath.*

peel-away sheath. A specially designed cannula used to facilitate the percutaneous introduction of catheters such as pacing leads. Once the cannula has been introduced, the catheter or lead is passed through the cannula or introducer, which can then be partially withdrawn and split in half axially and peeled away for easy removal.

peeling-back refractoriness. The normalization of antegrade conduction by premature depolarization of the affected tissue with a retrograde impulse. The refractory period of the tissue is reset by the retrograde impulse, thus allowing time for recovery so that the tissue will depolarize normally in response to the next antegrade impulse.

PEGASUS-CRT. See *Pacing Evaluation-Atrial Support in Cardiac Resynchronization Therapy.*

PEI. Abbreviation for *preejection interval.*

Pellethane. Trademark for a polyurethane that has long segments of soft aliphatic polyether (-CH2CH2CH2CH2-) connected to relatively short segments of hard aromatic polyurethane (Dow Chemical Company, Midland, Michigan). Altering the ratio of the ether segments and urethane segments varies the physical properties of polyurethane. Pellethane 2363-80A has a high soft (ether) to hard (urethane) segment ratio and Pellethane 2363-55D has less ether segments and is thus stiffer. See also *polyurethane, shore rating.*

percutaneous. Through the skin. Temporary pacing catheters frequently are placed percutaneously.

percutaneous coronary venoplasty (PCV). As it relates to device implantation, balloon dilation of a central vein or coronary vein to enlarge the vessel to the point that a pacing lead can be inserted.

percutaneous introducer. See *lead introducer.*

percutaneous radiofrequency catheter ablation (RFCA). See *radiofrequency catheter ablation.*

perforation. A puncture wound. In pacing, perforation may occur when the pacing lead punctures the myocardium. As a complication of lead implantation, myocardial perforation may manifest during lead placement or within the first 24 hours after implantation. On rare occasions, perforation occurs at a later date. Some

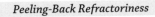

Peeling-Back Refractoriness

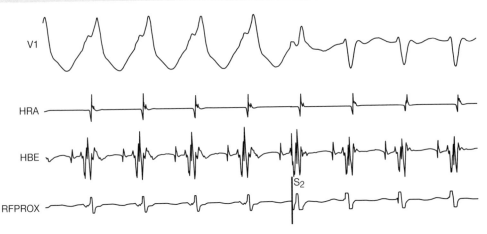

cases of perforation are asymptomatic and pacing continues at an elevated threshold. Others are associated with intermittent failure of pacing or sensing, diaphragmatic or abdominal muscle twitching, distant heart sounds, pericardial rub, and, in extreme situations, cardiac tamponade.

pericardium. The fibroserous sac that surrounds the heart and the roots of the great vessels entering and leaving the heart. The pericardium consists of an external layer of fibrous tissue and an inner serous layer. The inner serous layer of the pericardium is called the epicardium.

permanent atrial fibrillation. Sometimes also called chronic atrial fibrillation. In a more narrow sense, permanent atrial fibrillation cannot be cardioverted or it recurs within seconds of attempted cardioversion. More generally, atrial fibrillation that has been present for years with or without attempts at cardioversion is said to be permanent atrial fibrillation.

permanent form of junctional reciprocating tachycardia (PJRT). A type of atrioventricular reentrant tachycardia involving an accessory pathway that possesses atrioventricular nodal-like properties and is located in the posteroseptal region. Permanent junctional reciprocating tachycardia is a narrow-complex tachycardia and has a long RP interval. The accessory pathways can conduct in the antegrade direction when the normal atrioventricular node is not conducting. Patients with permanent junctional reciprocating tachycardia often present with incessant tachycardia, and the condition may cause tachycardia-induced cardiomyopathy.

permanent lead. An endocardial or epicardial pacing lead designed for long-term use. See also *endocardial lead, epicardial lead*.

permanent pacemaker. A pacemaker designed for implantation and long-term use to support or maintain rate support. See also *pacemaker*.

persistent atrial fibrillation. Atrial fibrillation that requires chemical or electrical cardioversion to terminate. Linear ablation and pulmonary vein isolation are both often needed for ablative therapy. See also *paroxysmal atrial fibrillation*.

persistent left superior vena cava. The most common thoracic venous anomaly, in which the normally absent left superior vena cava remains and drains into the right atrium via the coronary sinus. There are several congenital variations of persistent left superior vena cava, including variable communication with right-sided superior vena cava, absence of right-sided superior vena cava, drainage into the left atrium creating a right-to-left shunt, and association with other congenital anomalies of the heart and great vessels. A persistent left superior vena cava can be problematic during device implantation. If this is encountered, options include aborting the procedure and placing the device from the right side (assuming the right superior vena cava is intact) or going through the persistent left superior vena cava, through the coronary sinus, and then into the right

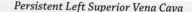

Persistent Left Superior Vena Cava

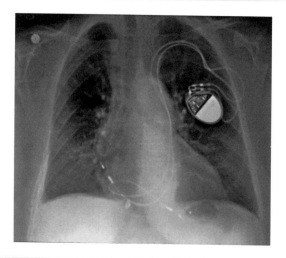

atrium for subsequent lead positioning in the right-sided chambers.

pervenous lead. See *endocardial pacing.*

PES. Abbreviation for *programmed electrical stimulus.*

phantom pacing. 1. The observation of pacing-related phenomena on either telemetry or interrogation of device function without actual pacing occurring. One example of this phenomenon is phantom crosstalk. Crosstalk usually occurs when events in one chamber (i.e., the ventricle) are sensed by a pacemaker lead in the other chamber (the atria). Sometimes, even when an atrial lead has been plugged (note pacing lead), crosstalk occurs because of parasitic capacitance changes at the circuit level. 2. Pacing in a torso phantom to evaluate lead and pacing function.

phantom programming. An errant or spurious change in the programmed parameters of a pacemaker. Phantom programming may be a result of intentional reprogramming not recorded in the patient's record. Phantom programming rarely is caused by an external signal sensed by the pacemaker. See also *dysprogramming, misprogramming.*

phantom shocks. Implantable cardioverter-defibrillator shocks that are felt by the patient but delivered therapies cannot be documented on device interrogation. This is a psychological phenomenon in which patients, during either the sleep or the awake state, have a strong and certain feeling that they have been shocked. This may be part of a posttraumatic stress syndrome from multiple prior shocks or a stand-alone occurrence.

Pharmacological Intervention in Atrial Fibrillation (PIAF). This study compared rate with rhythm control in patients with atrial fibrillation. The study found no superiority of either intervention in terms of atrial fibrillation-related symptoms (Hohnloser SH, Kuck K-H, Lilienthal J. Rhythm or rate control in atrial fibrillation: Pharmacological Intervention in Atrial Fibrillation [PIAF]: a randomised trial. Lancet. 2000;356:1789-94).

pharmacologic denervation. A combination of atropine and propranolol used in electrophysiologic testing to determine intrinsic heart rate. Pharmacologic denervation is used to assess sinus node dysfunction on the basis of comparison of the experimentally derived intrinsic

heart rate with the defined value anticipated for the patient's age. See also *intrinsic heart rate.*

pharmacologic treatment. Drug therapy. In electrophysiology, pharmacologic treatment refers to the use of drugs for the management of arrhythmias. See also *antiarrhythmic agent.*

phased radiofrequency energy. Experimental method of delivering radiofrequency energy from two or multiphased generators via two or more electrodes in an attempt to give rise to more uniform lesions.

phase 5 study. One of the final stages of a large study in which all collected information is analyzed.

phase singularity. A location in which all points have essentially the same phase. Mathematically, phase singularity occurs when each point in a field of view has an individual phase value but the phase is not deterministic. The integration along the minimum closed path encircling phase singularity is 2*pi. Phase singularity is an important concept in understanding reentry dynamics and finding the circuits and source of complex ventricular arrhythmia because the core of three-dimensional reentry circuits has the properties of phase singularity. Thus, a phase-singularity recognition algorithm can be applied in myocardial circuit studies to localize the reentry core.

phases of depolarization. See *depolarization phases.*

phenytoin. An anticonvulsant medication that has class IB antiarrhythmic drug activity. Phenytoin has little effect on refractoriness or conduction in normal atrial and ventricular tissue. It has been touted as an effective treatment for arrhythmias due to digitalis toxicity. Phenytoin is metabolized by the liver and has a plasma half-life of 24 hours. Side effects of phenytoin include central nervous system effects and, chronically, megaloblastic anemia, lupus syndrome, and gingival hyperplasia.

phrenic nerve stimulation. See *diaphragmatic stimulation.*

pH sensing. The determination of pH levels by the use of sensors that measure changes in the pH of the circulatory system or body tissues. A decrease in blood pH is caused by increased carbon dioxide production due to increased oxygen consumption during exercise. pH sensors have been used investigationally as a sensor for closed-loop rate-adaptive pacing.

physiologic heart rate. A heart rate that is appropriate for a specific activity or level of activity. An individual who is able to achieve an appropriate physiologic heart rate is said to be chronotropically competent.

physiologic pacing. Commonly used to refer to dual-chamber pacing that mimics, as closely as possible, normal cardiac conduction and contraction. Physiologic pacing occasionally may be used in reference to closed-loop rate-adaptive pacing systems that mimic normal cardiac responses to physiologic variables. Depending on the patient's underlying conduction system abnormality, pacing modes that may result in restoration of normal physiology include DDD, DDDR, VDD, and AAIR. See also *AAIR, DDD, DDDR, VDD.*

PI. Abbreviation for *preexcitation index.*

PIA. Abbreviation for *pacemaker-induced arrhythmia.*

PIAF. See *Pharmacological Intervention in Atrial Fibrillation.*

PIC. See *Pacing in Cardiomyopathy.*

piezoelectric crystal. A component of electronic circuitry that has the ability to generate a voltage from an applied mechanical force or to generate a mechanical force from an applied voltage. In pacing, piezoelectric crystals have been used for motion or activity sensing in rate-adaptive pacemakers.

pill electrode. A bipolar electrode in the shape of a pill so that it can be swallowed and used as an esophageal electrode to record or pace the left atrium.

pindolol. A nonselective, β-adrenoreceptor blocking agent with intrinsic sympathomimetic activity. Because of its intrinsic sympathomimetic activity, pindolol may less frequently cause problems with bradycardias and fatigue than some other β-adrenergic blocking agents. Pindolol is metabolized by both the liver and the kidneys. For side effects, see *β-adrenergic blocking drugs.*

PJRT. Abbreviation for *permanent form of junctional reciprocating tachycardia.*

planar wave front. Electrical wave front propagation may progress in a single plane in myocardial tissue. In a planar wave front there may be no orthogonal currents, and this parallel nature of wave-front propogation and current flow is responsible in part for the biomagnetic properties of wave-front propagation.

plateau early afterdepolarizations. See *early afterdepolarization.*

plateau phase. Phase of the cardiac action potential in which inward and outward current flows are nearly balanced. Calcium currents and potassium current flow are active in this phase. Phase 2 of the cardiac action potential.

platinization. The process by which a material is covered or plated with platinum. In pacing, platinization sometimes is used in the manufacturing process of porous-surfaced electrodes. Platinization creates a microtextured surface to increase the electrode surface area. See also *porous-surfaced electrode.*

platinum-iridium (Pt-Ir). A biocompatible metal alloy, typically composed of 90% platinum and 10% iridium. Platinum-iridium may be used in pacing systems as the anodal or cathodal electrode material. Platinum-iridium is corrosion-resistant. See also *alloy.*

pluripotent myocytes. Early stage in the differentiation of myocardial cells in which the cells retain the potential to differentiate into various tissues, including non-myocardial tissue. In canine experiments involving higher energy ablation, potent myocytes have been found to differentiate into cartilaginous, bone, and other tissues.

plutonium batteries. Plutonium is a radioactive source of energy that has been used for permanent pacemakers, so-called nuclear pacemakers.

PM. Abbreviation for *pacemaker.*

PMA. Abbreviation for *premarket approval.*

PMAA. Abbreviation for *premarket approval application.*

PMT. Abbreviation for *pacemaker-mediated tachycardia.*

PMT termination algorithm. See *pacemaker-mediated tachycardia protection.*

pneumothorax. An accumulation of air in the pleural cavity. Pneumothorax may occur as a complication of subclavian puncture.

pocket stimulation. The stimulation of muscle tissue surrounding a unipolar pacemaker by the concentration of current flow at the pacemaker case (the anode). Pocket stimulation also may be caused by current leakage at any site within the pocket, including the connector block, by a lead insulation break, by a lead conductor break, or by a defect in the protective undercoating of a unipolar pacemaker (see also *current leakage*). A classification of pocket stimulation has been described as follows:

Grade 0: No subjective sensation of detectable local muscle contraction

Grade 1: Subjective awareness of the stimulation in the vicinity of the pocket but no palpable muscle contraction

Grade 2: Contraction that is palpable but not visible in the vicinity of the pulse generator

Grade 3: Visible local muscle stimulation

Grade 4: Marked local muscle contraction that is visible even when the patient is dressed

Poincare plots. Graphical representation of heart rate variability. This method of illustrating heart rate variability has the benefit of allowing analysis of nonlinear variation in heart rate.

polarity. In electrical circuits, the sign (positive or negative) of the voltage relationship of one point relative to another. The electrical orientation of the electrodes determines the direction of current flow. When a resistive load is connected between the two terminals, an electrical current (defined as the flow of positive electrical charge) flows through the resistance from the positive terminal (anode) to the negative terminal (cathode). In pacing, the stimulating electrode typically is the cathode, which has negative polarity relative to the indifferent electrode (anode). See also *bipolar electrode system, electrode configuration, unipolar electrode system*.

polarization. The condition of an electrode wherein its electrical potential differs from its equilibrium potential, that is, the temporary change in the electrode potential due to current flow. Endocardial cells are polarized when the electrical charge on the interior of the cells is negative with respect to the outside of the cells. In pacing, polarization also refers to the concentration of ions on or near the stimulating electrode after a pacemaker output pulse. The polarization of the electrode must decay, that is, the electrode must return to its equilibrium potential before the next pacing stimulus. Polarization is directly proportional to pulse duration and inversely proportional to electrode size. See also *crosstalk*.

polished-surface electrode. In pacing, a distal-tip electrode that has been smoothed by the use of abrasive materials during manufacture. Polished-surface electrodes may cause increased polarization at the electrode-endocardial interface. An electrode with a polished surface also is referred to as a smooth electrode.

polyethylene. A biocompatible polymeric material that has a high resistance to tearing and cutting. Polyethylene has been used to insulate pacing leads.

polymer capacitors. In certain capacitors, the oppositely charged electrical plates may be separated by an insulator or dielectric made of polymers such as tantalum or polystyrene.

polymorphic ventricular tachycardia. Ventricular tachycardia with a changing QRS complex. When associated with a prolonged QT interval, polymorphic ventricular tachycardia is known as torsades de pointes. See also *monomorphic ventricular tachycardia*.

polyurethane. A polymer having two or more urethane linkages (-NHCOO-). Polyurethanes include a family of biocompatible, thermoplastic polymers with a high resistance to abrasion. Polyurethane is a strong, flexible, and lubricious insulating material. In pacing, some types of polyurethane are used to insulate pacing leads. See also *lubricity, shore rating*.

POR. Abbreviation for *power-on reset*.

porosity. The state or property of having multiple holes or open spaces through which matter may pass. In pacing, porosity of an electrode surface permits tissue growth into the microstructure of the electrode. Porosity enhances chronic lead stability and may contribute to improved electrical performance. See also *Pellethane, porous electrode, porous-surface electrode*.

porous electrode. An electrode in which the distal tip is composed of a network of interstices, which allow tissue ingrowth to enhance chronic stability and may contribute to improved electrical performance of the lead. Use of porous electrodes reduces the thickness of the fibrotic capsule formed at the electrode-myocardial interface and increases the effective surface area of the electrode. Porous electrodes provide decreased polarization and current drain and increased current density at the electrode-myocardial interface, thereby providing reduced chronic stimulation thresholds and improved sensing of intracardiac signals. Porous electrodes may be totally porous or porous only on the surface of the electrode. See also *porous-surface electrode*.

porous-surface electrode. An electrode in which a network of interstices are distributed uniformly on the surface of a solid electrode to facilitate tissue ingrowth. Porous-surface electrodes may be fabricated in several ways: by sintering a metal powder or alloy, such as platinum-iridium or cobalt-nickel, to a solid metal substrate; by coating the surface of the electrode with a metal alloy, such as in platinization; or by creating small pores in the surface of the electrode with a laser. See also *platinization, porous electrode, totally porous electrode.*

port. In relation to implantable devices, the opening(s) in the header of the pulse generator into which the leads are placed and secured.

port plug. A small plug that is made to fit a specific port of a pulse generator when a lead will not be placed in that specific port.

positive AV interval hysteresis. A programmable parameter in some pulse generators which allows a longer AV interval up to a predefined limit in an effort to facilitate intrinsic atrioventricular conduction.

positive AV/PV hysteresis with search. A programmable parameter in some pulse generators which will result in a periodic search for intrinsic conduction and subsequently adjust the AV/PV interval to facilitate intrinsic atrioventricular conduction.

positive hysteresis. In pacing, the lengthening of the escape interval after a spontaneous beat, which consequently lengthens the pacing interval. Positive hysteresis decreases the pacing rate, allows more time for the pacemaker to sense the intrinsic activity, and thus enhances intrinsic conduction. See also *hysteresis, negative hysteresis.*

postatrial ventricular blanking (PAVB) period. A programmable interval that occurs with an atrial paced event and subsequently prevents inappropriate sensing of the atrial output pulse on the ventricular lead (i.e., crosstalk). Synonymous with *ventricular blanking period.*

Post AV Nodal Ablation Evaluation (PAVE). This study was a prospective comparison of chronic biventricular pacing with right ventricular pacing in patients undergoing atrioventricular node ablation for the management of atrial fibrillation. Biventricular pacing resulted in a significant improvement in the 6-minute hall walk test and ejection fraction compared with right ventricular pacing. The benefits of cardiac resynchronization appeared to be greater in patients with impaired systolic function or with

symptomatic heart failure (Doshi RN, Daoud EG, Fellows C, Turk K, Duran A, Hamdan MH, et al, PAVE Study Group. Left ventricular-based cardiac stimulation post AV nodal ablation evaluation [the PAVE study]. J Cardiovasc Electrophysiol. 2005;16:1160-5).

posterior cardiac vein (PCV). One of the commonly used veins for left ventricular lead implantation done for cardiac resynchronization. The posterior cardiac vein runs parallel to the middle cardiac vein. Lateral branches of the posterior cardiac vein intertwine with tributaries of a lateral vein, if present, or an anterolateral vein. The distal portion of the posterior cardiac vein has various degrees of anastomosis with apical branches of the middle cardiac vein and anterior interventricular vein.

posterior left ventricular vein. One of the main tributaries of the coronary sinus used for left ventricular lead implantation. The posterior left ventricular vein often has large lateral branches that drain the lateral wall of the left ventricle. See also *posterior cardiac vein, posterior ventricular vein.*

posterior ventricular vein. The posterior ventricular vein either arises as a separate tributary running parallel to the middle cardiac vein or may be the first branch of the middle cardiac vein itself. Distal branches of the posterior ventricular vein anastomose with the similar branches of the anterior intraventricular vein. See also *posterior left ventricular vein.*

posterolateral vein. Important tributary of the coronary sinus used for left ventricular lead implantation. The posterolateral vein, when present, arises at the same distance from the coronary sinus ostium as the vein of Marshall (see *vein of Marshall*). The Vieussens valve (see *Vieussens valve*) sometimes guards the opening of the posterolateral vein. In some hearts, a distinct posterolateral vein may not be present, the posterolateral wall being drained by lateral branches of the posterior vein or a more anteriorly located lateral vein.

postmarket surveillance. Ongoing surveillance of pulse generator and lead performance as required by the Safe Medical Devices Act of 1990. At the time of this publication, the protocol that manufacturers will be required to follow has not been determined.

postpacing interval. To determine the circuit responsible for reentrant tachycardias, entrainment is performed. With entrainment, pacing is done at a rate slightly faster than the rate of the tachycardia. On cessation of pacing, the time taken for the next (return) electrogram seen on the pacing catheter is termed the postpacing interval.

postshock pacing (PSP). A period of sinus slowing or sinus arrest with failure of junctional escape after delivery of shocks by an implantable cardioverter-defibrillator. This period is relatively short, but in some patients it may give rise to symptoms. Also, in the immediate postshock period, escape ventricular contractions may occur and reinitiate tachycardia. For these reasons, most devices pace the heart after delivery of shocks by an implantable cardioverter-defibrillator. Because of a transient increase in pacing threshold after shocks, postshock pacing is usually at high output.

postural orthostatic tachycardia syndrome (POTS). Syndrome complex due to autonomic dysfunction in which patients, most commonly young females, have inappropriate sinus tachycardia and related symptoms that occur primarily when the patient is in the upright position.

postvagal tachycardia. Paradoxic increase in heart rate during vagal stimulation. Some evidence suggests that vasoactive intestinal peptide, which is stored in association with acetylcholine in postganglionic vagal fibers, is responsible for this phenomenon. Postvagal tachycardia also is known as vagally induced tachycardia.

postventricular atrial blanking (PVAB) period. A programmable feature in some dual-chamber pulse generators. During the period specified (in milliseconds), the atrial events are blanked from the atrial channel and therefore not considered when the atrial rate interval is calculated. The postventricular atrial blanking period is initiated with a ventricular paced or sensed event.

postventricular atrial refractory period (PVARP). In dual-chamber pacemakers, that portion of the timing cycle during which the atrial channel is refractory after a paced or sensed ventricular event. The postventricular atrial refractory period prohibits the atrial channel of the pacemaker from sensing the far-field ventricular depolarization or the afterpotential of the ventricular pacing impulse. If the postventricular atrial refractory period is sufficiently long, it can prevent pacemaker-mediated tachycardia by prohibiting sensing of premature atrial beats or retrograde atrial depolarizations after ventricular ectopic or paced ventricular beats. However, extension of the postventricular atrial refractory period limits the maximum tracking rate of the pacemaker.

postventricular atrial refractory period extension. A function of most pacemakers that provides an extension of the atrial refractory period after a sensed premature ventricular contraction. The pacemaker usually recognizes premature ventricular contraction as two consecutive sensed events on the ventricular channel without an intervening sensed atrial event. The atrial refractory extension is designed to prevent the sensing of retrograde P waves and to prevent the potential initiation of a pacemaker-mediated tachycardia. See also *DDX, pacemaker-mediated tachycardia protection.*

Postventricular Atrial Refractory Period

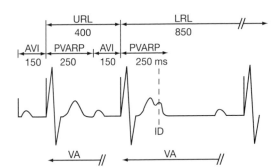

Modified from Hayes DL, Levine PA. Pacemaker timing cycles. In: Ellenbogen KA, editor. Cardiac pacing. Boston: Blackwell Scientific Publications; 1992. p. 263-308. Used with permission.

potassium channels. Any ionic channel that conducts potassium. For specific examples, see I_K, I_{K1}, and so on.

potassium currents. A very important set of transmembrane currents related to the flow of potassium into and out of the myocardial cell (see also I_{K1} and other I_K entries). Potassium currents are the main repolarizing current associated with the cardiac action potential (see also I_{Kr}, I_{Ks}, *inward rectifier*).

potential difference (PD). The difference in the relative voltage between two points. Current will flow when potential differences exist if a finite impedance joins the two points. Physiologically, the potential difference refers to the polarization of the membrane of a living cell, that is, the difference between the charged state inside the cell and the charged state outside the cell. See also *Ohm's law, resting potential, voltage*.

POTS. Abbreviation for *postural orthostatic tachycardia syndrome*.

pouch. A knitted mesh bag into which the pacemaker may be placed at the time of implantation. At one time a pouch was used to promote tissue ingrowth and interlacing within the mesh in an effort to anchor the pacemaker in the pocket more quickly. Use of a pouch was thought to possibly reduce the risk of wound hematoma, pacemaker migration, inversion, erosion, and manipulation by the patient. The pouch also is referred to as a Dacron pouch or a Parsonnet pouch. Pouches are rarely used today. See also *twiddler's syndrome*.

power. The rate of doing work or transmitting energy. Power is calculated as the product of voltage and current and usually is expressed in watts.

power-on reset (POR) mode. Power-on reset can occur when the pacemaker circuitry transiently loses power. Causes include battery depletion, externally applied electrical charge (i.e., electrocautery), cardioversion, or defibrillation. When power-on reset occurs, the programmed parameters may change and the rate or mode likely will revert to preset values. Synonym for electrical reset.

power source. In pacing, the term generically refers to the pacemaker battery, which consists of electrochemical cells capable of producing electrical energy. Two different chemical substances (poles), immersed in an electrolyte, cause electrons to flow in a circuit between them. See also *battery*.

PPI. Abbreviation for *postpacing interval*.

PP interval. The amount of time between one intrinsic atrial depolarization and the next, as measured from one P wave to the next on the surface electrocardiogram.

ppm. Abbreviation for *pulses per minute*.

PR. Sensed native atrial event to sensed native ventricular event.

preamendment devices. Devices that were commercially available at the time the U.S. Medical Devices Amendment was enacted in May 1976.

Predictors of Response to Cardiac Resynchronization Therapy (PROSPECT). The aims of this prospective, multicenter, nonrandomized study were to identify echocardiographic measures of dyssynchrony and to evaluate their ability to predict response to cardiac resynchronization. The primary response criteria are improvement in the heart failure clinical composite score and left ventricular reverse remodeling (Yu C-M, Abraham WT, Bax J, Chung E, Fedewa M, Ghio S, et al, PROSPECT Investigators. Predictors of response to cardiac resynchronization therapy [PROSPECT]: study design. Am Heart J. 2005;149:600-5).

preejection interval (PEI). A cardiac interval measured from the onset of ventricular depolarization to the beginning of ventricular ejection.

preejection interval sensing. Monitoring of the right ventricular preejection interval. This has been used as a parameter for a permanent rate-adaptive sensor.

preexcitation. Activation of all or part of the ventricular myocardium by an accessory pathway at an earlier time than if conduction had occurred only through the normal atrioventricular conduction system. Preexcitation yields a delta wave and usually a short PR interval on the surface electrocardiogram. Electrophysiologic studies may be used to define the predominant preexcitation pathway. See also *accessory pathway, Wolff-Parkinson-White syndrome*.

preexcitation index (PI). A measurement attained during atrioventricular reentrant tachycardia or atrioventricular nodal reentrant tachycardia while introducing single ventricular extrastimuli at gradually decreasing coupling intervals. The latest coupled extrastimulus (V2) that preexcites the atrium is used to calculate the preexcitation index (PI). PI = V1V1 – V1V2 where V1V1 is the cycle length of the tachycardia and V1V2 is the coupling interval of the latest ventricular extrastimulus to preexcite the atrium. The preexcitation index is useful for distinguishing between concentric retrograde atrial activation due to an accessory pathway rather than the atrioventricular node.

preexcitation syndrome. See *Wolff-Parkinson-White syndrome.*

preexcited tachycardia. Type of wide complex tachycardia in which ventricular activation occurs wholly or partly via an antegradely conducting accessory pathway. Types of preexcited tachycardia include any form of supraventricular tachycardia (atrioventricular node reentry, atrial tachycardia, atrial flutter, atrial fibrillation, sinus tachycardia) with antegrade conduction via an antegrade accessory pathway and antidromic tachycardia in which a reentrant tachycardia occurs with antegrade conduction via an accessory pathway and retrograde conduction via either the atrioventricular node or another retrogradely conducting accessory pathway.

preexcited wide QRS tachycardia. Wide QRS tachycardia in which the abnormal QRS morphology is caused by antegrade conduction across an accessory pathway, resulting in abnormal ventricular myocardial activation. Preexcited wide QRS tachycardia may be caused by any form of supraventricular tachycardia with partial or whole conduction to the ventricle occurring via an antegradely conducting accessory pathway.

premarket approval (PMA). In the United States, the process required by the Food and Drug Administration to introduce a class III device into commercial distribution which is not substantially equivalent to a device that was marketed before May 28, 1976, or for which the Food and Drug Administration has called for premarket approvals.

premarket approval application (PMAA). In the United States, application to the Food and Drug Administration for premarket approval to release a drug or device for commercial distribution.

premarket evaluation. The investigation of a clinical product by a regulatory agency before market release of the product (e.g., investigation of a pacemaker, defibrillator, or drug before its approval for general use).

premarket notification. An application submitted to the U.S. Food and Drug Administration to demonstrate that a medical device to be marketed is substantially equivalent to a device that was or currently is on the U.S. market. Sometimes referred to as a 510(k) application, derived from the section of the law that allows this process—Section 510(k) of the U.S. Federal Food, Drug, and Cosmetic Act as amended by the U.S. Medical Devices Amendment of 1976.

premature atrial complex (PAC). A depolarization of the atria from an ectopic focus that produces a P wave earlier than normal. A premature atrial complex also is known as an atrial premature complex or as a premature atrial contraction.

premature atrial contraction (PAC). See *premature atrial complex.*

premature stimulus. In electrophysiology, a programmed electrical stimulus critically timed from either a preceding stimulus or an intrinsic spontaneous event. Premature stimuli are used to assess the conduction system, to assess the refractoriness of various structures, and to initiate or terminate tachycardias. A single premature stimulus may stop a tachycardia if the stimulus is precisely timed to fall within the tachycardia termination zone. See also *premature atrial complex, premature ventricular complex, programmed electrical stimulus.*

premature ventricular beat (PVB). See *premature ventricular complex.*

premature ventricular complex (PVC). A depolarization of the ventricle out of sequence with the normal intrinsic rhythm. A premature ventricular complex usually is initiated by an ectopic focus and occurs earlier than the expected next normal sinus or nodal beat. Electrocardiographically, a premature ventricular complex must be distinguished from a supraventricular complex with aberration. In dual-chamber pacing, premature ventricular complexes are the most common cause of pacemaker-mediated tachycardia. A premature ventricular complex also is known as a premature ventricular contraction, a premature ventricular event, or a ventricular premature complex.

premature ventricular contraction (PVC). See *premature ventricular complex.*

premature ventricular event (PVE). See *premature ventricular complex.*

premature ventricular stimulus. A programmed electrical stimulus delivered to the ventricle. In electrophysiologic studies, premature ventricular stimuli are used to assess ventriculoatrial conduction and to induce arrhythmias. Premature ventricular stimuli are indicated by V2, V3, V4, and so on. See also *premature stimulus*.

preset. Fixed or unalterable before use. Early pacemakers were preset, and parameters were established at the time of manufacture. See also *nonprogrammable pacemaker*.

pressoreceptor. See *baroreceptor*.

presyncope. A near fainting sensation without total loss of consciousness.

printed circuit board. A circuit design that connects discrete and integrated components. Interconnecting conductors of the printed circuit board are formed by copper runs within or on an insulating material such as fiberglass. The copper runs usually are etched onto the insulation and covered or coated to prevent oxidation. The components usually are then individually mounted onto the circuit board. Flex circuits, frequently used in pacemaker circuitry, are a type of printed circuit board. See also *discrete component, flex circuit*.

PR interval. The amount of time from the onset of the intrinsic atrial depolarization (P wave) to the beginning of the next consecutive intrinsic ventricular depolarization (QRS complex), as measured on the surface electrocardiogram. Normal values of the PR interval are 120 to 200 milliseconds.

PR Logic. Trademark for a method of distinguishing supraventricular from ventricular tachycardia in implantable cardioverter-defibrillators (Medtronic, Inc., Minneapolis, Minnesota). The relationship between the ventricular and atrial electrograms (R and P) is analyzed when the ventricular and atrial electrograms are simultaneous and junctional tachycardia is considered likely. When the atrial electrogram occurs more than midway between two consecutive ventricular electrograms, a supraventricular tachycardia is considered likely. When the atrial electrogram occurs closer to the preceeding ventricular electrogram rather than to the next ventricular electrogram during tachycardia (short RP interval), ventricular tachycardia is considered likely. The interval between the ventricular electrogram and atrial electrogram at which supraventricular tachycardia (or ventricular tachycardia) is diagnosed is programmable.

proarrhythmia. Aggravation of underlying arrhythmias or the creation of new arrhythmias. The creation of new arrhythmias is more correctly called arrhythmogenesis. Proarrhythmia must be distinguished from spontaneous variability. Most often, proarrhythmia is used in relation to antiarrhythmic drugs.

probability density function (PDF). In some pacing systems, a calculation of myocardial electrical activity indicated by the slew rate of the intracardiac deflection between two amplitude limits, as measured on an intracardiac electrogram. In other pacing systems, probability density function is a calculation of myocardial activity indicated by the area above and below the isoelectrical line. Probability density function often is used as a criterion for data processing in an algorithm of the circuitry in an arrhythmia control device. For example, a specific range of probability density functions is defined in the algorithm used in some implantable cardioverter-defibrillators to distinguish normal sinus rhythm from ventricular tachycardia.

probe. A slender, small device brought into contact with, or inserted into, a system to take measurements of the system. A probe usually is designed to not disturb the system significantly. In electrophysiology, probes frequently are used during testing to sense intrinsic activity for the recording of an intracardiac electrogram. Probes also are used during surgical treatment of arrhythmias; for example, a cryoprobe may be used for ablation. See also *cryoprobe, finger probe*.

procainamide. A class IA antiarrhythmic agent that prolongs refractoriness in atrial, atrioventricular nodal, ventricular, and accessory pathway tissue. Procainamide has efficacy in the treatment of supraventricular and ventricular arrhythmias. It is metabolized in the liver to *N*-acetylprocainamide (NAPA), and both the parent compound and the NAPA are excreted by the kidneys. Side effects of procainamide include nausea, a lupus-like syndrome, proarrhythmia, and agranulocytosis.

programmability. The capability to send radiofrequency signals from an external programmer. Simple programmability suggests that the capability to noninvasively alter pacing is limited to one or two pacing parameters, usually the rate or output; this was the design of some of the earliest programmable devices. Contemporary devices are multiprogrammable. See also *multiprogrammability*.

programmable polarity. A pulse generator feature that allows the polarity configuration to be programmed (i.e., bipolar or unipolar). In some devices, pacing and sensing configurations are "tied," and in others it is possible to program them independently (i.e., paced unipolar-sensed bipolar configuration).

programmable shocking vector. In some devices, the vector used for shocks delivered by an implantable cardioverter-defibrillator is programmable, usually with the option of including or excluding the superior vena cava coil. See also *shocking vector*.

programmed atrial stimulation. During electrophysiologic study, a series of standard maneuvers performed with atrial pacing. These include, for example, decremental atrial pacing and atrial extrastimulus testing.

programmed electrical stimulus (PES). The delivery of one or several electrical stimuli at specifically timed intervals. Programmed electrical stimuli are used extensively in electrophysiologic testing. Examples of programmed electrical stimuli are premature stimuli, burst stimuli, and decremental or incremental stimuli. See also *burst stimulation, decremental pacing, premature stimulus*.

programmed stimulation. During electrophysiologic study, standard pacing maneuvers are utilized to induce arrhythmia and assess the integrity of the conduction system. These maneuvers include decremental (incremental) pacing, extrastimulus testing including multiple extrastimuli testing, and burst pacing.

programmed ventricular stimulation. During electrophysiologic study, ventricular pacing in a relatively standard format is performed to induce tachycardia and assess retrograde conduction to the atrium. Maneuvers performed include decremental ventricular pacing (incremental pacing) and ventricular extrastimulus testing.

programmer. A device used to noninvasively interrogate, monitor, and alter the operating parameters of a pacemaker, defibrillator, or cardiac resynchronization device. Early programmers used electromagnetic pulses. Programmers also receive, by means of telemetry, information stored within the implanted pulse generator and real-time signals via the electrodes implanted within the heart. See also *telemetry*.

programmer-commanded shock (PC shock). During device interrogation or electrophysiologic study, a programmer-demanded shock may be delivered if the operator wants the device to deliver a shock before meeting detection or for an undetected arrhythmia.

programmer head. That part of the programmer traditionally placed over the pulse generator to create the link needed for bidirectional programming. Newer technology will allow programming to be done at a distance via a radiofrequency link to the specific pulse generator. It may still require that the programmer head (or wand) is passed across or near the pulse generator to establish identification and the link.

programming. The noninvasive adjustment of programmable parameters. An external programmer is used to transmit coded information by means of radiofrequency signals or electromagnetic pulses from the programmer to a pacemaker or cardioverter-defibrillator. See also *programmer, telemetry*.

programming wand. See *programmer head*.

propafenone. A class IC antiarrhythmic agent that prolongs refractoriness in atrial, atrioventricular nodal, ventricular, and accessory pathway tissue. Propafenone has efficacy in the treatment of supraventricular and ventricular arrhythmias. It also has some β-adrenergic and calcium channel blocking activity. Propafenone is metabolized by the liver, and some of the metabolites produced are active. In patients who metabolize it rapidly, propafenone has a half-life of 5 to 6 hours. In patients who metabolize it slowly, propafenone has a half-life of about 17 hours. Side effects include bradycardias, proarrhythmia, constipation, metallic taste, exacerbation of asthma, congestive heart failure, increased hepatic enzyme values, and central nervous system effects.

propagation. In electrophysiology, the effective conduction of an impulse from one point to another point remote from the source, as exemplified by conduction from the sinus node through the atrioventricular conduction system to the ventricular myocardium. Propagation is evidenced by a wave of depolarization.

propranolol. A nonselective, β-adrenoreceptor blocking agent without sympathomimetic activity. Like most other β-adrenergic blocking agents, propranolol decreases sinus node automaticity and increases atrioventricular nodal refractoriness and conduction time, but it has no effect on atrial, ventricular, or accessory pathway refractoriness. Propranolol has efficacy in the treatment of supraventricular and some ventricular arrhythmias. It is metabolized by the liver. For side effects, see *β-adrenergic blocking drugs*.

PROSPECT. See *Predictors of Response to Cardiac Resynchronization Therapy*.

protein kinase. The most important of a group of signaling enzymes that modify other proteins in a signal transduction cascade. For example, cyclic adenosine monophosphate (cAMP) activates cAMP-dependent protein kinase that, in turn, activates a calcium channel that represents an effector protein. Protein kinases are a large and diverse group of enzymes that includes protein kinases A (activated by cAMP), protein kinases G (activated by cyclic guanosine monophosphate), protein kinases C (activated by phospholipids), and calcium/calmodulin-dependent kinases (activated by calcium and calmodulin).

protein kinase A. Important enzyme that participates in functional signaling. Protein kinase A is cyclic adenosine monophosphate-activated and is made up of two catalytic subunits: one that transfers the terminal phosphate of adenosine triphosphate to an effector protein and one that regulates these subunits by inhibiting its own activity under basal conditions. See also *protein kinase*.

protein kinase C. Cyclic guanosine monophosphate-activated protein kinase. See also *protein kinase, protein kinase A*.

protein kinase G. Protein kinase that is activated by phospholipids rather than cyclic adenosine monophosphate or cyclic guanosine monophosphate. See also *protein kinase, protein kinase A*.

protocol. A specified sequence of events or plan of action, such as that used for scientific studies. In electrophysiologic studies, the protocol is the order in which programmed electrical stimulation is performed. See also *programmed electrical stimulus*.

proximal. Closer to a given point of reference.

For example, in anatomy, if the shoulder is used as the point of reference, the elbow is proximal to the wrist, and the wrist is distal to the elbow. In pacing, the pacemaker case typically is used as the point of reference. For example, the terminal pin of a pacing lead is located at the proximal end of the lead, and the stimulating electrode is located at the distal tip of the lead. In an endocardial bipolar lead, the cathode typically is located at the distal tip of the lead and the anodal ring is located several millimeters proximal to the lead tip. Thus, the cathode is referred to as the distal-tip electrode and the anode is referred to as the proximal-ring electrode, even though the two electrodes are located only a few millimeters apart and both are some distance from the pacemaker case. See also *distal*.

proximal-ring electrode. The anode of an endocardial bipolar pacing lead. The proximal-ring electrode encircles the lead, usually several millimeters away from the distal-tip electrode. The charge usually flows from the distal-tip electrode to the proximal-ring electrode. However, the proximal-ring electrode also may be used as the cathode, in which case pacing and sensing occur through the proximal ring. The proximal-ring electrode also is referred to as the anodal band.

PRR. Abbreviation for *pulse repetition rate*.

PR sensitivity (or P/R sensitivity). Term used for the setting that dictates the sensitivity of the pulse generator when it detects a P wave or an R wave. A signal greater than the programmed sensitivity in millivolts will be detected. A lower millivolt value increases the sensitivity; a higher millivolt value decreases the sensitivity.

PSA. Abbreviation for *pacemaker systems analyzer*.

pseudoatrial exit block. With a dual-chamber pacing system, if a premature atrial depolarization occurs during the postventricular atrial refractory period (PVARP), the next atrial pacemaker stimulus will not result in atrial depolarization. This situation may become repetitious in that the next ventricular stimulus will likely result in retrograde ventriculoatrial conduction. This atrial activation again occurs within the PVARP such that atrial pacing continues but without atrial depolarization and resulting atrioventricular dyssynchrony. See also *exit block*.

Pseudofracture

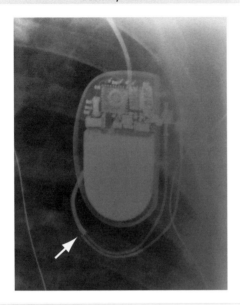

pseudofracture. This term is used most correctly to describe the radiographic appearance of some bifurcated bipolar pacing leads in which the anodal and cathodal conductors come together. Without close inspection, there appears to be discontinuity of the conductor. The term also has been used to describe a compression defect of endocardial pacing leads in which the conductor coils are distorted without losing electrical continuity. Often this is caused by encircling tight ligatures used to secure the lead(s) to adjacent subcutaneous tissue. See also *conductor fracture.*

pseudofusion beat. The electrocardiographic waveform that occurs when a pacemaker stimulus is superimposed on a spontaneous P wave during atrial pacing or upon a QRS complex during ventricular pacing. When pseudofusion occurs, the pacing stimulus is ineffective and the native P wave or QRS complex is not altered. The tissue around the electrode already has spontaneously depolarized and is in its absolute refractory period. See also *fusion beat, pseudopseudofusion beat.*

pseudohysteresis. A rarely used term to describe pauses in the paced electrocardiogram which have the appearance of hysteresis. Pseudohysteresis can result from an event that is inappropriately sensed, such as a retrograde P wave or a T wave that resets the pacemaker timing and results in a pause. See also *hysteresis.*

pseudomalfunction. Unusual, unexpected, or eccentric electrocardiographic findings that appear to result from pacemaker malfunction but which are, in fact, due to normal pacemaker function.

pseudopacemaker syndrome. Also called pacemaker syndrome without a pacemaker. This can occur when there is marked PR interval prolongation to the point that effective atrioventricular synchrony is lost and symptoms of pacemaker syndrome are present.

pseudopseudofusion beat. A type of pseudofusion beat that can occur when the atrial output artifact is superimposed on an intrinsic QRS complex, as seen on an electrocardiogram. The atrial pacing stimulus is ineffective because atrial depolarization already has occurred spontaneously and the output pulse is not capable of directly contributing to ventricular activation. Pseudopseudofusion beats occur most often in the atrioventricular sequential ventricular-inhibited pacing mode (DVI). See also *fusion beat, pseudofusion beat.*

pseudo-supernormal conduction. Several factors may cause phenomena appearing to result from supernormal conduction. For example, if a bundle branch block pattern paradoxically resolves with more rapid pacing, supranormality may be considered. However, these phenomena may in fact be due to various other reasons, including 1) resolution of bradycardia-related block, 2) appearance of bundle branch block in the previously conducting bundle resulting in near equal bilateral bundle branch delay and eventual conduction with a narrow QRS complex, 3) coincidental simultaneous premature

Pseudopseudofusion

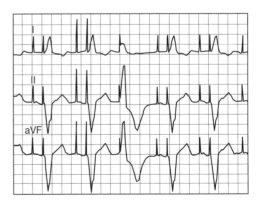

ventricular complex from the ventricle on the same side of the bundle branch block, and 4) proximal gap phenomenon. These conditions may be referred to as producing pseudo-supernormal conduction.

pseudo-Wenckebach response. An upper rate response of some dual-chamber pacemakers. The pseudo-Wenckebach response occurs when the spontaneous intrinsic atrial rate increases above the programmed upper rate limit of the pacemaker. The ventricular output pulses are delivered at the upper rate limit, which causes an effective prolongation of the atrioventricular interval. An intermittent block occurs when an intrinsic atrial event falls within the postventricular atrial refractory period of the pacemaker. The P wave is not sensed by the pacemaker and, therefore, a ventricular output pulse is not synchronized to this atrial event. As the atrial rate increases above the upper rate limit of the pacemaker, a progressively higher degree of pseudo-Wenckebach block is observed until 2:1 block occurs. See also *upper rate response*.

PSP. Abbreviation for *postshock pacing*.

PSVT. Abbreviation for *paroxysmal supraventricular tachycardia*.

PTER. Abbreviation for *patient-triggered event record*.

Pt-Ir. Chemical symbol for *platinum-iridium*.

P-type adenosine triphosphatases (ATPases). An important large protein family essential to creation and maintenance of normal ionic gradients across plasma membranes. The P-types are so-named because they form a phosphorylated intermediate product during transfer. Members include the sodium-potassium ATPases and calcium ATPases in the ceroplastic ventricular membrane.

public access defibrillation. The presence of external defibrillation equipment in public places to allow rapid response by lay public. Thus, when a passerby witnesses a sudden collapse in a patient, possibly from ventricular arrhythmia, access to a semiautomated defibrillator in a public place allows prompt defibrillation, if required.

pulmonary artery (PA). Great artery that arises from the right ventricle and transports blood to the lung. Outflow tract ventricular tachycardia may arise from myocardial extension into the pulmonary artery.

pulmonary vein (PV). Vein that drains the pulmonary venous blood back to the left atrium. The pulmonary venoatrial junction and, likely, musculature within the pulmonary vein are important sources for the initiation and possibly maintenance of atrial fibrillation. Typically, four pulmonary veins, two on the left and two

Pseudo-Wenckebach Response

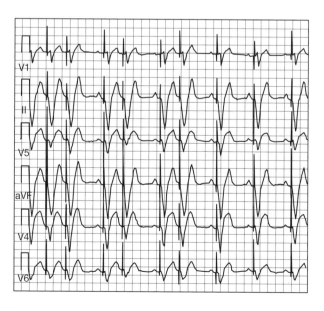

on the right, are present. Sometimes, anomalous drainage of the pulmonary vein may occur in which a particular pulmonary vein may drain into the superior vena cava, right atrium, inferior vena cava, azygos vein, or coronary sinus instead of the left atrium.

pulmonary vein isolation. Catheter ablation technique in which sequential radiofrequency or other energy-source ablations are performed at or near the pulmonary venoatrial junction. A result of this circumferential or near circumferential ablation is that the musculature of the pulmonary vein is electrically isolated from the left atrium. The premise for this type of procedure is that now the focal source of atrial fibrillation within the pulmonary vein is no longer able to exit to the heart. During sinus rhythm, pulmonary vein isolation is realized when pulmonary venous potentials are no longer seen (entrance block).

pulmonary vein, left inferior (LIPV). Left-sided pulmonary vein that drains the lower lobe of the left lung. The left inferior vein has an important anatomic relationship with the descending aorta. The left inferior and left superior veins may arise from a common ostium or be separated by a margin of tissue called the carina. See also *pulmonary vein.*

pulmonary vein, left superior (LSPV). Pulmonary vein entraining the upper lobe of the left lung. It has a tributary that usually drains the lingula of the left lung. The left superior pulmonary vein has an important relationship with the left atrial appendage, which is located anterior to this vein. The left superior pulmonary vein and the left inferior pulmonary vein may arise from a common vein or may have a small rim of tissue separating them called the carina. See also *pulmonary vein.*

pulmonary vein, right inferior (RIPV). Vein draining the lower lobe of the right lung. Also called right lower vein. See also *pulmonary vein.*

pulmonary vein, right superior (RSPV). Pulmonary vein that drains the upper lobe of the right lung, usually via a branch of the middle lobe of the right lung. The right superior pulmonary vein runs from the right upper lobe to the left atrium just posterior to the right atrium and the posterior surface of the superior vena cava. The right middle lobe vein may drain directly to the left atrium.

pulmonary venoatrial junction. Junction between the pulmonary vein and the left atrium. This is a site of conduction delay and may be important to the initiation and maintenance of atrial fibrillation. Pulmonary vein isolation is a procedure performed with ablation at or near the pulmonary venoatrial junction. See also *pulmonary vein, pulmonary vein isolation.*

pulse amplitude. The peak (maximum), average, or effective magnitude of an electrical waveform or pulse. In pacing, pulse amplitude typically indicates the magnitude of the voltage or amperage level reached during a pacemaker output pulse. With respect to pacemaker output pulses, pulse amplitudes usually are expressed in volts (V) or milliamperes (mA).

pulse deficit. The absence of an arterial pulse when an apical beat and ventricular contraction are present. Pulse deficit is a hemodynamic consequence of ventricular contraction that is insufficient to open the aortic valve and give rise to a peripheral arterial pulse.

pulse duration. In pacing, the amount of time during which an electrical stimulus is applied to the myocardium by a pacemaker or defibrillator. Pulse duration also may be referred to as pulse width. Pulse duration is expressed in milliseconds. See also *tilt.*

pulsed-wave Doppler (PWD). Method of Doppler imaging of blood flow or tissue Doppler, in which a pulse volume or a relatively small area is used for sampling. See also *Doppler echocardiography.*

pulse generator. The portion of the pacing, defibrillation, or cardiac resynchronization system that contains the power source and electronic circuitry and produces the output stimuli. The pulse generator does not include the pacing leads and electrodes. See also *implantable cardioverter-defibrillator, pacemaker.*

pulse interval. The amount of time between corresponding points of successive pulses. In pacing, the pulse interval is the amount of time between identical points of consecutive pacemaker impulses. The pulse interval is expressed in milliseconds.

pulse oximetry. Method of measuring oxygen saturation, sometimes used during catheter ablation, tilt-testing, or prolonged device-implantation procedures.

pulse pressure. Difference between systolic and diastolic blood pressures. A wide pulse pressure occurs in aortic regurgitation and in the elderly. The perceived pulse volume on palpation is an indirect measure of the pulse pressure.

pulse rate. In pacing, the number of pacemaker output pulses per unit of time. Pulse rate is expressed in pulses per minute (ppm). Pulse rate may be used more generically to refer to the number of intrinsic ventricular depolarizations per minute, or beats per minute.

pulse repetition rate (PRR). The number of times per second that a pulse is transmitted. In pacing, the pulse repetition rate is the amount of time between pacemaker discharges. The pulse repetition rate is controlled by the timing circuitry.

pulses per minute (ppm). The number of pacemaker impulses delivered to the heart within 60 seconds. In pacing, the number of pulses per minute describes the stimulation rate of the heart by pacemaker output pulses.

pulse width (PW). See *pulse duration*.

Purkinje fibers. See *Purkinje system*.

Purkinje network. Network of specialized conducting fibers located in the ventricle. The Purkinje network is responsible for rapid conduction from the His bundle, right bundle, and left bundle to the myocardium.

Purkinje potential. During catheter ablation of certain forms of ventricular tachycardia, such as fasicular tachycardia, a discrete potential likely arising from the Purkinje network may be found at the site of origin or part of the circuit of these arrhythmias.

Purkinje potentials in left ventricular tachycardia. During certain forms of left ventricular tachycardia, such as left posterior fascicular tachycardia (Belhassen's tachycardia), discrete near field potentials are found at successful ablation sites. These likely represent potentials arising from the Purkinje tissue at or near the left posterior fascicle. Purkinje potentials apparently initiating tachycardia also have been found during catheter ablation procedures for ventricular fibrillation. Purkinje potentials may be found at many sites not responsible for tachycardia, and pacing maneuvers are required to make a distinction between arrhythmogenic and non-arrhythmogenic Purkinje potentials in patients with left ventricular tachycardias. See also *Purkinje potential*.

Purkinje system. Specialized, rapidly conducting fibers in the ventricular portion of the atrioventricular conduction system which transmit excitation impulses from the bundle branches to the myocardium. The Purkinje system also is known simply as Purkinje fibers.

PV. Abbreviation for *pulmonary vein*.

PVAB. Abbreviation for *postventricular atrial blanking*.

PVARP. Abbreviation for *postventricular atrial refractory period*.

PVARP extension. See *postventricular atrial refractory period extension*.

PVB. Abbreviation for *premature ventricular beat*.

PVC. Abbreviation for *premature ventricular complex*.

PV delay. See *PV interval*.

PVE. Abbreviation for *premature ventricular extrasystole*. See *premature ventricular complex*.

PV interval. In pacing, the amount of time from the onset of a P wave to the next consecutive ventricular output pulse, as measured on an electrocardiogram. The PV interval may appear to be longer than the programmed atrioventricular interval if atrial sensing does not occur at the leading edge of the P wave.

P wave. The wave preceding a QRS complex during sinus rhythm, as seen on an electrocardiogram. The P wave represents atrial depolarization.

P-wave inhibited pacing. See *atrial-inhibited pacing mode (AAI)*.

P-wave synchronous pacing. Pacing in which sensing occurs in the atrium and pacing occurs in the ventricle with a triggered mode of response. Intrinsic atrial activity is sensed, a preset programmable atrioventricular interval is initiated, and the ventricle is paced at the end of the atrioventricular interval. P-wave synchronized pacing maintains atrioventricular synchrony. Pacing modes capable of P-wave synchronized pacing include VDD, VDDR, DDD, and DDDR (and historically VAT).

P-wave triggered pacing. See *atrial-triggered pacing mode (AAT)*.

PWD. Abbreviation for *pulsed-wave Doppler, pulse width duration*.

q

Q-A interval. Interval between the onset of the QRS complex and the Doppler A wave in the mitral valve inflow Doppler recording. Interval used in optimizing the atrioventricular interval with biventricular pacemakers and defibrillators. See also *Ritter method (and formula)*.

QOL. Abbreviation for *quality of life*.

QRS. The surface electrocardiographic waveform that is produced by right and left ventricular depolarization. See also *QRS complex*.

QRS alternans. Significant beat-to-beat variation, usually by more than 25% of the QRS complexes. This variation may be in the R-wave amplitude (positive deflections) or the S-wave amplitude (negative deflections) or represent true alternation, with an R wave being present in one beat and an S wave in the next. Causes of QRS alternans include large pericardial effusions and rapid tachycardias, including atrioventricular reentrant tachycardia.

QRS axes. The vector of depolarization of the ventricular myocardium. The usual QRS axis is downward and to the patient's left in a normal heart.

QRS complex. The surface electrocardiographic waveform produced by ventricular depolarization. The QRS complex is composed of the Q wave, the R wave, and the S wave. The duration of a normal QRS complex ranges from 60 to 100 milliseconds in adults.

QRS duration. Interval between the onset of the Q wave on the surface electrocardiogram and the termination of the S wave. This interval is normally 60 to 120 milliseconds. This is a reflection of intraventricular and interventricular conduction time. See also *QRS prolongation*.

QRS morphology. The morphologic pattern of the surface QRS allows distinction among various types of myocardial and conduction abnormalities. For example, when the right bundle branch does not conduct, the QRS morphology usually is an R wave followed by an S wave, followed by a second R wave in electrocardiographic lead V_1. The QRS morphology during ventricular tachycardia also may help to localize the site of origin of the tachycardia. For example, during ventricular tachycardia, a QRS morphology with a deep S wave in lead V_1 and a positive R wave in lead V_6 suggests an origin in the right ventricle.

QRS prolongation. When the time between the initial portion of the Q wave and terminal portion of the S wave is prolonged (typically more than 120 milliseconds), conduction abnormality in either the cardiac conduction system or the intraventricular conduction is present. QRS prolongation often is associated with abnormal myocardial contraction properties. See also *QRS duration*.

QRS tachycardia. Tachycardias sometimes are distinguished on the basis of their QRS duration. Tachycardias with QRS duration less than 120 milliseconds are referred to as narrow QRS tachycardia, and those with QRS duration more than 120 milliseconds are referred to as wide QRS tachycardia. Narrow QRS tachycardias are almost always supraventricular in origin, although certain rare forms of ventricular tachycardia also may manifest with a narrow QRS complex. Wide QRS tachycardias may be from ventricular tachycardia, supraventricular tachycardia with aberrant conduction from bundle branch block, or supraventricular tachycardia with aberrant conduction via an accessory pathway.

QT. See *QT interval*.

QTc interval. The corrected QT interval. As the QT interval changes with heart rate, the QTc tries to adjust for this. The QTc is calculated most commonly with Bazett's formula, in which QTc is equal to QT divided by the square root of RR. A value more than 440 milliseconds is considered long for the QTc.

QT interval. The amount of time from the onset of ventricular depolarization (the QRS complex) to the end of ventricular repolarization (the T wave) as measured on the surface electrocardiogram. The QT interval typically ranges from 270 to 430 milliseconds.

QT interval prolongation. Prolongation in the amount of time from the onset of ventricular depolarization (QRS complex) to the end of ventricular repolarization (the T wave). The QT interval tends to be normally somewhat longer in women. QT intervals more than 430 milliseconds, particularly after correction for the heart rate (see also *QTc interval*), are abnormally prolonged. See also *QT interval*.

QT interval sensing. A method for rate-adaptive pacing that responds to changes in the duration of the QT interval, that is, the interval from the paced ventricular depolarization to the subsequent T wave. A decrease in the QT interval during exercise is due in part to an increase in catecholamine level and in part to increased heart rate. Therefore, QT interval sensing has proved to be a reliable parameter for long-term rate-adaptive sensing.

QT prolongation. See *QT interval prolongation*.

QT-sensing pacing systems. See *QT interval sensing*.

quadripolar electrode. A catheter containing four electrical poles for stimulation and sensing of intracardiac events.

quality of life (QOL). A frequent outcome measurement (primary end point) for congestive heart failure and cardiac resynchronization trials. There are many tools to assess quality of life, but one of the most commonly used for device trials in recent years is the Minnesota Living With Heart Failure quality-of-life assessment.

quartz crystal. A natural or artificial crystal of piezoelectric quartz cut in a particular configuration to provide a specific resonant frequency of high accuracy. Such crystals are used in precision oscillators that control microcomputer timing. See also *quartz-crystal oscillator*.

quartz-crystal oscillator. An electronic circuit in which a cut quartz crystal, enclosed in a vacuum, vibrates at its resonant frequency. Quartz-crystal oscillators are reliable timing devices, and failure is likely to occur only with severe mechanical shock. In pacing, quartz-crystal oscillators are used in the pacemaker timing circuitry. Specific numbers of crystal oscillations, counted by digital circuitry, are set equal to the various pacing intervals. Thereafter, the quartz-crystal oscillator controls the frequency at which the pacemaker output pulses are delivered. Quartz-crystal oscillators also provide the capability for recording real-time values that can be retrieved by telemetry.

quinidine. A class IA antiarrhythmic agent that prolongs refractoriness and slows conduction in atrial, ventricular, and accessory pathway tissue. It has efficacy in the treatment of supraventricular and ventricular arrhythmias. Quinidine is predominantly metabolized in the liver, but 20% is excreted unchanged by the kidneys. Its plasma half-life is 5 to 8 hours. Quinidine has α-adrenergic blocking activity that may cause orthostatic hypotension. It also is vagolytic. Side effects include gastrointestinal distress, central nervous system effects, thrombocytopenia, and prolonged QT syndrome.

Q wave. The first negative wave of the QRS complex not preceded by a positive R wave, as seen on an electrocardiogram. Typically, Q waves are said to be normal if they are less than 30 milliseconds in duration.

r

R. Abbreviation for *resistance*.

R (rate modulation). Fourth position in the NBG code, indicating presence of rate-adaptive capability. See the table *NBG code*.

RAAVD. Abbreviation for *rate-adaptive AV delay*.

RACE. See *Rate Control Versus Electrical Cardioversion*.

radiofrequency (rf). An alternating electrical current in the range of 100 kHz to 5 MHz, which is within the portion of the electromagnetic radiation spectrum of energy suitable for communication. In pacing, radiofrequency signals are used to transmit programming codes from an external programmer to an implanted pacemaker or cardioverter-defibrillator and to transmit information from the pacemaker or cardioverter-defibrillator to the programmer by telemetry.

radiofrequency ablation (RFA). Destruction of arrhythmogenic tissue with radiofrequency energy delivered through an electrode catheter. Lesion size is related to power (wattage), contact pressure of the electrode, and duration of application. Typical lesions range from 3 to 5 mm in diameter. Radiofrequency may be delivered with minimal or no discomfort to patients who are awake. See also *ablation*.

radiofrequency catheter ablation (RFCA, RCA). The use of radiofrequency (alternating electrical current in the range of 100 kHz to 5 MHz within the electromagnetic spectrum of energy) energy to destroy arrhythmogenic tissue (either a focal source or part of a reentrant circuit) in the treatment of cardiac arrhythmias. Radiofrequency catheter ablation may be performed either from the percutaneous route (i.e., via femoral, subclavian, internal jugular, or other percutaneous venous access) or from an open chest, extracardiac, or transcardiac approach. The vast majority of catheter ablation procedures are performed via the percutaneous route. See also *ablation, radiofrequency energy*.

radiofrequency energy (RF). Alternating current energy in the range of 100 kHz to 5 MHz. A portion of the electromagnetic spectrum used for communication. Radiofrequency energy is used for the most common type of catheter ablation. Radiofrequency signals are also used in pacemakers and implantable cardioverter-defibrillators for transmission of information from the device to the programmer by telemetry.

radiofrequency generator. Device used to generate radiofrequency energy. See also *radiofrequency catheter ablation, radiofrequency energy*.

radiographic evaluation. Evaluation of pacemaker systems with x-rays, often done after implantation to assess adequacy of lead location and for evidence of procedural trauma (pneumothorax) from the procedure. Specific types of pacemakers and implantable cardioverter-defibrillators and evidence of lead fractures can sometimes be identified.

radiographic identification. Identification of an implanted pacemaker or cardioverter-defibrillator with x-rays. See also *pacemaker radiography, radiopaque identification letters*.

radiopaque identification letters. The letters imprinted within the pacemaker case to identify the manufacturer or the model number of the pacemaker. The radiopaque identification letters are not appreciably penetrable by x-rays or other forms of radiation and thus can be read on a chest radiograph. See also *pacemaker radiography, radiographic identification*.

RAM. Abbreviation for *random-access memory*.

ramp. Type of progressive pacing used in an attempt to terminate reentrant arrhythmias by implantable cardioverter-defibrillators. There is a progressive decrease in the coupling interval between one extrastimulus and the next during the train of stimuli.

ramping. The incremental changing of the interval between one coupling of extrastimuli and the next. Ramping may be automatic or controlled, preset or programmable, and incremental or decremental. See also *coupling interval*.

ramp pacing. The progressive changing of the coupling interval between one extrastimulus and the next during a train of stimuli. Ramp pacing may be automatic or controlled, preset or programmable, and incremental or decremental.

ramp pacing in tachycardia termination. With progressive shortening of the coupling interval during pacing by an implantable cardioverter-defibrillator, the reentrant arrhythmias can be terminated. Automatic arrhythmias may be temporarily suppressed (overdrive suppression) with ramp pacing, and triggered automatic arrhythmias may be accelerated with ramp pacing. For ramp pacing to be effective, the reentrant circuit must have a significant excitable gap. See also *ramp*.

random-access memory (RAM). A data storage design in microcomputer systems which provides rapid access to stored data and facilitates rapid entry of data. Data are stored as electrical charges that can be altered after programming. See also *read-only memory*.

rapid atrial pacing. A type of overdrive pacing of the atrium at an accelerated rate to terminate recurrent supraventricular tachycardia or atrial flutter.

rapid pacing. Rapid and sometimes progressive pacing is performed during electrophysiologic studies and by implantable cardioverter-defibrillators to terminate reentrant arrhythmias. Rapid pacing in the electrophysiology laboratory can be used to distinguish automatic arrhythmias (which show overdrive suppression) from triggered automatic arrhythmias (which may show acceleration) and reentrant tachycardias (which may terminate with rapid pacing).

rate. The speed of a rhythm expressed in beats per minute. In contrast, cycle length is expressed in milliseconds. Rate is equal to 60,000 divided by the cycle length.

rate adaptation. In a rate-adaptive pacemaker, the capability of the pacemaker to arbitrate between the patient's intrinsic rate and the sensor-determined rate. The faster of the two will predominate.

rate-adaptive AV delay (RAAVD). See *rate-variable AV interval*.

rate-adaptive AV interval. See *rate-variable AV interval*.

rate-adaptive pacemaker. A pulse generator in which the pacing rate is changed automatically by rate modulation. Rate-adaptive pacemakers are useful in patients with chronotropic incompetence, a condition in which the spontaneous rate does not change sufficiently or fast enough

with exercise or emotional stress. See also *rate-adaptive pacing*.

rate-adaptive pacing. Pacing in which the paced rate changes in response to one or more sensors incorporated into the pacemaker. Sensors used in rate-adaptive pacemakers monitor and react to changes in measurable parameters such as body movement, minute ventilation, temperature, and stroke volume. Dual-chamber pacemakers that track the intrinsic sinus rate also are rate-adaptive, but the term generally is used to refer to sensor-driven rate adaptation. See also *AAIR, AATR, closed-loop control system, rate modulation, sensor, VVIR*.

rate-adaptive postventricular atrial refractory period. A programmable feature that progressively shortens the postventricular atrial refractory period as the rate increases during rate-adaptive pacing.

rate arbitration. In dual-chamber rate-adaptive pacing, automatic determination of whether to track spontaneous atrial depolarizations (atrial-synchronous ventricular pacing) or to provide dual-chamber pacing (atrioventricular synchronous pacing) at a faster rate determined through measurements of an auxiliary physiologic variable. See also *rate-adaptive pacing, rate modulation*.

Rate Control Versus Electrical Cardioversion (RACE). This study assessed the influence of rate control or maintenance of sinus rhythm in patients with atrial fibrillation. The study found that treatment strategy does not affect quality of life but that patients with complaints related to atrial fibrillation may benefit from rhythm control if sinus rhythm can be maintained (Hagens VE, Ranchor AV, Van Sonderen E, Bosker HA, Kamp O, Tijssen JG, et al, RACE Study Group. Effect of rate or rhythm control on quality of life in persistent atrial fibrillation: results from the Rate Control Versus Electrical Cardioversion [RACE] Study. J Am Coll Cardiol. 2004;43:241-7).

rate-dependent block. Bundle branch block occurring either with increasing or decreasing heart rate. See also *acceleration-dependent bundle branch block, deceleration-dependent bundle branch block*.

rate drop response (RDR). A programmable feature that detects a predefined dramatic drop in heart rate and results in pacing at a significantly faster rate for a defined period. The algorithm is

Rate Smoothing

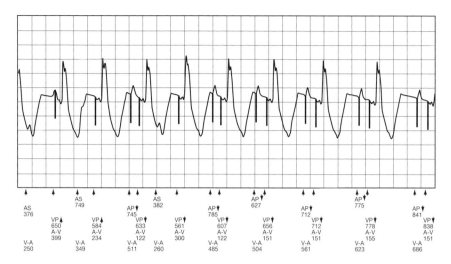

used in patients with cardioinhibitory vasovagal syncope. Rapid pacing may help to minimize the blood pressure fall that often accompanies the cardioinhibitory response. Several manufacturers have variations of this algorithm, for example, "sudden brady response (SBR)".

rate histogram. See *heart rate histogram*.

rate hysteresis. See *hysteresis*.

rate-modulated pacing. See *rate-adaptive pacing*.

rate modulation. In pacing, automatic modification of the pacing rate on the basis of measured values of an auxiliary physiologic variable such as mechanical vibration, cardiac stroke volume, or minute ventilation. The values of the auxiliary variable are measured via a sensor. See also *rate-adaptive pacing*.

rate-response curves. A graphic representation of a rate-adaptive pulse generator's rate response, based on sensor input(s) from physiologic parameters.

rate-response factor (RRF). A programmable feature in some rate-adaptive pulse generators which sets the expected change in pacing rate in response to increasing levels of exercise.

rate-response optimization. A programmable parameter in some rate-adaptive pulse generators which automatically adjusts the slope in the event of change in a patient's condition.

rate-responsive pacing. See *rate-adaptive pacing*.

rate-responsive ventricular refractory period. Ventricular refractory period that shortens as the paced rate increases, a programmable feature in some pulse generators.

rate smoothing. A programmable option of some pacemakers that prevents the atrial or ventricular paced rate from changing by more than a programmed percentage from one cardiac cycle to the next. This prevents large changes in cycle-to-cycle intervals. The ventricular paced rate will increase or decrease only by the programmed percentage from one ventricular depolarization to the next. For example, if an atrial tachycardia occurs at a rate of 120 beats per minute and rate smoothing is on at 6%, then the paced ventricular cycle length after the onset of the tachycardia will be 940 milliseconds, that is, 1,000 milliseconds (60 beats per minute) minus 6% (60 milliseconds). See also *sensor-driven rate smoothing, smoothing constant*.

rate-variable AV interval. A function of some dual-chamber pacemakers whereby the AV interval shortens as the ventricular cycle length shortens. The method of AV interval shortening varies with the pacemaker and may be progressive and directly related to the ventricular rate, or a shortening may occur at fixed ventricular rates. See also *differential AV interval*.

RBBB. Abbreviation for *right bundle branch block*.

RB-I$_{Kr2}$. One of the channels responsible for the inward rectifying potassium current (I_{K1}). The α subunit for this member of the potassium channel family is Kir2.2 and is coded for by the gene *KCNJ12*. See also *inward rectifier*.

RCA. Abbreviation for *radiofrequency catheter ablation*.

RD-CHF. A randomized trial that included patients with a standard pacemaker with right ventricular pacing and New York Heart Association class III or IV heart failure, an aortic pre-ejection delay of more than 180 milliseconds, or an interventricular delay more than 40 milliseconds. Patients were randomized to 3-month crossover periods to right ventricular pacing or biventricular pacing to determine whether patients with a pacemaker who meet criteria for cardiac resynchronization therapy would benefit from upgrade to cardiac resynchronization. The study concluded that in patients with heart failure with poor left ventricular function who have a pacemaker, upgrading from right ventricular to biventricular pacing significantly improves symptoms and exercise tolerance. The study also presented data showing that hospitalizations for heart failure were reduced in the biventricular pacing group (Leclercq C, Cazeau S, Lellouche D, Fossati F, Anselme F, Davy JM, et al. Upgrading from single chamber right ventricular to biventricular pacing in permanently paced patients with worsening heart failure: the RD-CHF Study. Pacing Clin Electrophysiol. 2007;30 Suppl 1:S23-30).

RDR. Abbreviation for *rate drop response*.

reaction time. A programmable parameter in some rate-adaptive pacemakers which determines how quickly the pacing rate will increase via sensor activation.

read-only memory (ROM). A data storage design in microcomputer systems which permits permanent storage of data. The data are non-erasable but can be read out for use by the computer or referenced by the user. However, existing data cannot be altered and new data cannot be added. The read-only memory usually is used to store programs essential for the operation of the central processing unit. The program provides the translation from high-level commands to a series of detailed control codes recognizable by the microprocessor for execution. The size of the read-only memory varies, according to use requirements, within the maximum-allowed capacity of the microprocessor. See also *random-access memory*.

real-time position management (RPM) system. Electrophysiology mapping system that allows electrical and anatomical correlation three-dimensionally and in real-time. One of the available electroanatomic mapping systems.

real-time telemetry. The transmission of information, quantified at the time of interrogation, from a pacemaker to a programmer. Real-time telemetry provides on-line access to measured performance, parameters, and detected signals of an implanted pacemaker such as lead impedance, battery voltage, marker channels, and intracardiac electrograms.

recall. Action taken by a firm or a regulatory agency either to remove a product from the market or to conduct a field correction. In the United States, recalls may be conducted on a firm's own initiative, at the request of the Food and Drug Administration, or by order of the Food and Drug Administration under statutory authority. In a class I recall, there is a reasonable probability that the use of or exposure to a violative product will cause serious adverse health consequences or death. In a class II recall, use of or exposure to a violative product may cause temporary or medically reversible adverse health consequences or the probability of serious adverse health consequences is remote. In a class III recall, use of or exposure to a violative product is not likely to cause adverse health consequences (U.S. Food and Drug Administration [homepage on the Internet]. Rockville (MD): U.S. Food and Drug Administration [updated 2005 Dec 19; cited 2007 Feb 5]. Learn About Medical Device Recalls. Available from: http://www.fda.gov/cdrh/recalls/learn.html). See also *device recall*.

rechargeable battery. A battery that generates energy and, after discharge, may be restored to a charged condition by sending a current through the cell(s) in the appropriate direction. Rechargeable batteries, such as nickel-cadmium, have been used in some pacemakers. These batteries provide a theoretical longevity of 70 to 80 years but must be recharged every 6 to 8 weeks. See also *nickel-cadmium*.

reciprocal beat. The return of an impulse to its chamber of origin due to the wave front traversing a reentrant pathway. Reciprocal beats may be spontaneous or induced. See also *echo beat*.

reciprocating tachycardia. Any mechanism of reentrant tachyarrhythmias. Usually refers to supraventricular tachycardia that requires the reciprocation that is reentry to the atrium via either a second atrioventricular nodal pathway or an accessory pathway connecting the atrium and ventricle. Common forms of reciprocating tachycardia include atrioventricular reentrant tachycardia (both orthodromic and antidromic) and atrioventricular nodal reentrant tachycardia. More generally, reciprocating tachycardia also includes pacemaker-mediated tachycardia, bundle branch reentrant tachycardia, and other forms of reentrant ventricular tachycardia.

reciprocation. See *echo beat, reciprocal beat*.

recommended replacement time (RRT). As pulse generator battery depletion occurs, the point in time when the pulse generator should be replaced. The projected time from recommended replacement time to true battery depletion varies between manufacturers but should be a period of at least 3 months.

reconditioning. The process of treating an explanted pacemaker in preparation for reuse. Reconditioning necessitates cleaning, testing, packaging, and sterilization of the pacemaker but not disassembly or reassembly. Reconditioning currently is not permitted by the U.S. Food and Drug Administration. See also *refurbishing, reuse*.

recovery time. A programmable parameter in some rate-adaptive pacemakers that determines how quickly the sensor-driven pacing rate will decrease once the sensor is no longer activated.

rectification of Kir2.x channels. See *inward rectifier, Kir channels, potassium channels*.

rectifier. An electrical circuit that converts a signal possessing both positive and negative components into a signal with only positive or negative components. A rectifier is used before a comparator to allow signals on both sides of the isoelectric line to be sensed using the one comparator reference level.

recycle. In pacing, the resetting of a pacemaker timing cycle from a specific paced or intrinsic event. For example, in a dual-chamber pacemaker with a ventricular-based timing system, a premature ventricular contraction resets the timing cycle and initiates the ventriculoatrial interval. See also *timing cycle*.

redetection. When programmed, implantable cardioverter-defibrillators may, on completion of charging, reanalyze the ventricular electrograms to determine whether detection criteria for the ventricular arrhythmia that prompted the charge are still present. Redetection may be programmed "off"; if this is done, the therapies are referred to as committed.

redundancy. The deliberate duplication of essential components or functions in a system to decrease the probability of a system failure by providing an alternative arrangement for use on failure of the primary arrangement. In pacing, redundancy is incorporated into the pacemaker circuitry and lead design. See also *circuit redundancy, lead redundancy*.

reed switch. A small switch that consists of two metal strips (reeds) sealed in a glass tube. The switch is sensitive to magnetic fields, and the reeds make contact with each other to form a conductive pathway on application of a magnetic field. In pacing, a reed switch is the component in some pacemakers that activates the predetermined magnet rate. In some programmable pacemakers, the reed switch also detects the initiation and implementation of a programmer and causes the reed switch to complete or disrupt the pathway through which the binary programming codes are received. New pacemakers use solid-state magnet detectors that are telemetry-based and are more reliable than reed switches.

reed switch bounce. An oversensitive reed switch that has a tendency to display extra opening and closing when a magnetic field is introduced. See also *reed switch*.

reed switch chattering. See *reed switch bounce*.

reed switch inhibition. In pacing, the temporary inhibition of normal pacemaker function due to incomplete or intermittent closure of the pacemaker reed switch when a magnet is positioned inappropriately over the switch. Inhibition of the pacemaker function occurs only if the pacemaker interprets this signal as intrinsic cardiac activity. See also *reed switch*.

reentrant arrhythmia. An arrhythmia caused by an impulse that depolarizes the myocardium and is perpetuated by a circuit that consists of a loop surrounding a central region of functional or anatomic block. Reentrant arrhythmias can be initiated and terminated by programmed stimulation. See also *reentrant circuit*.

reentrant circuit. A loop of tissue that may perpetuate conduction and thereby cause repetitive beats or tachycardias. Reentrant circuits can occur when three functional or structural conditions exist in the myocardium: 1) the impulse must be conducted through two pathways that have different conduction velocities and refractoriness, 2) the pathways must be joined proximally and distally to form a continuous loop, and 3) unidirectional block must occur in one pathway. The initial impulse is conducted through the unblocked pathway of the loop. As the impulse reaches the end of that pathway, it is conducted in the retrograde direction through the alternate, unidirectionally blocked pathway. The depolarizing impulse then reenters the perpetuating circuit at the top of the circuit. Reentrant circuits may occur within the sinus node, the atria, the atrioventricular node, the His-Purkinje system, or areas of the myocardium adjacent to a ventricular infarct or aneurysm and via accessory pathways. Reentrant circuits may cause echoes, repetitive beats, or sustained tachycardias. See also *circus movement tachycardia, reentrant arrhythmia.*

reentrant premature contractions. Contractions in either the atrium or the ventricle resulting from an intramyocardial reentrant circuit. Examples include reentrant premature ventricular contractions, which may involve only the ventricular myocardium (often related to ischemic or scarred tissue) or portions of the bundle branch system. Another example is reentrant atrial contractions, usually referring to echo beats involving abnormal atrial myocardium but also may more generally refer to atrioventricular nodal single reentrant beats. See also *echo beat, premature atrial complex, premature ventricular complex.*

reentrant supraventricular tachycardia. General term referring to many varieties of supraventricular tachycardia, including atrioventricular node reentry, atrioventricular reentry, and intra-atrial reentrant tachycardia. Reentrant supraventricular tachycardias often start and stop abruptly and generally are amenable to both antiarrhythmic therapy and catheter ablation.

reentrant tachycardias. See *reentrant circuit, reentrant supraventricular tachycardia, ventricular tachycardia.*

reentrant ventricular tachycardia. General term referring to various mechanisms of ventricular tachycardia. Examples include reentrant tachycardia related to prior myocardial infarction, bundle branch reentrant tachycardia, and interfascicular tachycardia.

reentry. An arrhythmia mechanism in which an impulse is conducted in one direction and returns via another pathway. If the earlier site has

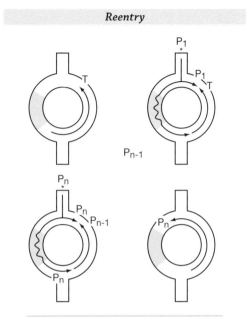

Reentry

Entrainment of tachycardia by pacing. The tachycardia impulse (T) travels around the reentrant circuit in the orthodromic direction (upper left panel). The first pacing impulse (P1) enters the reentrant circuit in the antidromic direction and collides with the last impulse of tachycardia, but it also travels in the orthodromic direction so as to continue the tachycardia (upper right panel). Each subsequent paced impulse produces the same effect as the first one until the last paced impulse (Pn) collides in the antidromic direction with the next-to-the-last paced impulse (Pn-1, bottom left panel) and also in the orthodromic direction where, finding no subsequent paced impulse with which to collide, it continues around the circuit as the next tachycardia impulse (lower right panel). From Stanton MS. Programmed electrical simulation: elucidation of mechanisms. In: Fisch C, Surawicz B, editors. Cardiac electrophysiology and arrhythmias. New York: Elsevier; 1991. p. 264.

recovered from refractoriness and can be reactivated, a reentrant circuit results. See also *intrinsic automaticity, reentrant circuit, triggered activity.*

reentry tachycardia. See *reentrant arrhythmia.*

reflection. A potential mechanism of arrhythmias that is a variation of reentry. An area of depressed conduction exists between the proximal and distal normal tissue and slowly conducts electronically to the distal tissue of the fiber. When the distal normal tissue is excited, the area of depressed conduction can then passively conduct a depolarizing current back to the proximal portion, where another action potential is generated. Alternatively, adjacent cells with markedly different action potential durations cause the fibers to respond differently to the same stimulus. This variation in action potential duration may cause a completely recovered (excitable) fiber to be reexcited by the adjacent fiber that is still depolarized.

reformation. The process of regenerating the oxide layers of an aluminum electrolytic capacitor by application of high voltage to maintain good charge time in an implantable cardioverter-defibrillator. Reformation may be performed via telemetry during patient follow-up visits or may be done automatically by the defibrillator itself. Reformation typically is performed every 2 months.

refractory period. 1. Physiologically, the amount of time after onset of an action potential during which the myocardium cannot respond at all to either intrinsic or extrinsic stimulation (the absolute refractory period) or can be depolarized only by supranormal stimuli (the relative refractory period). 2. In pacing, the refractory period is an interval in the pacemaker timing cycle(s) that follows a sensed or paced event. During the atrial and ventricular refractory periods, the respective sensing amplifiers are unresponsive to all input signals from the heart. Pacemaker refractory periods often are programmable parameters and independent values can be set for the atrial and ventricular channels. See also *absolute refractory period, atrial refractory period, blanking period, effective refractory period, functional refractory period, postventricular atrial refractory period, relative refractory period, total atrial refractory period, ventricular refractory period.*

refractory time generator. A component of the pacemaker sensing circuitry that protects the system from errant sensing by initiating a period of time during which the sensing amplifiers are insensitive to input signals and waveforms. The refractory time generator, therefore, regulates the blanking period or the refractory periods of a pacemaker.

refractory zone. The portion of a reentrant circuit during an arrhythmia which is unexcitable at any given time. The remainder of the circuit is the excitable gap.

refurbishing. The process by which an explanted pacemaker is treated in preparation for reuse. Refurbishing requires some degree of

pacemaker disassembly and reassembly, that is, replacement of the connector or reassembly of the outer housing. Refurbishing is currently not permitted by the U.S. Food and Drug Administration. See also *reconditioning, reuse.*

regional dyssynchrony. In the evaluation of left ventricular dyssynchrony, tissue Doppler and strain techniques often show specific regional areas of greatest loss of synchrony. Defining the areas of regional dyssynchrony may allow more effective lead placement and subsequent programming of cardiac resynchronization devices.

reinnervation. Regrowth of nerve fibers into a region that previously underwent denervation. Sympathetic reinnervation may occur after denervation caused by myocardial infarction.

relative refractory period (RRP). 1. In cell physiology, the period of time after the absolute refractory period and before repolarization, during which the myocardium can be depolarized prematurely by stimulus of supranormal intensity. The excitability threshold of the tissue is higher than normal during the relative refractory period, and depolarization (phase 0) is slower than normal. Thus, in tissues, the relative refractory period is the time during which conduction delay occurs. 2. In pacing, the relative refractory period is that portion of the total refractory period during which the pacemaker circuitry is sensing for external interference that does not meet the criteria of an intracardiac signal. The relative refractory period in pacing also is referred to as the noise sampling period. See also *atrial relative refractory period, AV nodal relative refractory period, His-Purkinje system relative refractory period, VA conduction system relative refractory period, ventricular relative refractory period.*

remote monitoring. Various systems by which a patient with an implanted cardiac rhythm device can be monitored long distance. Although transtelephonic monitoring is technically a type of remote monitoring, this term more specifically applies to newer techniques and systems that are capable of interfacing with the patient's device and retrieving and sending data for review. The current trend is for the data to be downloaded to a remote server and then made available for caregiver review. Current remote monitoring systems include products from Biotronik, Berlin, Germany (Home Monitoring),

Boston Scientific, Natick, Massachusetts (Latitude), Medtronic Inc., Minneapolis, Minnesota (CareLink), and St. Jude Medical, St. Paul, Minnesota (Housecall Plus). See also *telemetered information, telemetry*.

remote patient management. See *remote monitoring*.

repetitive monomorphic ventricular tachycardia (RMVT). A form of ventricular tachycardia that typically occurs in young people with normal hearts. Repetitive monomorphic ventricular tachycardia usually presents with light-headedness, or it may be asymptomatic but observable during electrocardiographic monitoring. The morphology most commonly is left bundle branch block with a normal axis or right-axis deviation. The arrhythmia slows before spontaneous termination. Repetitive monomorphic ventricular tachycardia usually has a benign course. If treatment is necessary, β-adrenergic blockers and calcium channel blockers frequently are effective.

repetitive nonreentrant ventriculoatrial synchronous (RNRVAS) rhythm. Repeated retrograde ventriculoatrial conduction in patients with dual-chamber pacemakers may result in ventriculoatrial synchrony. In one mechanism, pacemaker-mediated tachycardia results, in which retrograde ventriculoatrial conduction occurs after a paced beat is sensed in the atrium, which triggers another ventricular paced beat after the program-sensed atrioventricular interval (see also *endless-loop tachycardia*). In another mechanism, also referred to as atrioventricular dyssynchronization arrhythmia, the retrograde P wave is not sensed and the atrial-paced stimulus falls in the atrial refractory period. Thus, although the atrial and ventricular stimuli are synchronous, unfavorable hemodynamic effects result from atrioventricular dyssynchronization.

repetitive nonreentrant ventriculoatrial synchrony. See *repetitive nonreentrant ventriculoatrial synchronous rhythm*.

repolarization. The restoration of excitable tissue to its initial resting state after depolarization. Ventricular repolarization is represented on the electrocardiogram by the T wave, and the atrial repolarization waveform is buried in the QRS complex. Both atrial and ventricular repolarization can be identified, however, on their respective intracardiac electrograms.

repolarization alternans. Beat-to-beat alteration of the T-wave amplitude, termed T-wave alternans, is a measure of electrical instability in the heart and a marker for susceptibility to sudden cardiac death. The physiologic basis for this electrocardiographic phenomenon is repolarization alternans at the level of the ventricular myocyte. Repolarization alternans is likely related to impairment of intracellular calcium cycling. See also *T-wave alternans*.

repolarization dispersion. Because of the hydrogenous distribution of ion channels in ventricular muscle, spatial variation in the action potential duration occurs primarily during the repolarization phase. Although this contributes to the normal repolarization sequence in healthy hearts, enhanced dispersion or variant of repolarization underlies certain ventricular arrhythmias, including torsades de pointes.

repolarized state. The condition of the myocardium in which the membrane potential is restored to its resting state. During the repolarized state, the myocardium can be depolarized by intrinsic or extrinsic stimuli of adequate strength and duration.

rescue pacing spike. In autocapture algorithms, if failure to capture occurs at a lower output, the device triggers an automatic backup safety pulse to ensure capture, sometimes designated as a rescue pacing spike.

rescue shock. With an implantable cardioverter-defibrillator, if an initial shock fails to terminate ventricular fibrillation, a second, usually maximal voltage shock, termed rescue shock, is delivered. Rescue shock may be required either because the initial shock was programmed to deliver energy lower than the defibrillation threshold or because the shock itself may have induced a second episode of arrhythmia.

resettable refractory period. A period of time after a sensed event during which the pacemaker sensing circuitry is unresponsive. The resettable refractory period is restarted each time a sensed event is detected outside the blanking period. Resettable refractory periods are used to detect interference, such as noise.

resetting. Advancement of the tachycardia by the introduction of a premature complex, either spontaneous or extrinsic. May occur in automatic, triggered, or reentrant rhythms. In reentry, resetting occurs when a premature impulse enters the reentrant circuit in its excitable gap.

Resetting

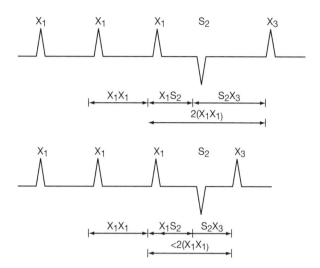

Response of tachycardia to a single extrastimulus (S_2). The tachycardia cycle length is X_1X_2. The coupling interval of the extrastimulus is X_1S_2. The return cycle length of the first complex of tachycardia after the extrastimulus is S_2X_3. In the top portion of the figure, the extrastimulus does not affect the tachycardia circuit and a compensatory pause occurs. Resetting of the tachycardia is shown in the bottom portion of the figure. From Stanton MS. Programmed electrical simulation: elucidation of mechanisms. In: Fisch C, Surawicz B, editors. Cardiac electrophysiology and arrhythmias. New York: Elsevier; 1991. p. 262. Used with permission.

Entrainment is continuous resetting by a pacing train. See also *entrainment, excitable gap.*

reset zone. The portion of a reentrant tachycardia cycle in which an intrinsic pulse or programmed electrical stimulus penetrates the excitable tissue of a tachycardia and causes the tachycardia to be advanced. The reset zone is used for calculation of sinus node conduction time. See also *resetting.*

resistance (R). Electrically, the opposition to the flow of direct (constant) current through a material or device that is resistive due to its physical properties, dimensions, and geometric configuration. The resistance of a material or device is equal to the voltage drop across it divided by the current through it. Resistance does not take reactive components (capacitance or inductance) or phase relationships into account because these factors play no role in direct-current phenomena, and thus resistance can be expressed as a single number. Resistance is related to voltage (V) and current (I) by Ohm's law, R = V/I. Resistance is measured in ohms. See also *impedance.*

resistor. An electronic circuit component used to limit or determine current flow or to provide a voltage drop. A resistor is designed to have a specific, predetermined amount of resistance.

respiration sensing. The determination of the respiratory rate by the use of sensors that measure changes in intrapleural pressure or in thoracic impedance. Respiration sensors may be used in rate-adaptive pacemakers to control pacing rate.

response time. A term used with rate-adaptive pacemakers to determine the time it takes for the sensor to respond to activity. In an open-loop rate-adaptive pacing system, the response time is usually a programmable parameter.

Resistance

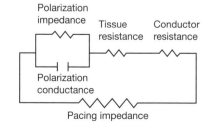

resting membrane potential. With reference to cardiac cells, the resting membrane potential is the voltage gradient across the myocyte membrane. The resting membrane potential is by convention described with the inside of the cell negative and the outside positive at rest. Normal resting membrane potentials for ventricular myocardial cells are between –80 mV and –90 mV; for the sinus node, between –50 and –60 mV; for atrial myocardial cells, between –80 and –90 mV; and for the atrioventricular node, between –60 and –70 mV.

resting potential. The voltage gradient that exists between the inside (negative) and the outside (positive) of cells at rest. Normal resting potentials vary for different cell types. Those for the sinus node are –50 to –60 mV; for the atrium, –80 to –90 mV; for the atrioventricular node, –60 to –70 mV; for the His-Purkinje system, –90 to –95 mV; and for the ventricle, –80 to –90 mV. See also *depolarization phases*.

resting state. According to the modulated receptor hypothesis, ion channels exist in three states: activated, inactivated, and resting. The channel is closed while in the resting state and cannot conduct ions until it is activated. The channel must return to the resting state before it can be activated. Resting state blockers, such as tetradotoxin, are not clinically useful. See also *modulated receptor hypothesis*.

restitution curve. A graphic representation of the time course of recovery (restoration) of a given electrophysiologic phenomenon, usually cellular. For example, a restitution curve of action potential duration as a function of time at a given pacing cycle length can be generated by pacing a cell at that cycle length for a fixed number of beats and then coupling an extrastimulus at progressively increasing intervals until the action potential duration reaches a plateau.

Resynchronization Reverses Remodeling in Systolic Left Ventricular Dysfunction (REVERSE). This trial includes patients with New York Heart Association class I congestive heart failure who were previously symptomatic and patients with class II congestive heart failure and a QRS duration of 120 milliseconds or more, left ventricular ejection fraction of 40% or less, left ventricular end-diastolic dimension of 55 mm or more, without bradycardia, with or without an indication for an implantable cardioverter-defibrillator and receiving optimal medical therapy to determine whether cardiac resynchronization will limit the clinical progression of heart failure. The primary end point is a clinical composite response (Linde C, Gold M, Abraham WT, Daubert J-C, REVERSE Study Group. Rationale and design of a randomized controlled trial to assess the safety and efficacy of cardiac resynchronization therapy in patients with asymptomatic left ventricular dysfunction with previous symptoms or mild heart failure: the REsynchronization reVErses Remodeling in Systolic left vEntricular dysfunction [REVERSE] study. Am Heart J. 2006;151:288-94).

resynchronization therapy. See *cardiac resynchronization therapy*.

Resynchronization Therapy In Normal QRS (RethinQ). This is a multicenter trial evaluating the safety and efficacy of cardiac resynchronization in patients with an approved indication for an implantable cardioverter-defibrillator, New York Heart Association class III congestive heart failure, and a QRS duration of less than 130 milliseconds but evidence of mechanical dyssynchrony by echocardiography. The primary efficacy end point is peak oxygen consumption, and secondary end points include assessment of quality of life and New York Heart Association functional class.

retention wires. See *J retention wire*.

RethinQ. See *Resynchronization Therapy In Normal QRS*.

retriggerable postventricular atrial refractory period. In some dual-chamber pacemakers used before the current forms of automatic mode switch capability, retriggerable atrial refractory periods were used to deal with supraventricular tachycardia occurring faster than the programmed double rate. An atrial signal detected in the postventricular atrial refractory period beyond the initial postventricular atrial blanking period does not start a programmed atrioventricular interval but rather retriggers a new total atrial refractory period. Thus, during supraventricular tachycardia the retriggered total atrial refractory periods continue to be reinitiated and overlap until the P-P interval lengthens beyond the duration of the total atrial refractory period, at which time normal atrioventricular synchrony results. In effect, the dual-chamber pacemaker has converted to a nonatrial tracking mode such as DVI or DVIR. Similar but more refined algorithms are now used in pacemakers with automatic mode switch capability.

retrograde atrial activation sequence. The order in which the electrical wave front approaching in the retrograde direction from the ventricles spreads throughout the atrial myocardium. The retrograde atrial activation sequence gives information regarding the presence of accessory pathways and dual atrioventricular nodal physiology.

retrograde atrioventricular conduction. During ventricular pacing or a spontaneous ventricular rhythm, conduction to the atrium may occur. This retrograde ventriculoatrial conduction may occur via either the atrioventricular conduction system or an accessory pathway. Retrograde conduction across the atrioventricular node or an accessory pathway may occur in the absence of antegrade conduction from the atrium to the ventricle.

retrograde block to atrium. During ventricular pacing or a spontaneous ventricular rhythm, block to the atrium (i.e., cessation of ventriculoatrial conduction) occurs when the retrograde refractory period of the conducting structure is reached.

retrograde capture of His bundle. 1. During ventricular pacing on the interventricular septum near the base, direct capture of the His bundle may occur at high-output pacing. This phenomenon is utilized to analyze the nature and mechanism of retrograde ventriculoatrial conduction (parahisian pacing). 2. In patients with an antegrade conducting accessory pathway that connects directly to the His bundle or proximal right bundle during atrial pacing, the His bundle is directly captured via the accessory pathway instead of antegrade conduction via the atrioventricular node or retrograde conduction from the ventricular myocardium via the accessory pathway.

retrograde conduction. The transmission of a depolarizing impulse from the ventricular myocardium to the atrial myocardium. Retrograde conduction may occur via normal conduction pathways of the heart (i.e., the His-Purkinje system and atrioventricular node) or via accessory pathways such as those found in the Wolff-Parkinson-White syndrome, but it is not limited to pathways in which antegrade conduction occurs. The incidence of retrograde conduction is highest in patients with normal antegrade conduction. However, it may occur in patients with antegrade complete heart block. Retrograde conduction also is referred to as ventriculoatrial conduction. See also *antegrade conduction*.

retrograde coronary venography. 1. Coronary venography is sometimes required for left ventricular lead placement. In retrograde coronary venography, coronary arteriography is performed and prolonged fluoroscopy after arterial injection is used to image the late phase of the coronary veins. Although this term is frequently used, the filling in the coronary veins is actually in the usual or antegrade fashion. 2. Retrograde venography of the coronary vein (i.e., against the natural flow of blood in the coronary vein) may be performed with balloon occlusion of the proximal coronary sinus and injection via an end-hole catheter into the coronary vein.

retrograde P waves. A P wave that results from retrograde conduction. The P wave may be inverted or partially or totally obscured by the QRS. See also *retrograde conduction*.

retrograde refractory period. The longest ventricular pacing interval during which each ventricular paced beat results in retrograde activation of the atrium. The retrograde refractory period may be calculated separately for the atrioventricular node and an accessory pathway conducting in the retrograde direction, if present.

retrograde Wenckebach point. In electrophysiologic testing, the lowest rate in decremental ventricular pacing at which 1:1 ventriculoatrial conduction no longer is possible through the normal conduction pathway and Wenckebach-type block occurs. See also *Mobitz type I second-degree atrioventricular block*.

retromammary pacemaker placement. A surgical technique that has been uncommonly used for pulse-generator placement. The technique was used for cosmetic purposes (i.e., the incision was made inframammary and the device was "hidden" behind the breast tissue, leaving no obvious incision or evidence of the device).

retropectoral veins. 1. Generally refers to veins located below the pectoralis major muscle which are used during implantation of a pacemaker or implantable cardioverter-defibrillator. These include the extrathoracic portion of the subclavian vein and most of the axillary vein. 2. Sometimes

Ritter Method

Short AV delay 50 ms

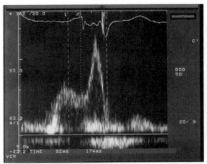

Long AV delay 160 ms

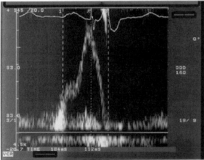

Optimized AV delay 100 ms

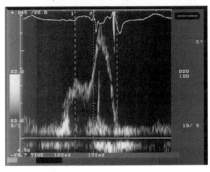

specifically used in reference to dilated collateral retropectoral veins that may be entered either directly with contrast venography or with a surgical cutdown procedure, which allows device implantation when the subclavian venous system is occluded.

reuse. In pacing, the implantation of a pacemaker that was previously implanted in a different patient. Reuse currently is not permitted by the U.S. Food and Drug Administration. See also *reconditioning, refurbishing.*

REVERSE. See *Resynchronization Reverses Remodeling in Systolic Left Ventricular Dysfunction.*

reversed polarity. When an implantable cardioverter-defibrillator delivers shocks, an antegrade polarity of initial polarity that defines the vector of shock delivery is programmed. When defibrillation thresholds are increased, the polarity for the shocks can be reversed and sometimes results in effective defibrillation.

reverse remodeling. Beginning of normalization of a cardiac chamber that has structural changes as a result of a pathologic process. As it relates to device therapy, trials of cardiac resynchronization have found left ventricular reverse remodeling in many patients after cardiac resynchronization, as shown by a decrease in left ventricular diastolic dimension and improvement in left ventricular ejection fraction.

reversion. 1. The point at which a tachycardia terminates. 2. In some pacemakers, the automatic suspension of sensing capability that occurs when the patient is exposed to certain electromagnetic fields. This type of reversion is a safety feature that allows the pacemaker to continuously pace, rather than inhibit, in the presence of continuous electromagnetic interference.

RF. See *radiofrequency energy.*

RFA. Abbreviation for *radiofrequency ablation.*

RF ablation. See *radiofrequency ablation.*

RF catheter ablation (RFCA, RCA). See *radiofrequency catheter ablation.*

rheobase. The value, derived from a strength-duration curve, that indicates the minimum intensity of the steady cathode current that will stimulate the myocardium irrespective of the pulse duration. Rheobase indicates the point at which capture of myocardial tissue with a pacemaker output pulse will not be improved by an increase in the pulse duration. See also *chronaxie, strength-duration curve.*

ri. Abbreviation for *internal longitudinal resistance.*

right atrial linear ablation. One of the ablation techniques used in the treatment of atrial fibrillation and multiple atrial flutters. Catheter ablation is performed in a linear point-to-point fashion to create lines of block, usually connecting to electrically inert structures such as the superior vena cava and inferior vena cava or the tricuspid anulus and the inferior vena cava. Light atrial linear ablation is used to complete the right atrial maze procedure. Also used typically in part of a biatrial endocardial maze procedure for atrial fibrillation. Incomplete lines during right atrial linear ablation may constitute the substrate for proarrhythmic atrial flutters.

right bundle branch. The division of the bundle of His that travels down the right side of the septum to activate the right ventricle.

right bundle branch block (RBBB). A disruption of conduction in the right bundle branch of the His-Purkinje system. Cardiac activation occurs by initial activation of the septum in the normal left-to-right direction. Lead V_1 displays an rSR' pattern. The QRS interval is prolonged because of an activation of the right ventricular myocardium by cell-to-cell conduction. Because the initial deflection of the QRS is unaffected, the pathologic Q waves can still be interpreted.

right bundle branch block and ST-segment elevation syndrome. See *Brugada syndrome.*

right inferior pulmonary vein (RIPV). Vein draining the lower lobe of the right lung. Also called right lower vein. See also *pulmonary vein.*

right superior pulmonary vein (RSPV). Pulmonary vein that drains the upper lobe of the right lung, usually via a branch of the middle lobe of the right lung. The right superior pulmonary vein runs from the right upper lobe to the left atrium just posterior to the right atrium and the posterior surface of the superior vena cava. The right middle lobe vein may drain directly to the left atrium.

right ventricular apex (RVA) electrogram. The electrical activity recorded by a catheter located in the apex of the right ventricle.

right ventricular disconnection. Surgical procedure rarely performed for the treatment of intractable ventricular tachycardia in patients with arrhythmogenic right ventricular dysplasia. The right ventricle is incised and resutured so as to electrically isolate the dysplastic right venticule.

right ventricular dysplasia (RVD). See *arrythmogenic right ventricular dysplasia.*

right ventricular outflow tract (RVOT). Portion of the right ventricular myocardium in the vicinity of the pulmonic valve. This region of the heart is a common site of origin for ventricular tachycardia in otherwise healthy patients.

right ventricular outflow tract pacing. Technique of placing the pacing lead somewhere on the right ventricular outflow tract or septum. Although the data are still limited, some investigators believe that pacing from this position may be hemodynamically advantageous to pacing the right ventricular apex. Many portions of the outflow tract or septum could theoretically be paced.

right ventricular outflow tract tachycardia. Common form of tachycardia in patients with structurally normal hearts. Patients with right ventricular outflow tract tachycardia often present with palpitations and rarely presyncope. Symptoms usually occur with exercise but also may occur with rest. The ventricular myocardium in relation to the pulmonary valve is the site of origin for this arrhythmia. The prognosis is generally good, and this arrhythmia is particularly amenable to catheter ablation.

right ventricular septal (RVS) pacing. See *right ventricular outflow tract pacing.*

right ventricular stimulation. Pacing from the right ventricle to induce ventricular tachycardia during electrophysiologic studies. See also *electrophysiologic study, programmed stimulation.*

ring electrode. See *contact ring, proximal-ring electrode.*

RITE protocol. Ramping incremental treadmill exercise (RITE) protocol, used to optimize minute ventilation rate-adaptive pacemakers. Specifically, the protocol was designed to assess the correct HR/VE (heart rate and minute ventilation) slope below the anaerobic threshold (Lewalter T, MacCarter D, Jung W, Bauer T, Schimpf R, Manz M, et al. The "low intensity treadmill exercise" protocol for appropriate rate adaptive programming of minute ventilation controlled pacemakers. Pacing Clin Electrophysiol. 1995;18:1374-87).

Ritter method (and formula). An echocardiographic technique used to determine the optimal atrioventricular interval (at rest).

Ritter technique. See *Ritter method (and formula)*.

RMS. Abbreviation for *root mean squared* (voltage).

RMVT. Abbreviation for *repetitive monomorphic ventricular tachycardia*.

RNRVAS. Abbreviation for *repetitive nonreentrant ventriculoatrial synchronous* (rhythm).

rolling-trend event counters. A diagnostic counter that continues to collect the material and store it over a defined period (e.g., a 6-month rolling trend will continue to collect and display the data but delete information from day 1 when day 181 is reached; for this example, consider 6 × 30 days).

ROM. Abbreviation for *read-only memory*.

Romano-Ward syndrome. Congenital long QT syndrome not associated with hearing deficit. The Romano-Ward syndrome has autosomal dominant transmission.

R-on-T pattern. The electrocardiographic waveform that occurs when a premature ventricular complex occurs during the T wave of the preceding complex. In pacing, an R-on-T pattern also may occur when a ventricular output pulse falls on the T wave, such as during magnet application or during loss of ventricular sensing. An R-on-T pattern may cause ventricular tachycardia or ventricular fibrillation due to stimulation during the vulnerable period. R-on-T waveforms almost never cause arrhythmias in normal hearts. See also *vulnerable period*.

root mean squared (RMS) voltage. One of the three parameters analyzed at the time domain signal-averaged electrocardiogram. It is the average voltage in the terminal 40 milliseconds of the signal-averaged electrocardiogram. The typical normal value for root mean squared voltage is 20 mV or more.

RP interval. Measurement of the time from the onset of the QRS to the earliest onset of the P wave in any lead. Tachycardias are divided into long RP (RP greater than PR) and short RP (RP less than PR) tachycardias.

RPM. Abbreviation for *real-time position management* (system).

RRF. Abbreviation for *rate-response factor*.

RR interval. The amount of time from the onset of one QRS complex to the onset of the next QRS complex, which represents the duration of one cardiac cycle. The RR interval usually is measured from one R wave to the next and is expressed in milliseconds.

RRP. Abbreviation for *relative refractory period*.

RRT. Abbreviation for *recommended replacement time*.

RSPV. Abbreviation for *right superior pulmonary vein*.

R-S-R morphology. The QRS morphology in right bundle branch block consists of an initial upward deflection R followed by a negative deflection S and then a second upward deflection. The second upward deflection gives rise to the R-S-R morphology. By convention, rSR' reflects the situation in which the first upward deflection is smaller than the second and is typical of right bundle branch block. When the first deflection is as large or larger than the second (RSR pattern), atypical right bundle branch block or ventricular tachycardia should be suspected.

R2 patch. A cutaneous patch used for pacing or external cardioversion-defibrillation.

runaway pacemaker. A pacemaker that exceeds the rate limitation protection, usually due to circuit malfunction or damage to the circuitry. Rates are so rapid that the situation can be life-threatening. The phenomenon was more common in early pacemakers without rate-limitation protection. Runaway pacemakers are now uncommon but still can result from damage to the pacemaker from therapeutic radiation. See also *pace limit*.

runaway protection. An independent circuit that monitors the pacing output and intervenes to block pacing in a runaway pacemaker.

RVA. Abbreviation for *right ventricular apex* (electrogram).

RVD. Abbreviation for *right ventricular dysplasia*.

RVOT. Abbreviation for *right ventricular outflow tract*.

RVS. Abbreviation for *right ventricular septal* (pacing).

R wave. The first positive deflection of a QRS complex as seen on an electrocardiogram. The R wave represents a portion of ventricular depolarization. See also *QRS complex*.

R-wave amplitude. Height, in millivolts, of the measured R wave.

R-wave inhibited pacing. See *ventricular-inhibited pacing mode (VVI)*.

R-wave triggered pacing. See *ventricular-triggered pacing mode (VVT)*.

ryanodine receptor. A calcium channel, located on the sarcoplasmic reticulum, that releases calcium from the sarcoplasmic reticulum in response to calcium influx into the cell through

L-type calcium channels. Ryanodine receptors are so-named because they can be blocked by the experimental drug ryanodine.

ryanodine-receptor calcium-release channel. This important calcium-release channel is located on the foot process (processes of the sarcoplasmic reticulum). The ryanodine receptor releases calcium from the sarcoplasmic reticulum in response to a small amount of calcium that enters the cell through the L-type calcium channels located on the plasma membrane. The plant alkaloid ryanodine blocks this calcium-release channel.

ryanodine-receptor disease. See *ryanodine right ventricular cardiomyopathy*.

ryanodine right ventricular cardiomyopathy. Form of right ventricular cardiomyopathy presenting with exercise-induced palpitations. A defective sarcoplasmic reticulum calcium-release channel is responsible for this condition. Also referred to as catecholamine-sensitive polymorphic ventricular tachycardia syndrome. Ryanodine right ventricular cardiomyopathy has a poor prognosis; up to half of patients succumb to this illness without treatment.

RyR1. Ryanodine receptor 1. See *ryanodine-receptor calcium-release channel*.

RyR2. Ryanodine receptor 2. See *ryanodine-receptor calcium-release channel*.

RyR3. Ryanodine receptor 3. See *ryanodine-receptor calcium-release channel*.

S

S (single). Generic abbreviation for "single" that manufacturers use to label single-chamber pacing devices that may be used for either atrial or ventricular applications (i.e., SSI or SSIR pacing mode).

S_1. The electrical stimulus of the basic drive cycle. The drive cycle length is the S_1S_1 interval. If S_1 captures the heart, its response is termed A_1 in the atrium and V_1 in the ventricle.

S_1-A_1 interval in refractory periods. The interval between the last electrical stimulus of the basic drive train (see S_1) and the atrial electrogram resulting from atrial capture associated with that stimulus. The S_1-A_1 interval is a measure of capture latency and intra-atrial conduction time.

S_1-H_2 interval in refractory periods. The interval between the last stimulus of the basic drive train (see S_1) and the His-bundle electrogram associated with a coupled extrastimulus.

S_1-S_2 interval in refractory periods. Interval between the last stimulus of the basic drive train (see S_1) and the first electrical extrastimulus introduced after the drive train (see S_2). Also called coupling interval.

S_2. The first electrical extrastimulus introduced either after a drive train (S_1) or during spontaneous rhythm. The second extrastimulus is termed S_3, the third is termed S_4, and so on.

S_2-A_2 interval in refractory periods. Interval between the first electrical extrastimulus and the atrial electrogram associated with this first extrastimulus (see S_2). The S_2-A_2 interval is a measure of capture latency and intra-atrial conduction time in the atrium.

SA. Abbreviation for *sinoatrial*.

SACT. Abbreviation for *sinoatrial conduction time*.

SAECG. Abbreviation for *signal-averaged electrocardiography*.

Safe Medical Device Act (SMDA) of 1990. A congressional act passed in the United States during 1990 which mandates that physician and institutional reports be filed with the U.S. Food and Drug Administration about any serious injury or death that is the result of a faulty or failed medical device. The act also requires postmarket surveillance of implantable devices.

safety advisory. See *device recall, recall*.

safety alert. Any communication issued by a manufacturer, distributor, or other responsible party, or by the U.S. Food and Drug Administration, to inform health professionals or other appropriate persons or firms regarding a risk of substantial harm from a medical device in commercial use. Notifications are issued at the request of the U.S. Food and Drug Administration. Safety alerts are voluntarily issued. See also *recall*.

safety margin. The difference between the value of the stimulation threshold and the programmed value of the pacemaker output. The safety margin provides an output that is greater than the output needed to capture the myocardium. Its purpose is to avoid the loss of capture that might otherwise occur due to physiologic changes. Safety margin also can be applied to the sensing threshold (i.e., the difference between the threshold value at which sensing in a specific chamber occurs and the more sensitive value programmed to allow a margin to ensure sensing).

safety margin test. An automatic output function of some pacemakers, usually magnet-initiated, that allows confirmation of an appropriate safety margin. The pacemaker automatically decreases output, and simultaneous observation of the electrocardiogram permits verification that capture has occurred. The presence of capture by pacemaker output stimuli that occur within the safety margin confirms that the pacemaker output is sufficient to allow for slight variations in the pacing threshold. See also *safety margin*. •

safety pace interval. A preset or programmable interval in the first portion of the atrioventricular interval following an atrial output pulse. A signal sensed in the ventricular channel during the safety pace interval causes the delivery of a ventricular output pulse and terminates the interval. The safety pace interval is designed

Safety Margin Test

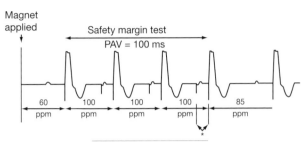

Atrial and ventricular pulse duration is reduced by 25% for these two pulses only.
Modified and used with permission of Medtronic, Inc., Minneapolis, Minnesota.

to prevent inhibition of ventricular output due to crosstalk. The safety pace interval also is referred to as the nonphysiologic atrioventricular interval and the 110-millisecond phenomenon. See also *safety pacing*.

safety pacing. In dual-chamber pacemakers, the delivery of a ventricular output pulse, following atrial pacing, if a signal is sensed by the ventricular channel during the early portion of the atrioventricular interval. It is used to ensure that ventricular depolarization occurs if the sensed event was something other than an intrinsic ventricular depolarization. See also *safety pace interval*.

Safety Pacing, Ventricular

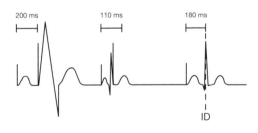

From Hayes DL, Levine PA. Pacemaker timing cycles. In: Ellenbogen KA, editor. Cardiac pacing. Boston: Blackwell Scientific Publications; 1992. p. 263-308. Used with permission.

sandwich beat. An intrinsic ventricular depolarization immediately preceded and followed by a pacemaker output pulse and thus sandwiched between two consecutive pacemaker output pulses. The intrinsic depolarization occurs during the refractory period of the first pacemaker output pulse and is not sensed by the pacemaker.

SA node. See *sinus node*.

SA node conduction time. See *sinoatrial conduction time*.

sarcoglycans. Family of membranes spanning glycoproteins whose isoforms interact with the dystrophin glycoprotein complex in the plasma membrane.

sarcoidosis. A disorder characterized by the presence of epithelioid cell tubercles, without caseation. Older lesions have a hyaline, fibrous appearance. Cardiac involvement by sarcoidosis can result in conduction disturbances that require permanent pacing.

SAV. Abbreviation for *sensed AV interval*.

sawtooth waves. Baseline variations seen in several forms of atrial flutter that represent continuous atrial activation in these reentrant arrhythmias. This term is most commonly specifically used to describe the flutter waves seen in typical cavotricuspid isthmus-dependent flutter.

SCA. Abbreviation for *sudden cardiac arrest*.

scanning pacemaker. A term that was used with an older-generation antitachycardia pacemaker that automatically searched for the pacing interval most likely to terminate a tachycardia. The scanning mechanism is activated when a tachycardia is sensed. The extrastimuli are delivered at the critical coupling interval that successfully terminated the last tachycardia. Initially, the coupling intervals of the extrastimuli are programmed. However, the coupling intervals can change automatically to the critical coupling intervals that are successful in breaking the tachycardia.

scar-based ablation. Technique used when the target arrhythmias are multiple and associated with hemodynamic instability. Ablation is performed between two scars and between scars and anatomical obstacles such as the mitral valve.

SCD. Abbreviation for *sudden cardiac death*.

SCD-HeFT. See *Sudden Cardiac Death in Heart Failure Trial*.

Schizotrypanum cruzi. The organism responsible for Chagas' disease. Chagas' disease is a common cause of cardiomyopathy and conduction disorders in certain South American countries.

SCL. Abbreviation for *sinus cycle length*.

SCN5A. Gene that codes for the cardiac sodium channel. Mutations associated with this gene are responsible for Brugada syndrome, long QT syndrome 3, progressive conduction system disease, and progressive cardiac dilatation.

scopolamine. A competitive antagonist of acetylcholine and other muscarinic agonists. Scopolamine is structurally similar to atropine but permeates the blood-brain barrier to a much greater degree. Scopolamine can be delivered transcutaneously by a slow-release patch.

screw-in lead. An active fixation endocardial or sutureless epicardial lead with a metal helical coil at the distal tip of the lead. Although the specific configuration of screw-in leads varies, all screw-in leads can be manipulated during implantation for penetration of the myocardium. Some screw-in leads have a retractable helical coil to avoid vascular complications during transvenous insertion. The helical coil may or may not be electrically active, depending on the specific design of the lead.

scuba diving. See *hyperbaric pressure recommendations*.

SCV. Abbreviation for *superior caval vein*.

search AV. Parameter in some pacemakers and implantable cardioverter-defibrillators that use the patient's intrinsic atrioventricular conduction time to adjust sensed and paced atrioventricular intervals, either longer or shorter, to promote intrinsic ventricular activation.

search (AV) hysteresis. A mechanism whereby the atrioventricular interval is lengthened or searched to a certain programmable maximum length in an effort to minimize ventricular pacing. If the programmed maximum atrioventricular interval is reached during a search cycle, the atrioventricular interval reverts to a shorter interval for a specified number of cycles until another search occurs.

secondary pacemaker. See *ectopic focus*.

second-degree AV block. A partial disruption of the conduction system in which some, but not all, atrial impulses pass through the atrioventricular node and are conducted to the ventricles. Second-degree AV block is classified by the method of conduction of atrial impulses through the atrioventricular node. In type I second-degree AV block, the PR interval lengthens progressively until one atrial impulse is not conducted through the AV node. Type II second-degree AV block is characterized by intermittent conduction of atrial impulses through the atrioventricular node with no lengthening of PR interval before the blocked beat. Type I second-degree AV block also is called Mobitz type I second-degree AV block or Wenckebach block. Type II second-degree AV block also is called Mobitz type II second-degree AV block. See also *AV block, first-degree AV block, Mobitz*

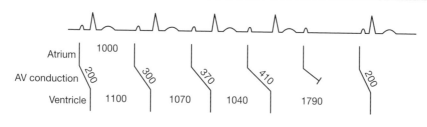

Second-Degree AV Block (Type I, Wenckebach)

Atrium	1000				
AV conduction	200	300	370	410	200
Ventricle	1100	1070	1040	1790	

The sinus rate is constant at a cycle length of 1,000 milliseconds. AV conduction (PR interval) gradually prolongs from 200 to 410 milliseconds before block of the fifth P wave. The RR interval shortens before the blocked P wave. This occurs because although the PR interval is lengthening, it does so by decreasing increments. Note that the RR interval encompassing the blocked P wave equals two times the sinus cycle length minus the amount that the PR interval is prolonged (210 milliseconds).

Second-Degree AV Block (Type II)

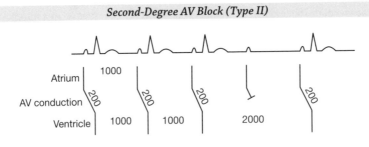

The sinus cycle length is constant at 1,000 milliseconds. The PR interval remains constant before block of the fourth P wave. The RR interval encompassing the blocked P wave measures two times the sinus cycle length.

type I second-degree AV block, Mobitz type II second-degree AV block, third-degree AV block.

second-degree pacemaker block. Prolongation of the period of time between an atrial output spike and the subsequent QRS complex to such a degree that a Wenckebach block or 2:1 block phenomenon occurs. See also *latency*.

second-degree sinus node exit block. A disruption in sinus node conduction manifested on the surface electrocardiogram by pauses or irregularity in the sinus rhythm. Second-degree sinus node exit block is analogous to second-degree AV block and is subclassified into type I (Wenckebach) and type II second-degree sinus node exit block. In type I second-degree sinus node exit block, the PP interval gradually shortens until a pause occurs without a P wave. This is analogous to the progressive shortening of the RR interval in type I second-degree AV block. Type II sinus node block is diagnosed when the PP interval encompassing the pause is a multiple of (usually twice) the basic sinus cycle length. See also *sinus node exit block*.

segmental circumferential ablation. Method of ablation for atrial fibrillation, usually paroxysmal atrial fibrillation. Ablative lesions are placed segmentally along the circumference of the pulmonary vein to be isolated. After this ablation, pulmonary vein potentials are no longer seen in sinus rhythm.

segmental ostial catheter ablation (SOCA). Method of ablation for atrial fibrillation. Ablative lesions are placed segmentally at the ostium of the pulmonary vein or just atrial to the pulmonary vein ostium. The end point for this ablation is conduction block into the vein during sinus rhythm (loss of pulmonary vein potentials).

segmented signal. A notched or broken depolarization waveform that may cause apparent undersensing by a pacemaker. The notch may cause the sensing circuit to reset. The slew rate of the waveform is evaluated segmentally and is too small to be identified by the sensing circuitry as a depolarization.

self-discharge. An electrochemical reaction that takes place between battery electrodes without the delivery of energy to an external load. Self-discharge reduces the amount of usable charge in the battery from the theoretical battery capacity to the maximum available capacity. See also *battery capacity*.

self-terminated arrhythmias. Cardiac arrhythmias that, once initiated, terminate spontaneously. This often occurs in arrhythmias that have enhanced automaticity or triggered automaticity as their underlying mechanism. In contrast, reentrant arrhythmias frequently terminate as a result of a premature beat, either atrial or ventricular.

semiconductor. An element in electronic circuitry that conducts electricity better than an insulator but not as well as a conductive metal, which is the building block of integrated circuits. Semiconductors provide electrical amplification and rectification and usually control the flow of electrical current in one direction. See also *complementary metal-oxide semiconductor*.

sense amplifier. Sensing circuit component of a pulse generator that allows detection, amplification, and processing of incoming signals. See figure *Circuit (Simplified) of a Pacemaker*.

sensed AV interval (SAV). The programmed interval from an intrinsic (sensed) P wave to a paced ventricular event.

sensed event marker. A temporary programmable option of some pacemakers that results in a marker appearing on the electrocardiogram,

Second-Degree Sinus Node Exit Block (Type I, Wenckebach)

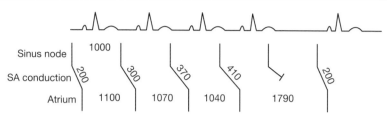

The sinus node fires at a constant cycle length of 1,000 milliseconds. There is increasing delay as the sinus impulse exits to activate the atrium. The fifth sinus impulse blocks in the perinodal region. Note that the PP interval gradually shortens because, although the sinus node conduction time is increasing, it is doing so by progressively smaller increments. The pause emcompassing the blocked sinus impulse equals two times the sinus cycle length minus the increase in perinodal delay.

Second-Degree Sinus Node Exit Block (Type II)

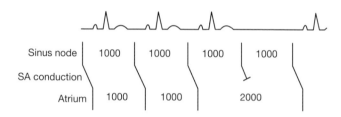

The sinus node is firing at a cycle length of 1,000 milliseconds. The fourth sinus impulse is blocked while trying to exit the sinus node and, thus, no P wave is generated. The next sinus impulse fires on time and leads to a P wave that closes a pause equal to two times the sinus cycle length.

generated by the programmer, which indicates points of sensing of events by the pulse generator. This feature may be helpful to determine the appropriate sensing and to assist in programming sensitivity values.

sensing assurance. Parameter in some devices that automatically adjusts sensitivity, within defined limits, based on device monitoring of peaked amplitude of sensed signals. Can increase or decrease atrial or ventricular sensitivities.

sensing circuit. The portion of a pacemaker or defibrillator circuit used to identify incoming signals for additional signal processing. The sensing circuit is composed of several circuit elements: the amplifier, the bandpass filter, and the level detector. Each of these circuit elements has a preset range of functionality that is determined during the circuit design.

sensing configuration. Refers to the polarity configuration for sensing. Options may be bipolar, unipolar tip, or unipolar ring.

sensing impedance. The opposition to alternating current flow by the electrode of a pacing system during sensing. Sensing difficulties occur if the sensing impedance increases because of a resultant decrease in the signal voltage. Sensing impedance is higher than stimulating impedance.

sensing safety margin. Safety margin (see definition) as it applies to sensing. For example, if the measured R wave is 10 mV, programming the sensitivity to 5 mV would give a sensing safety margin of 100%.

sensing threshold. The minimum atrial or ventricular intrinsic electrical signal, expressed in millivolts, required for consistent sensing by the pacemaker sensing amplifier. Failure to sense, intermittent sensing, and loss of sensing have several different causes. These include intrinsic signals that are too low for the pacemaker sensing circuit to detect, loss of contact between the electrode and responsive myocardial tissue, lead or conductor fracture, and an improper connection between the lead terminal pin and the connector block. Sensing thresholds of the atria and ventricles typically differ.

sensing threshold test. A capability of most contemporary pulse generators whereby the sensitivity level is modified to determine a safety margin for sensing intrinsic cardiac activity.

sensitivity. In pacing systems, the ability to sense an intrinsic electrical signal, which depends on the amplitude, slew rate, and frequency of the signal. The sensitivity setting of the pulse generator indicates the minimum intracardiac signal amplitude that will be sensed by the device to initiate the device response (inhibited or triggered). Terminology is somewhat confusing in that when sensitivity levels are programmed, a high sensitivity is indicated by a low setting

pacing, respiration sensing, stroke volume sensing, temperature sensing.

sensor crosscheck. When dual sensors are incorporated in a pulse generator, one sensor can verify that a rate change indicated by the other sensor is indeed appropriate. For example, if a pulse generator included both an activity sensor and a minute ventilation sensor, if the patient were to tap on the pulse generator the mechanical motion would activate the activity sensor. However, in the absence of any change in minute ventilation, the other sensor would indicate that a rate increase was not appropriate.

Sensor Crosscheck

QT interval

		Rate ↑	Rate ↓
Activity	Rate ↑	Exercise confirmed Increase pacing rate	Exercise NOT confirmed False-positive activity sensing Ignore activity sensor
	Rate ↓	Emotional or isometric stress confirmed Limited increase in pacing rate	Recovery confirmed Decrease pacing rate

such as 0.5 mV and a low sensitivity is indicated by a high setting such as 5.0 mV. Sensitivity corresponds to the reference level set for the sensing comparator.

sensor. A device that monitors an event or condition by sensing the absolute value of, or a change in, a physiologic or nonphysiologic parameter. The sensor converts the monitored values into a useful response signal that is delivered to a control system. The input provided by the sensor is the basis from which the event or condition can be measured or from which a control action can be initiated. Sensors can be used in rate-adaptive pacemakers to measure mechanical or physiologic parameters associated with changes in heart rate. The measured information is processed through the pacemaker circuitry to automatically adjust the pacing rate. See also *body motion sensing, closed-loop control system, dP/dt sensing, minute volume sensing, open-loop control system, oxygen saturation sensing, pH sensing, preejection interval sensing, rate-adaptive*

sensor-driven rate smoothing. The capability of a rate-adaptive pacemaker to minimize variation in ventricular cycle length, especially at the maximum tracking rate, by sensor-driven pacing. In a DDD pacemaker, there may be marked variations in cycle length when the sinus rate exceeds the maximum tracking rate with pseudo-Wenckebach or 2:1 rate behavior. In an optimally programmed DDDR pacemaker, ventricular cycle length is minimized because sensor-driven atrioventricular sequential pacing may occur before the longer pseudo-Wenckebach or 2:1 cycle is completed.

sensor histogram. A graphic display of the sensor rates. In some devices, a display is available for the sensor rates achieved, and in other devices a display is also available for what the sensor would have achieved had it been programmed "on." It also may be possible to alter sensor settings and the sensor histograms will show what the sensor-indicated rates would be had the new values been programmed.

Sensor-Driven Rate Smoothing

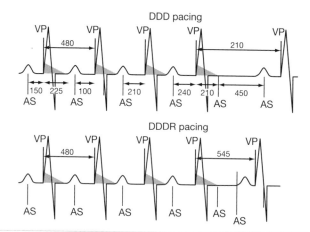

AP, atrial paced event; AS, atrial sensed event; VP, ventricular paced event. Modified from Markowitz HT. Dual chamber rate responsive pacing (DDDR) provides physiologic upper rate behavior. Physiopace. 1990;4:1-4.

sensor-indicated rate. Rate that the rate-adaptive sensor dictates based on the activation of the sensor. If the patient has chronotropic incompetence, the sinus-indicated rate and the sensor-indicated rate may appropriately be significantly different. If the sensor is programmed too aggressively, the sensor-indicated rate may be inappropriate for a given level of exercise.

sensor-mediated tachycardia. In a rate-adaptive pacing system, an abnormally high heart rate mediated by the sensor, that is, a sensor-indicated rate that is inappropriately high for the concurrent physiologic state of the patient. For example, in a patient with an activity-sensing rate-adaptive pacemaker, pressure applied to the pacemaker while the patient is at rest may cause sensor-mediated tachycardia, depending on the sensor settings of the pacemaker and degree of pressure applied. See also *pacemaker-mediated tachycardia.*

sensor optimization. Programming the rate-adaptive sensor such that the sensor-indicated rate is appropriate for a given level of activity. Many pulse generators have the capability of auto-optimization of the sensor.

sensor threshold. A programmable value for rate-adaptive pacemakers which determines, in part, the level of activity necessary to activate the sensor. Programming the sensor threshold is not consistent across manufacturers. In some devices, the higher the sensor threshold is set, the greater the level of activity required to increase the pacing rate, and vice versa in others.

sensor-varied postventricular atrial refractory period. Feature of a pacemaker or implantable cardioverter-defibrillator that determines a value for postventricular atrial refractory period according to the sensor-indicated rate.

septal flutter. Type of atrial flutter in which the slow zone and most of the circuit are on the interatrial septum, typically on the right atrial aspect of the septum. Septal flutters may occur in patients with patch repair of an atrial septal defect or after right atrial maze procedures.

septal isthmus tissue. Atrial myocardium between the tricuspid valve and the inferior vena cava located on the interatrial septum. The septal isthmus constitutes part of the cavotricuspid isthmus. See also *cavotricuspid isthmus.*

septal pacing. See *right ventricular septal pacing.*

septal-posterior wall motion delay (SPW-MD). A measurement derived from M-mode echocardiography that indicates ventricular synchrony or lack of synchrony. It has been suggested that this relatively simple measurement can be used as a measurement of dyssynchrony before implantation of a cardiac resynchronization device. Data are mixed regarding the usefulness of this measurement.

septolateral delay. Term used in biventricular pacing for cardiac resynchronization, referring to the delay in mechanical activation of the intraventricular septum in comparison with the free wall of the left ventricle. Septolateral mechanical delay usually reflects electrical delay between septal left bundle branch activation at propagation of the impulse to the lateral wall. Septolateral delay is an important cause for septolateral dyssynchrony. See also *septolateral dyssynchrony.*

septolateral dyssynchrony. An important cause of inefficient cardiac contraction that is targeted with therapy with left ventricular lead implantation. In extreme forms of septolateral dyssynchrony, the left ventricular free wall contracts so late after septal contraction that blood flow resulting from lateral wall contraction is toward the septum instead of effective output through the aortic valve. Septolateral electrical and mechanical delay and local myocardial ischemia or infarction of the lateral wall are the causes of septolateral dyssynchrony.

sequential shock. Delivery of two shocks in close sequence, that is, delivery of two shocks separated by less than 1 millisecond. Sequential shock also is known as sequential pulse defibrillation.

ser-1928. A binding site for cyclic adenosine monophosphate-dependent protein kinase (PKA) located on the L-type calcium channel ($Ca_v1.2$). PKA is an important up-regulator of this calcium channel and acts via the ser-1928 binding site. This phosphorylation relation site is the central pore-forming $\alpha_1 1.2$ subunit of $Ca_v1.2$.

SERCA2 (sarcoplasmic reticulum-adenosine triphophatase). Plays a major role in the contraction-relaxation cycle and is responsible for transporting calcium into the lumen of the sarcoplasmic reticulum.

SERCA2a. Form of SERCA2, also referred to as cardiac slow-twitch isoform. This sarcoplasmic reticulum adenosine triphosphatase form is regulated by phospholamban and has gained importance in understanding the pathogenesis of heart failure. SERCA2a is deficient in some forms of heart failure, and its overexpression has been found to be protective against heart failure and to have a survival benefit in animal models. See also *SERCA2*.

serial drug testing. Use of a given test, such as programmed ventricular stimulation, to assess the efficacy of several different drugs. Typically, once a drug is found that fulfills the criteria for success, that drug can be prescribed as the appropriate therapy for a patient.

series circuit. A circuit in which the components are connected in succession, end to end, to form a single path for current flow. In pacemakers with more than one power source, the batteries are connected in series to provide the voltage necessary for myocardial stimulation. The positive pole of one battery cell is connected in series to the negative pole of another cell, and the resulting battery voltage is the sum of the voltage of individual cells.

setscrew. A small screw with a recessed hexagonal socket. Setscrews are used to hold electrical circuit components in place. In pacing, setscrews often are used to secure the lead terminal pin within the connector block. To prevent a short circuit, the setscrew is insulated from body tissues by a sealing mechanism or silicone elastomer stopper. See also *Allen setscrew, lead terminal pin.*

shelf life. The maximum amount of time that materials and devices retain their performance characteristics, without evidence of deterioration, during storage. In implantable cardiac rhythm devices, shelf life is an indication of the performance characteristics of the device with respect to the battery status. Shelf life also may be used to indicate the sterility condition of the device packaging. Once the shelf life has elapsed, use of the product is not recommended.

shelf settings. The configuration settings of the pulse generator as it is stored or "on the shelf" before implantation. Many of the hardware functions may be disabled as shelf settings, and these may or may not be the same as the shipped settings or nominal values.

shifting burst. A type of burst stimulation in which the extrastimuli are coupled to a tachycardia at an independently scanned value. See also *burst scanning mechanism.*

shipped settings. Pulse generator-programmed nominal values at which the device is shipped. These may or may not be the same as the shelf settings. See also *shelf settings.*

shock-energy programming. Programming the delivered energy for detected ventricular fibrillation when shocks are programmed. Typically, shock energy is programmed to the maximal energy delivery possible in that device. Another typical shock-energy programming sequence is programming the first shock at a lower energy close to the defibrillation threshold and subsequent shocks at the maximal possible energy.

shocking vector. In implanted cardioverter-defibrillators, the delivered shock usually occurs in a biphasic form in a vector between a negative and a positive electrode, coil, or can. The shocking vector can be changed noninvasively in some devices when defibrillation thresholds are high (usually by taking out the superior vena cava coil). In difficult cases with intractably high defibrillation thresholds, the shocking vector is changed by placing a coil in nontraditional sites such as the coronary sinus or azygos vein or subcutaneously.

shock-on-T fibber. Method of inducing ventricular fibrillation during defibrillation threshold testing at implantation or reprogramming of an implantable cardioverter-defibrillator. This specific method is used in devices made by St. Jude Medical (St. Paul, Minnesota).

shock-on-T wave. Method of induction of ventricular fibrillation during defibrillation threshold testing with implantable cardioverter-defibrillators. A low-energy shock, typically between 0.6 and 1 J, is delivered at the peak of the T wave (vulnerable) to initiate ventricular fibrillation. With most devices, the coupling interval of the shock with reference to the QRS complex and the delivered energy are programmable. Once ventricular fibrillation is induced, both the sensing function and the ability of the device to terminate ventricular fibrillation can be observed. See figure *Fibrillation Induction.*

shock-wave lithotripsy. See *lithotripsy.*

shore rating. The scale used to categorize and classify different materials, such as plastics and elastomers, on the basis of their hardness. In pacing, shore ratings are used in the selection of appropriate segmented polyurethanes or silicones for use as pacing lead insulation. See also *polyurethane.*

short circuit. A direct low-resistance connection across a voltage source or between the anode and the cathode of an electrical system which diverts current flow around the circuit. A short circuit prevents the output of any effective voltage even though there is excessive current flow. In pacing, a short circuit is a persistent or transient malfunction in which the pacemaker output pulses are shunted away from the myocardium. Current is drained from the pacemaker battery but an effective voltage is not delivered, thus capture does not occur. Short circuits may be caused, for example, by the looping of a bipolar lead, which can bring the distal-tip electrode in contact with the proximal-ring electrode, or by a defective insulator between the conductors of a bipolar lead and subsequent contact between the conductors.

shortest preexcited RR interval. A measure of the fastest conduction that can occur over an accessory pathway during atrial fibrillation, that is, the shortest cycle length between two consecutive ventricular complexes activated over an accessory pathway. A shortest preexcited RR interval during atrial fibrillation greater than 250 milliseconds identifies patients who are at very low risk for development of ventricular fibrillation and sudden death. The positive predictive value of a shortest preexcited RR interval less than 250 milliseconds has been reported to be 12% to 19%.

short QT syndrome. Disease associated with increased risk of sudden cardiac death with a characteristic electrocardiographic finding is a short QT interval, usually less than 300 milliseconds. The probable cause for this syndrome is increased activity of the outward potassium current in phase 2 and phase 3 of the cardiac action potential. When this disorder, inherited as an autosomal dominant trait, is recognized, it is usually treated with implantation of a defibrillator. Patients with short QT syndrome also may experience atrial fibrillation.

short-wave diathermy. See *diathermy.*

shunting circuit. A conductive pathway that connects two points of a main circuit and serves to divert a portion of the electrical flow from the main circuit. In pacing, a shunting circuit is used to maximize protection of the implanted pacemaker against electrical damage from the delivery of large levels of energy, as in defibrillation countershocks. See also *zener diode.*

sick sinus syndrome (SSS). See *bradycardia-tachycardia syndrome, sinus node dysfunction.*

sidearm lock. A mechanism for securing the terminal end of pacing leads within the connector block. The sidearm lock is used in lieu of the more commonly used setscrew.

side-lock connector. A lead connector that uses a wedging element to fix the lead and prevent inadvertent withdrawal from the connector block. The lead can be locked in place by simple finger pressure. A release mechanism is present, if needed.

sigmoid coronary sinus. Anatomic variation in the coronary sinus anatomy, usually in severe cardiomyopathy or after valve surgery. The name is derived from an S-shaped curve caused by initial posterior and atrial curvature followed by the more usual curvature around the mitral anulus seen in the coronary sinuses.

signal-averaged electrocardiography (SAECG).
A technique used to search for late potentials, which may be a marker of an arrhythmogenic substrate and may identify patients who are at risk for life-threatening arrhythmias. By averaging approximately 200 QRS complexes, random noise is greatly reduced so that fine, intrinsic characteristics of conduction patterns can be revealed in the QRS morphology. The orthogonal leads are then filtered, amplified, and combined into a single vector, which is analyzed for three parameters: total duration of the filtered QRS, duration of low-amplitude signals (less than 40 μVs) in the terminal QRS, and root mean squared voltage of the terminal 40 milliseconds of the QRS. Normal values vary among investigators. A signal-averaged electrogram may show, for example, a filtered QRS of less than 120 milliseconds, low-amplitude signals less than 38 milliseconds, and root mean squared voltage less than 20 μV. Requiring more of these parameters to be abnormal increases the specificity of the test but decreases sensitivity. Signal-averaged electrocardiograms have not been shown to be useful for analyzing right bundle branch block.

signal-averaged P wave. The signal-averaged P wave uses technology similar to that of signal-averaged electrocardiography for the QRS complex to study and identify abnormalities associated with late atrial activation. An abnormal signal-averaged P wave may be a predictor for occurrence and recurrence of atrial fibrillation. See also *signal-averaged electrocardiography*.

signal-to-noise analyzer. A component of pacemaker sensing circuitry that analyzes the signal-to-noise ratio. The signal-to-noise analyzer is activated for noise detection during the final portion of the pacemaker refractory period. See also *noise, signal-to-noise ratio*.

signal-to-noise ratio (SNR). The ratio of the signal voltage amplitude at any point to the noise voltage amplitude at the same point. In pacing, the signal-to-noise ratio is a design characteristic of the sensing circuit. It allows measurement of performance during the elimination of ambient noise in an intrinsic cardiac signal. The signal-to-noise ratio often is expressed in decibels. See also *noise, signal-to-noise analyzer*.

Silastic. Trademark for a biocompatible, heat-stable polymer of silicone (Dow Corning Corp.,

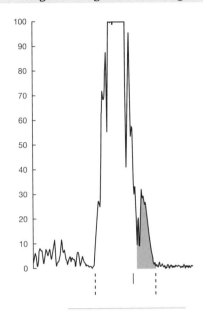

Signal-Averaged Electrocardiogram

Signal-averaged electrocardiogram positive by all three criteria. Duration of filtered QRS = 126 milliseconds (time between the two broken vertical lines). Duration of low-amplitude signals (<40 μV) at the terminal end of QRS = 47 milliseconds (terminal end of QRS to solid vertical line). Root mean square of the voltage of the terminal 40 milliseconds = 19 μV (shaded region). Each small division on the X axis is 5 milliseconds.

Midland, Michigan) used to insulate some pacing leads. See also *silicone elastomer*.

silent atria. With silent atria, no discernible atrial activation is found either on the surface electrocardiogram (absent P wave) or with intracardiac electrodes. Patients with silent atria have sinus node arrest and absent retrograde activation from an ensuing junctional or ventricular escape rhythm (or ventricular paced rhythm). Silent atria can be very difficult to distinguish from fine atrial fibrillation, and an invasive electrophysiologic study may be required to make this distinction. Patients with silent atria may be helped with placement of an atrial pacing lead. See also *atrial standstill*.

silicone chip. See *integrated circuit*.

silicone elastomer. A biocompatible, heat-stable, water-repellent, polymeric compound. Silicone elastomer is used as a pacing lead insulator because it is soft and flexible and allows easy manipulation of the lead within the venous system and the heart.

silicone rubber insulation. See *silicone elastomer*.

silver-vanadium cell chemistry (AgLiVO5). A battery technology that characteristically has low impedance and is used in implantable cardioverter-defibrillators to ensure adequate charging current. Silver-vanadium cell chemistry also is referred to as lithium-silver-vanadium oxide, lithium-silver pentoxide, and silver-vanadium oxide.

single-chamber pacing. The application of electrical stimuli to one chamber of the heart to artificially restore myocardial contraction. Single-chamber pacing requires the use of one pacing lead in the chamber to be paced or sensed. Single-chamber pacing modes include VVI, VVIR, VVT, AAI, AAIR, AAT, VOO, and AOO.

single-loop reentry. Most common form of reentrant tachycardia in which a single loop involving the entrance limb, the exit limb, and the slow zone is sufficient for initiation and maintenance of the reentrant arrhythmia.

single-pass lead. An endocardial lead that contains the atrial and ventricular electrodes in a single lead body. The atrial electrode is positioned in the middle of the atrium and is capable of sensing intrinsic atrial activity. The ventricular electrode is positioned against the ventricular endocardium and can pace and sense. This configuration allows P-synchronous pacing (VDD) with a single lead.

single-pulse cardioversion or defibrillation. Termination of a ventricular tachycardia or ventricular fibrillation with a single high-voltage pulse.

sinoatrial arrest. See *sinus arrest*.

sinoatrial block. See *sinus node exit block*.

sinoatrial conduction time (SACT). The amount of time for conduction of an impulse through the perinodal tissue of the sinus node. Sinoatrial conduction time is determined by indirect testing. It is measured during the delivery of premature atrial stimuli and generation of a resetting curve for the sinus node.

sinoatrial electrogram. See *sinus node electrogram*.

sinoatrial nodal reentry. Mechanism of an uncommon form of supraventricular tachycardia. The atrial tissue around the sinoatrial node and the sinoatrial node itself participate in the reentrant circuit responsible for this arrhythmia (sinoatrial nodal reentrant tachycardia). The P-wave morphology with reentry beats or tachycardia from this mechanism is similar to or identical with the P-wave morphology and intra-atrial activation sequence obtained in sinus rhythm. There is some debate whether this mechanism actually exists or whether intra-atrial reentry with an exit site close to the sinus node is the actual cause of this mechanism of arrhythmia.

sinoatrial (SA) node. See *sinus node*.

sinoatrial node recovery time. See *sinus node recovery time*.

sinoatrial Wenckebach. See *second-degree sinus node exit block*.

sinus arrest. A halt in sinus node firing caused either by a failure of automaticity in the sinus node or by repetitive exit block in the perinodal tissue. Sinus arrest is indicated by an abnormally prolonged time between atrial depolarizations. See also *sinus node block*.

sinus arrhythmia. A normal variant, especially in younger individuals, that is characterized by a variability in the sinus cycle length, especially at slower rates. In some individuals it can be shown to relate to the respiratory cycle with slight slowing of the sinus rate during expiration and a slight increase in rate during inspiration.

sinus bradycardia. A sinus rate of less than 60 beats per minute.

sinus cycle length (SCL). The length of time between two consecutive impulses initiated by the sinus node.

sinus node. A group of specialized myocardial cells located epicardially at the junction between

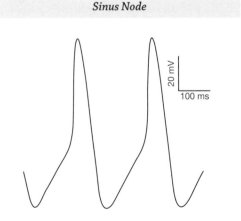

Sinus Node

20 mV

100 ms

Normal spontaneous automaticity in a sinus nodal cell.

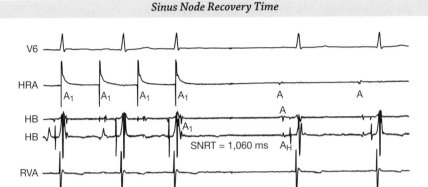

Sinus Node Recovery Time

the high right atrium and the superior vena cava. The sinus node is the natural pacemaker of the heart and initiates electrical impulses in the myocardium at a more rapid rate than other myocardial cells. It receives its blood supply from the sinus nodal artery in approximately 60% of cases. The sinus node also is referred to as the sinoatrial node or SA node. See also *depolarization, intrinsic automaticity*.

sinus node block. See *sinus node exit block*.

sinus node dysfunction. Abnormalities in sinus node activity or conduction that result in slow or irregular heart rates or intermittent tachycardia. Sinus node dysfunction also is called sick sinus syndrome, bradycardia-tachycardia syndrome, or tachy-brady syndrome. Sick sinus syndrome is a common indication for permanent pacing.

sinus node electrogram (SNE). The intracardiac electrogram of the sinus node recorded via a bipolar catheter placed in the high right atrium. Sinus node electrograms are useful for analyzing sinus node function because they give direct measurements of sinus node recovery time and sinoatrial conduction time. A sinus node electrogram is not routinely recorded in a standard electrophysiologic study. See also *sinoatrial conduction time, sinus node recovery time*.

sinus node exit block. Prolonged sinus node conduction time or disruption of conduction of sinus node impulses in the perinodal tissue. See also *first-degree sinus node exit block, second-degree sinus node exit block, third-degree sinus node exit block*.

sinus node recovery time (SNRT). The amount of time that it takes for the sinus node to recover after the discontinuation of sustained atrial pacing. Sinus node recovery time is measured as the longest pause after a period of atrial pacing (usually 30 seconds) at different constant cycle lengths. The sinus node pause after an atrial output pulse is caused by overdrive suppression of the sinus node. Sinus node recovery time is primarily a test of sinus node automaticity, standardized to a corrected value by subtracting the basic sinus cycle length. The normal corrected sinus node recovery time typically is less than 550 milliseconds. See also *corrected sinus node recovery time*.

sinus node reentry. A relatively slow paroxysmal arrhythmia that involves sinus nodal tissue and has a P wave identical to the sinus P-wave morphology. Sinus node reentry may be initiated by extrastimuli and may be terminated by extrastimuli or vagal maneuvers.

sinus node Wenckebach. See *second-degree sinus node exit block*.

sinus of Valsalva. Aortic sinus that houses the ostium of the coronary arteries (right coronary cusp, left coronary cusp, and noncoronary cusp; no coronary artery ostium). Some forms of left ventricular outflow tract tachycardia and premature ventricular contractions that initiate ventricular fibrillation may arise from the sinus of Valsalva.

sinus pause. An unexpected prolongation of the sinus cycle length.

sinus preference pacing. Programmable parameter in certain pulse generators that attempts to maintain sinus rhythm, when possible, by allowing the tracking of a sinus rate that is slower than the sensor rate by periodically searching for the intrinsic rhythm.

sinus rhythm. Normal cardiac rate set by the sinus node, which is in turn influenced by the autonomic nervous system. See also *intrinsic heart rate*.

sinus tachycardia. A sinus rate of more than 100 beats per minute.

site of earliest activation. During cardiac mapping, the portion of the myocardium activated first during a tachycardia. The site of earliest activation is one criterion used to assess sites for ablation.

site of origin. The exit point of an impulse from a tachycardia circuit as determined by various mapping techniques.

situational syncope. Syncope, usually of a neurocardiogenic basis, that occurs in certain situations. Cough syncope, micturition syncope, and syncope associated with public speaking are examples of situational syncope. Cough syncope, a common form of situational syncope, has both neurocardiogenic and central nervous system factors responsible for its occurrence.

6-minute walk. Test of functional capacity frequently used as a functional end point in many randomized trials of congestive heart failure. The measured outcome is the distance walked, and clinical trials compare distance walked at baseline with that after intervention.

sleep rate programming. A programmable option in some devices that allows the base rate to be lower during sleep. In some devices it is programmed based on time (i.e., the usual hours that the patient is at rest or asleep), and in other devices, if programmed "on" it will respond to inactivity of a rate-adaptive sensor over a certain period of time (i.e., based on sensor inactivation the pulse generator assumes that the individual is resting). Also called sleep mode, rest rate, or auto rest.

sleeve. See *suture sleeve*.

slew rate. The maximum rate at which the output voltage of an amplifier changes in response to a stepwise input. In electrophysiology and in pacing, slew rate is used to measure the amount of change in voltage that occurs, peak-to-peak, in a given segment of an intracardiac waveform divided by the period of time during which the voltage change occurs. Slew rate is one of the parameters of a sensed waveform used by the sensing circuit of a pacemaker to identify the signal as an intrinsic depolarization. Graphically, the slew rate is the slope of the recorded waveform on an intracardiac electrogram and usually is expressed in volts per millisecond. See figure *Intrinsic Deflection*.

slope. As it relates to pulse generators, the slope of a rate-adaptive pacemaker is a programmable value that determines the pacing increment over the base rate which will occur with different levels of sensor signal input. For example, if the patient has an inadequate sensor-indicated rate at a given level of activity, making the slope steeper may allow the patient to reach higher sensor-driven rates.

slow conduction mapping. Method of mapping in an electrophysiologic study and ablation procedures for ventricular tachycardia, in which conduction maps are obtained without induction of the tachycardia. A similar process also can be used to map potential reentrant circuits in the atrium, particularly with congenital heart disease. In that case, electroanatomic maps are obtained during either sinus rhythm or a paced rhythm to identify regions of scar and slow conduction. Slow conduction sites are targeted for ablation, often in a linear fashion, to prevent future inductions of tachycardia. Slow conduction mapping has the advantage

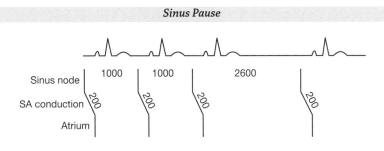

Sinus Pause

Sinus node

SA conduction

Atrium

1000   1000   2600

200   200   200   200

The sinus node is discharging at a cycle length of 1,000 milliseconds. After the third sinus impulse, the sinus node fails to generate an impulse for 2,600 milliseconds.

that potentially hemodynamically unstable arrhythmias need not be induced for the mapping procedure.

slow conduction zone. See *zone of slow conduction*.

slowly conducting accessory pathways. Typically, accessory pathways conduct in either the antegrade or the retrograde manner more rapidly than the atrioventricular node. Some accessory pathways conduct current slowly and often decrementally. Examples include antegrade conduction in a Mahaim fiber or retrograde conduction in pathways responsible for TJRT (permanent form of junctional reciprocating tachycardia).

slow pathway. One of the pathways involved in dual atrioventricular nodal physiology. Typically, the slow pathway participates in atrioventricular nodal reentrant tachycardia as the antegrade limb. Compared with the fast pathway, the slow pathway has a shorter effective refractory period and, probably, slower conduction. The slow pathway also is known as the α pathway.

slow pathway ablation. Ablation of the posterior atrial input to the atrioventricular node (slow pathway), performed to treat atrioventricular node reentry. Slow pathway ablation is highly effective for preventing recurrences of atrioventricular node reentry and is associated with a slow junctional tachycardic response during ablation.

slow pathway in atrioventricular nodal reentry. The atrial musculature that inputs to the atrioventricular node posteriorly in close association with the coronary sinus and right posterior septal atrial fibers located just ventricular to the eustachian ridge constitutes the slow pathway in the genesis of atrioventricular nodal reentry. More than one slow pathway may be present, and the slow pathway may be utilized for either antegrade or retrograde activation during atrioventricular nodal reentry.

slow pathway potentials. Mapping catheters placed inferior and posterior to the compact atrioventricular node in the vicinity of the ostium off the coronary sinus (slow pathway site) may show a characteristic electrogram with an early near field and later far field signal during sinus rhythm. Some ablationists target this potential for ablation for atrioventricular nodal reentry. The sensitivity and specificity of these potentials for successful ablation site are questionable because many locations near to the eustachian ridge and tendon of Todaro may show complex atrial signals. See also *AV nodal reentry, slow pathway*.

SMDA. Abbreviation for *Safe Medical Device Act*.

smooth electrode. See *polished-surface electrode*.

smoothing constant. The percentage of change permitted from one paced atrial or ventricular cycle to the next during the rate smoothing response to changes in intrinsic rate. The smoothing constant is a programmable value that controls the amount of lengthening or shortening of each successive paced interval as the intrinsic rate changes. See also *rate smoothing*.

SNE. Abbreviation for *sinus node electrogram*.

SNR. Abbreviation for *signal-to-noise ratio*.

SNRT. Abbreviation for *sinus node recovery time*.

SOCA. Abbreviation for *segmental ostial catheter ablation*.

sock electrode. An array of electrodes built into a fabric that fits over the ventricles and allows, by rapid computer acquisition, mapping of epicardial ventricular activation.

sodium-calcium exchange current. See I_{NaCa}.

sodium channel blockers. Class of antiarrhythmic drugs (and some local anesthetic and antiepileptic drugs) that block the cardiac sodium channel. Examples of sodium channel blockers include flecainide and quinidine. They are useful in the treatment of both atrial and ventricular arrhythmias. Sodium channel blockers are classified as class I antiarrhythmic drugs in the Vaughn-Williams antiarrhythmic drug classification scheme.

sodium channels. Important class of cardiac cell membrane channels that allow movement into the cell of the sodium ion. Sodium channels and the resulting sodium current are responsible for earlier depolarization (phase 0) of the cardiac action potential.

sodium current. See I_{Na}.

sodium-potassium pump. See I_{NaK}.

Sof-Grip hemostat. A tool for gripping the pacing or defibrillator lead without damaging the lead; often used during lead extraction (Cook Medical, Inc., Bloomington, Indiana).

software. A set of preset or programmable stored instructions, or binary code, that control a computer system. Depending on the type of memory used, software may be altered after it is manufactured, whereas hardware cannot. Software controls the performance of the hardware for a specific function. In pacing, software is used in microprocessor-based pacemakers to control pacing functions. Software also is used as an element of external programmers. See also *hardware*.

sotalol. A class III antiarrhythmic drug with nonspecific β-adrenergic blocking properties that increases atrial, atrioventricular nodal, ventricular, and accessory pathway refractoriness. Sotalol has efficacy in the treatment of supraventricular and ventricular arrhythmias. It is excreted by the kidneys and has a half-life of 10 to 15 hours. In addition to the general side effects listed under *β-adrenergic blocking drugs*, sotalol may cause proarrhythmia, including torsades de pointes.

spatial frequency of polarization. The polarization produced when an electrical field is supplied to tissue covers many differing spatial frequencies. This frequency variation is determined in large part on the myocardial fiber angle and may be important in the induction and maintenance of reentry in cardiac tissue.

spectral-temporal analysis. A method of analyzing the signal-averaged electrocardiogram using both the time and the frequency domains.

SPICED TEAS. See *Study of Pacemaker and Implantable Cardioverter Defibrillator Triggering by Electronic Article Surveillance Devices*.

spike. Used to describe the pacing artifact seen on a surface electrocardiogram (i.e., pacing spike).

spiral wave. Spiral waves appear as rotating waves of either electrical or chemical activity through stationary media. They were first described as patterns of nonlinear wave propagation in chemical reactions (Belousov-Zhabotinsky reaction). Spiral waves of electrical activity following stimulation occur three dimensionally in atrial and ventricular myocardium and are important in the understanding of complex ventricular arrhythmias, including ventricular fibrillation and torsades de pointes.

splicing. A technique of historical interest in which the implanter repaired or spliced a conductor coil fracture in a silicone-insulated lead.

split cathodal configuration. Configuration in which the tip electrodes of the cardiac venous lead and the right ventricular lead are used as a split cathode with the ring electrode of a bipolar right ventricular lead as the common anode (bipolar split cathodal configuration). If programmed to the unipolar configuration, the pulse generator casing becomes the common anode (unipolar split cathodal configuration).

split-sheath lead introducer. A lead introducer that can be partially withdrawn and then split in half for easy removal after introduction of the lead into a vein. See also *lead introducer, peel-away sheath*.

spontaneous cycle length. The period of time between one complete intrinsic complex and the next one.

spring electrode. A transvenous defibrillation electrode that usually is placed in the superior vena cava near the right atrial junction. Spring electrodes were used in a spring-patch configuration with an epicardial patch electrode for the delivery of therapy with an implantable cardioverter-defibrillator. See also *spring-patch*.

spring-loaded barb. An active-fixation endocardial pacing lead-tip configuration primarily of historical interest. The spring-loaded barbs are closed and are under tension in the catheter during transvenous insertion. Once the lead is positioned, the catheter is withdrawn and the barbs spring apart to become embedded in the myocardium.

spring-patch. A defibrillation electrode configuration in which both an epicardial patch electrode and an endocardial spring electrode are used. The epicardial patch electrode usually is placed on the apex of the left ventricle and the endocardial electrode usually is positioned in the superior vena cava near the right atrial junction. See also *patch electrode, patch-patch configuration, spring electrode*.

SPWMD. Abbreviation for *septal-posterior wall motion delay*.

SSI. In pacing, the abbreviation used for a single-chamber demand pacemaker that inhibits its output pulses when intrinsic activity is sensed. SSI pacing may appropriately be used for either atrial or ventricular pacing. SSI is a generic designation that is used primarily by pacemaker manufacturers and is not part of the NBG code.

SSIR. In pacing, the abbreviation used for a single-chamber demand pacemaker that has rate-adaptive capability. SSI pacing may appropriately be used for either atrial or ventricular pacing. SSI is a generic designation that is used primarily by pacemaker manufacturers and is not part of the NBG code.

SSS. Abbreviation for *sick sinus syndrome*.

SST. The abbreviation, rarely used, for a synchronous pacemaker that triggers a pacemaker output pulse when intrinsic activity is sensed. SST pacing may appropriately be used for either atrial or ventricular pacing. SST is a generic designation that is used primarily by pacemaker manufacturers and is not part of the NBG code.

st. In electrophysiologic testing, an abbreviation used to indicate the application of an applied stimulus.

stability. 1. The lack of cycle length variation in tachycardias. Automatic tachycardias are less stable than reentrant tachycardias. 2. In implantable cardioverter-defibrillators, a detection algorithm that helps distinguish atrial fibrillation with rapid ventricular conduction (less stable) from ventricular tachycardia (usually stable).

stability of detection. An arrhythmia detection algorithm in implantable cardioverter-defibrillators that aids in discriminating between atrial fibrillation and ventricular tachycardia by assessing the variability of the cycle lengths in a tachycardia.

standard load. A load that is preplanned with regard to dimensions, weight, and resistance and is designated by a specific number or classification. In pacing, the standard load is the resistance that is conventionally placed across the terminals of a pacemaker when operation of the device is being tested after manufacture and before implantation. The standard load used for testing is 500 ohms.

Staphylococcus. A genus of gram-positive cocci of the family Micrococcaceae, order Eubacteriales. This organism frequently is the cause of pacemaker-related infections. See also *Staphylococcus aureus, Staphylococcus epidermidis*.

Staphylococcus aureus. Coagulase-positive *Staphylococcus*. Pacemaker system infections that occur early (less than 4 weeks after implantation) may be due to various organisms, but *Staphylococcus aureus* is the most commonly identified organism.

Staphylococcus epidermidis. Coagulase-negative *Staphylococcus*. Pacemaker system infections that occur in the late postoperative period (more than 4 weeks after implantation) may be due to various organisms, but *Staphylococcus epidermidis* is the most commonly identified organism.

static burst. A type of burst stimulation in which the extrastimuli are coupled to a tachycardia at an independent, fixed value. See also *burst stimulation*.

stat set. A special function of some external programmers that can be used to rapidly reprogram a pacemaker to preset pacing parameters and values in one step. The stat set values provide adequate pacing for the majority of patients and can be activated in most programmers by pressing a single button on the programmer.

stat set values. The preset values to which a pacemaker can be reprogrammed in one step. For the majority of patients, stat set values provide adequate pacing until the patient-specific values are reprogrammed.

steerable stylet. A stylet that aids in defining and altering the curvature of the distal aspect of a transvenous lead in an effort to better direct to a specific implant site. There are models available that control the extension and retraction of the helix of an active fixation pacing lead.

Stereotaxis system. Trademark for a magnet-aided navigation system (Stereotaxis, Inc., St. Louis, Missouri) used in ablation, cardiac resynchronization, and other cardiac interventions. Remote manipulation, stability of catheter position, and reduced fluoroscopy are potential advantages of this technique.

sternocleidomastoid muscle. Muscle that divides the neck into anterior and posterior triangles and serves as a point of reference for accessing the internal jugular vein percutaneously.

sternotomy. A surgical incision through the sternum that yields maximum cardiac exposure.

steroid-eluting lead. An endocardial lead, the tip of which contains a silicone core impregnated with a steroid that is released into the tissue

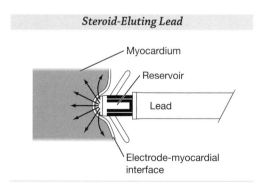

Steroid-Eluting Lead

adjacent to the pacing electrode at the electrode-myocardial interface. The steroid most commonly used is dexamethasone sodium phosphate. Steroid-eluting leads are designed to minimize the inflammatory response of the cardiac tissue at the electrode tip and thereby reduce the early peak thresholds that occur after pacemaker implantation and to minimize chronic thresholds. See also *porous electrode*.

stimulation threshold. The minimal amount of electrical stimulation that consistently produces a cardiac depolarization. The stimulation threshold can be expressed in terms of amplitude (milliamperes or volts), pulse duration (milliseconds), charge (microcoulombs), or energy (microjoules). See also *pacing threshold*.

stimulus. 1. Physiologically, an agent or action that initiates or alters an activity in a biological system. 2. In pacing, the pacemaker output pulse.

stimulus artifact. A deflection on an electrocardiogram or an intracardiac electrogram that coincides with the delivery of a pacemaker output pulse or other type of programmed electrical stimulation to the myocardium. A stimulus artifact also is referred to as a voltage deflection. See also *artifact*.

stimulus artifact amplitude. The measured height of the stimulus artifact. With digital recording systems (the type of recording systems used almost exclusively today), there is no diagnostic value of the stimulus artifact amplitude. With prior analog recording systems, the size and direction of the stimulus artifact could be meaningful.

stimulus duration. See *pulse duration*.

stimulus intensity. The amount of stimulation energy delivered by an extrastimulus.

stimulus-T interval. See *QT interval sensing*.

Stokes-Adams syndrome. The complex of symptoms and signs (dizziness, near-syncope, syncope, and possibly seizure activity) that result from transient complete heart block. Complete recovery typically occurs within a few seconds to a few minutes as a result of the return of normal conduction or resumption of ectopic ventricular focus. Stokes-Adams syndrome, the original indication for the use of permanent pacemakers, also is referred to as Stokes-Adams syncope and Adams-Stokes disease.

stored electrograms. Electrograms that are automatically stored or stored after the patient triggers the device for later display. Current pacemakers have up to 512 kilobytes of memory for diagnostic storage.

stored energy. The amount of power stored in a battery or defibrillator capacitor. Stored energy usually is expressed in watt-hours.

straight leads. Leads that are not preformed (e.g., preformed J leads).

strain imaging/mapping. Strain imaging is a method of echocardiographically analyzing myocardial deformation and is useful for assessing patients as potential candidates for left ventricular lead implantation. Strain is best described as local deformation and is the difference in velocity at two sites in relation to the distance separating these two sites. Strain can be measured as the integral of strain rate (see *strain rate imaging*). Strain rate has the problem of a high noise-to-signal ratio. This is less so with strain imaging, but strain is still sensitive

Strain Rate Imaging

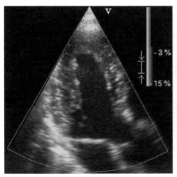 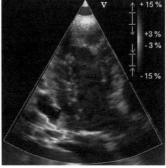

End-systolic shortening   End-systolic shortening and stretching

to nonrandom noise. Strain imaging is independent of translational and tethering effects on velocity. It is thus a method of assessing for the true location of regional dyssynchrony.

strain rate imaging. Strain rate imaging is an echocardiography-based method that represents a spatial derivation velocity. It is the equivalent of the rate at which strain changes (see *strain imaging/mapping*). Measuring algorithms remove effects on regional velocities such as translation and tethering. Both random and nonrandom noise are problems in the interpretation of the strain rate imaging. •

strength-duration curve. A graphic representation of the pulse amplitude, in voltage or current, required to produce an action potential in cells. The strength-duration curve is plotted as a function of pulse duration measured in milliseconds. At short pulse durations, greater voltage or current is required to depolarize the myocardium. As the pulse duration is increased, voltage or current requirements decline. The strength-duration curve levels out at a pulse duration of approximately 1 millisecond. This point is called rheobase, and an increase of pulse duration beyond this value does not provide more effective stimulation. See also *chronaxie, rheobase*.

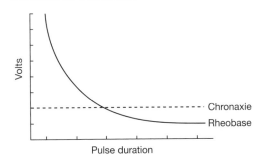

Strength-Duration Curve

strength-interval curve. The relationship between the strength of the stimulus needed to reach threshold and the time after onset of the action potential. The strength-interval curve demonstrates the time course of recovery of excitability.

stretch-activated ion channel. Cell deformation may evoke electrical signals in cardiac and noncardiac tissue. Stretch-activated current can be carried by potassium chloride and nonselective cationic channels.

stroke volume (SV). The quantity of blood pumped from the heart into the circulatory system during each ventricular contraction. Stroke volume is expressed in millimeters.

stroke volume sensing. The determination of the stroke volume by the use of a sensor that measures changes in intraventricular stroke volume impedance. The product of stroke volume impedance and ventricular rate is proportional to cardiac output, and thus stroke volume sensors may be used in rate-adaptive pacing systems to control the pacing rate. See also *closed-loop control system, rate-adaptive pacing*.

ST segment. On an electrocardiogram or intracardiac electrogram, the interval between completion of ventricular depolarization (QRS) and the onset of ventricular repolarization (T wave). The ST segment corresponds to the plateau (phase 2) of the Purkinje fiber and ventricular muscle action potential. Elevation of the ST segment represents the current of injury within the myocardium. It is seen frequently on the intracardiac electrogram when pacing electrodes contact the myocardium on implantation of a pacing system. Typical values of the ST segment range from 100 to 160 milliseconds. See also *current of injury*.

ST segment in Brugada syndrome. The ST segment in patients with Brugada syndrome shows a characteristic pattern of elevation with the maximal elevation occurring near the terminal portion of the QRS complex (J-point type elevation). This early ST-segment elevation resembles a broad R' and mimics right bundle branch block. See also *Brugada syndrome*.

Study of Pacemaker and Implantable Cardioverter Defibrillator Triggering by Electronic Article Surveillance Devices (SPICED TEAS). This study assessed the effect of antitheft devices on pacemakers and implantable cardioverter-defibrillators. The study found that interference can occur, although subsequent studies showed that electronic article surveillance equipment should not be of concern as long as patients "do not linger or lean" within or around the equipment (McIvor ME, Sheppard RC. SPICED TEAS manuscript: Study of Pacemaker and Implantable CardiovErter Defibrillator Triggering by Electronic Article Surveillance devices [letter]. Pacing Clin Electrophysiol. 1999;22:540-1).

stylet. A thin wire used to stiffen or provide

Subclavian Puncture

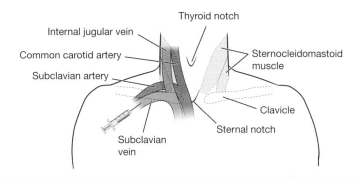

support to a cannula or catheter (such as a needle or a pacing lead) or to clear a passage for ease of insertion through the lumen of the cannula or catheter. Stylets may be preshaped to facilitate the placement of catheters or leads. For example, some stylets are J-shaped to facilitate atrial lead positioning.

stylet-driven leads. A standard pacing lead in which a stylet is used to advance and maneuver the lead. The stylet can be shaped in different ways in an attempt to deliver the lead to a specific location. These leads are in contrast to lumenless leads. See also *lumenless lead*.

subclavian crush. Pinching of a lead at the junction of the clavicle and first rib. In transvenous pacing, this can damage the conductor or insulation of a lead placed within the subclavian vein.

subclavian crush syndrome. When a lead is delivered via a subclavian puncture, it passes between the first rib and clavicle, an area that can be a relatively tight space, and, probably more important, may pass through the subclavius muscle. The muscle or the bony structures may pinch the lead and result in insulation damage or damage to the conductor coil.

subclavian puncture. A technique used for the percutaneous entry of the subclavian vein. In pacing, subclavian puncture commonly is used for the insertion of pacing leads. Subclavian puncture also is referred to as blind subclavian puncture because the vein is approached by anatomic landmarks or contrast venography and is not directly visualized. See also *contrast venography, cutdown*.

subclavian venipuncture. See *subclavian puncture*.

subcutaneous array. A lead placed subcutaneously along the left lateral aspect of the chest, sometimes extending posteriorly, in an effort to achieve acceptable defibrillation thresholds. Two types are currently available; one is a single coil, and the other has multiple coils all

Subcutaneous Array

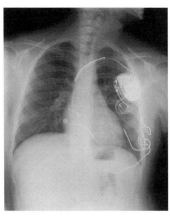 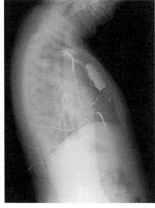

placed subcutaneously with the aid of a tunneling tool.

subcutaneous patch electrode. A defibrillation lead that may be used as part of a nonthoracotomy lead system. Typically, a subcutaneous patch electrode is placed under the skin of the left anterolateral chest wall over the cardiac apex.

subendocardial focal activity. Automatic arrhythmias have a focal source of early electrical activation. This site may be located in the mid myocardium, epicardium, or subendocardially. When subendocardial focal activation is noted, radiofrequency ablation from an endocardial approach has a higher chance of success.

subendocardial incision. See *subendocardial resection*.

subendocardial resection. A surgical procedure in which the subendocardial layers containing a ventricular tachycardia circuit are dissected and excised. Subendocardial resection usually is performed in conjunction with aneurysmectomy in patients who have ventricular tachycardia. Subendocardial resection, used in the treatment of ventricular tachycardia at sites of prior myocardial infarction, is much less traumatic than an endocardial encircling ventriculotomy. Subendocardial resection also is referred to as subendocardial incision. See also *endocardial encircling ventriculotomy*.

subpectoral pacemaker pocket. A space created deep to the pectoralis muscle for insertion of a pacemaker. More commonly, the pacemaker pocket is created superficial to the pectoralis muscle, that is, in the prepectoral area. The subpectoral pacemaker location is usually used because of body habitus (i.e., pediatric patients) or for cosmetic preference.

subsidary pacemaker. Cardiac sites capable of impulse initiation when the sinus node fails (e.g., atrioventricular junction, low right atrium).

substrate. A substance acted on. 1. In electronic circuitry, a substrate is a plate or wafer of some physical material onto which the components of a microcircuit are deposited or formed. A substrate is used in the manufacture of hybrid and integrated circuits primarily for mechanical support and insulation of the circuit components. 2. In electrophysiology, substrate refers to the anatomic basis for an arrhythmia. See also *hybrid circuit, integrated circuit*.

subthreshold stimulation. An extrastimulus delivered at a strength that is low enough to not cause a propagated response. Subthreshold stimuli may terminate ventricular tachycardias when delivered in the zone of slow conduction. Subthreshold stimulation is believed to result in local increase in intracellular calcium and is the mechanism for cardiac contractility modulation. See also *cardiac contractility modulation*.

sudden cardiac arrest (SCA). See *sudden cardiac death*.

sudden cardiac death (SCD). Death presumably caused by a lethal ventricular arrhythmia, that is, ventricular tachycardia or ventricular fibrillation. The definition varies widely among different investigators depending on the maximum amount of time from the onset of symptoms to death. See also *implantable cardioverter-defibrillator*.

Sudden Cardiac Death in Heart Failure Trial (SCD-HeFT). This mortality trial included patients with ischemic and nonischemic heart disease who had New York Heart Association class II or III congestive heart failure and left ventricular ejection fraction of 35% or less. They were randomized to receive conventional therapy plus placebo, implantable cardioverter-defibrillator, or amiodarone. Mortality was significantly reduced with an implantable cardioverter-defibrillator and the benefit occurred in both patients with ischemic and those with nonischemic disease (Bardy GH, Lee KL, Mark DB, Poole JE, Packer DL, Boineau R, et al, Sudden Cardiac Death in Heart Failure Trial [SCD-HeFT] Investigators. Amiodarone or an implantable cardioverter-defibrillator for congestive heart failure. N Engl J Med. 2005;352:225-37. Erratum in: N Engl J Med. 2005;352:2146).

sudden infant death syndrome. Syndrome that is likely multifactorial and associated with unexplained sudden death in infants, often occurring during sleep. Long QT syndrome is one of the recognized causes of sudden infant death syndrome. See also *long QT syndrome*.

sudden onset criteria. Criteria set to program the sudden onset function in defibrillators (see *sudden onset function*). The criteria to be met may be set as a percentage change in cycle length or as an absolute value in milliseconds change required for detection of ventricular tachycardia as opposed to sinus tachycardia.

sudden onset function. To minimize the occurrence of inappropriate therapy with an implantable cardioverter-defibrillator, some devices have a sudden onset function to help distinguish ventricular tachycardia from gradual-onset tachycardias such as sinus tachycardia. With this function, the cycle length of the sensed ventricular electrograms just before tachycardia detection is compared with the cycle length of the detected arrhythmia. If there is an abrupt (criteria programmable) change in the cycle length, the arrhythmia is detected as ventricular tachycardia and, if therapies were programmed, therapies are initiated. If the change in cycle length that occurs before meeting detection is gradual based on the programmed criteria, then sinus tachycardia is diagnosed and therapy is withheld.

superfast atrial recharge pulse. A circuit on the atrial channel of some dual-chamber pacemakers that is designed to recharge very quickly. The purpose of rapid recharge is to minimize the necessary length of the ventricular blanking period. If the recharge time is reduced, the blanking period can be shortened. However, a fast recharge time results in a recharge spike of greater amplitude. In some patients, the superfast atrial recharge pulse has resulted in pectoral muscle stimulation.

superior caval vein (SCV). One of the two main veins returning sustaining systemic blood to the right atrium musculature in the superior vena cava that drains blood from the head and neck back to the right atrium; may be responsible for tachyarrhythmia, including atrial fibrillation. The superior caval vein is traversed by pacing and defibrillator leads when leads are implanted via the subclavian vein into the atrium or ventricle.

superior cavoatrial junction. The junction of the superior vena cava with the right atrium. The superior cavoatrial junction may exhibit decremental conduction and be arrhythmogenic, including with respect to atrial fibrillation. The epicardial surface of the superior cavoatrial junction is the location of the sinus node, particularly in the posterolateral aspect.

superior limbus. Curved, thick band of atrial musculature that forms the superior boundary of the oval fossa. Bachmann's bundle is adjacent and superior to the superior limbus.

superior veins. Term used usually in reference to the right upper pulmonary vein and the left upper pulmonary vein collectively.

superior vena cava (SVC) syndrome. Symptoms related to significant obstruction or narrowing of the superior vena cava. There are multiple causes; in relation to device therapy, superior vena cava syndrome may develop as a result of placement of transvenous leads. It is more common when multiple transvenous leads are in place. Symptoms are due to impaired venous drainage from the head and upper extremities. Depending on the severity, surgery or percutaneous dilation may be necessary.

supernormal conduction. The propagation of electrical impulses at a rate faster than the expected conduction time. Supernormal conduction, best documented in the His-Purkinje tissue, can be determined by generating a strength-interval curve.

supernormal excitation. The supernormal period sometimes occurs at the end of the relative refractory period of the cardiac action potential. Supernormal excitation occurs when stimuli smaller than those typically needed to reach threshold produce a propagated action potential. The generated action potentials during the supernormal period are typically of lower amplitude.

supernormal phase. The phase of the action potential typically just at the end of the relative refractory period in which supernormal excitation or conduction of a generated impulse occurs. The supernormal phase occurs at about the same time as the vulnerable period (see *vulnerable period*) but is a different phenomenon; supernormality is characterized by a lower threshold, whereas in the vulnerable period there is an increased susceptibility to ventricular fibrillation. The supernormal period is best documented in the His-Purkinje system and is likely absent at other sites.

supraventricular tachycardia (SVT). An arrhythmia whose origin is above the ventricles. Supraventricular tachycardia is exemplified by sinus tachycardia, atrial flutter, and atrial fibrillation. The term is used broadly to include any tachyarrhythmia other than ventricular tachycardia and ventricular fibrillation.

surdocardiac syndrome. The congenital long QT syndrome associated with congenital deafness. Surdocardiac syndrome, also known as the Jervell and Lange-Nielsen syndrome, is transmitted by autosomal recessive inheritance.

Surethane. A polyether urea polyurethane that has been used for pacemaker lead insulation. Surethane differs from other polyurethanes by the addition of some urea linkages.

surface cracking. See *environmental stress cracking*.

surface mount. A type of electronic manufacturing technique in which components are soldered onto the surface of the pacemaker circuit board via flat connectors rather than via lead wires passed through the circuit board as in traditional methods. Surface mounts are more amenable to automated, high-yield production.

surgical ablation. The removal or destruction of arrhythmogenic tissue by surgery. See also *endocardial encircling ventriculotomy, endocardial resection, ventriculotomy*.

surveillance equipment/systems. See *antitheft surveillance equipment and electromagnetic interference*.

sustained duration timer. When discriminators for supraventricular tachycardia have been programmed on and there is a sustained arrhythmia for which therapies have been withheld by the implantable cardioverter-defibrillator because of a discrimination criterion for supraventricular tachycardia categorizing the tachycardia as not being ventricular tachycardia, there is some risk of continued sustained, possibly symptomatic, ventricular tachycardia. As a means to prevent this scenario for sustained arrhythmias, a sustained duration timer that is turned on will cause a cessation of the withholding of ventricular fibrillation therapy after a certain programmed period has elapsed and regardless of the discriminatory criteria for supraventricular tachycardia, therapies appropriate for that tachycardia zone will be delivered.

sustained monomorphic ventricular tachycardia. When ventricular tachycardia occurs with one morphology and is sustained (requiring cardioversion or antitachycardia pacing to terminate), there is likely a fixed abnormal substrate, often from prior myocardial infarction. Sustained monomorphic ventricular tachycardias are more amenable to catheter ablation than tachycardias that are nonsustained (inadequate for mapping) or polymorphic (changing morphology difficult to map). See also *monomorphic ventricular tachycardia*.

sustained tachycardia. A persistent accelerated heart rate, usually more than 100 beats per minute, that lasts longer than 30 seconds or is terminated by an intervention before that time because of hemodynamic compromise.

sustained VT timer. See *sustained duration timer*.

suture hole. A small hole near the edge of the pacemaker header through which a suture may be passed to secure the pacemaker to subcutaneous tissue within the pacemaker pocket and to prevent pacemaker migration.

sutureless lead. An epicardial lead secured to the myocardium by the use of a special fixation device rather than by the use of sutures. See also *epicardial lead*.

suture sleeve. A silicone elastomer or polyurethane sheath that fits around an endocardial pacing lead just proximal to the site of transvenous entry. The suture sleeve is used to protect the lead from damage when the securing suture is tightened to hold the lead in place. See also *lead fracture, pseudofracture*.

SV. Abbreviation for *stroke volume*.

SVC. Abbreviation for *superior vena cava*.

SVT. Abbreviation for *supraventricular tachycardia*.

SVT discrimination. Once a tachycardia has been detected in a programmed ventricular tachycardia zone based on cycle length, further discriminatory algorithms may be operative (if programmed "on") to distinguish rapid ventricular rates resulting from supraventricular tachycardia from the more malignant ventricular tachycardia. These discriminatory algorithms include onset criteria to help distinguish from sinus tachycardia, stability criteria to help distinguish from rapidly conducted atrial fibrillation, and wave or electrogram morphology to help distinguish ventricular tachycardia from conducted arrhythmias. SVT discrimination helps to prevent inappropriate implantable cardioverter-defibrillator therapies.

S wave. The negative deflection of a QRS complex that follows a positive R wave as seen on the surface electrocardiogram. See also *QRS complex*.

sympathetic denervation. Interruption of sympathetic nerves. Sympathetic denervation may occur after myocardial infarction in human beings. Sympathetic denervation has been shown to be arrhythmogenic in experimental studies.

sympathetic nervous system. The portion of the autonomic nervous system that causes increased chronotropic, inotropic, and dromotropic responses in the heart. In addition, the sympathetic nervous system generally shortens

Syncope: Differential Diagnosis		
Category	**Type**	**Comments**
Cardiogenic	Brady 　Sinus arrest 　Atrioventricular block	Diagnosis with monitoring treated by pacemaker
	Tachycardia 　Ventricular 　Preexcited atrial fibrillation 　Rarely, supraventricular 　　tachycardia	Diagnosed with monitoring or electrophysiologic study
Neurocardiogenic	Cardioinhibitory Vasodepressor	Diagnosis with tilt-table testing
Neural	Seizure	Diagnosed from history, electrocardiography, and long-term monitoring
Other	Hysterical conversion Malingering	Underlying psychological disorder

refractoriness in most tissues. In the ventricles, the sympathetic nerves course in a base-to-apex orientation within the subepicardium. Norepinephrine is the major neurotransmitter in the sympathetic nervous system. See also *parasympathetic nervous system*.

synchronous antitachycardia pacing. Pacing in which output pulses are delivered at a preset interval after an intrinsic depolarization is sensed. See also *burst pacing, critically timed stimulus, overdrive pacing, scanning pacemaker, underdrive pacing*.

syncope. Loss of consciousness with spontaneous recovery after a variable period of time. Syncope may occur suddenly or gradually and has multiple cardiovascular and noncardiovascular causes.

syncytium. Physiologically, a mass of cells that act as one functional unit. In the heart, the two atria form one functional syncytium and the two ventricles form another. A stimulus of sufficient strength and duration delivered anywhere within either atrium will cause both atria to contract. Similarly, a stimulus of sufficient strength and duration delivered anywhere in either ventricle will cause both ventricles to contract. This is the reason that pacing leads need to be placed in only one of the two atria or one of the two ventricles. The atrioventricular node and the His bundle, and sometimes accessory pathways, provide the pathway(s) for transmission of impulses from the atrial syncytium to the ventricular syncytium. Thus, if the intrinsic cardiac conduction system is normal, an impulse of sufficient strength and duration delivered to either atrium will cause contraction of the atria and ventricles in a normal sequence.

t

T. Abbreviation for "triggered" in the NBG code. Used in the third position for the mode of response, "T" indicates triggered or tracked. For a single-chamber pacemaker, for example, VVT, "T" indicates that if intrinsic ventricular activity is sensed, the device will trigger an output immediately, that is, it is delivered when the chamber is refractory. For a dual-chamber pacemaker, for example, VAT, the "T" indicates that the mode of response is to track sensed atrial activity, which will trigger a ventricular output at the programmed atrioventricular interval. See the table *NBG code*.

tachyarrhythmia. See *tachycardia*.

tachy-brady syndrome. See *bradycardia-tachycardia syndrome, sick sinus syndrome, tachycardia-bradycardia syndrome*.

tachycardia. An abnormally rapid heart rate, inappropriate for the tissue involved and inappropriate for metabolic need. Tachycardias usually have a rate more than 100 beats per minute but may be less, such as in junctional tachycardias, which are any junctional rhythms faster than 60 beats per minute.

tachycardia-bradycardia syndrome. Paroxysms of supraventricular tachycardias such as atrial tachycardia, atrial fibrillation, and atrial flutter interposed with other periods of bradycardias such as sinus bradycardia or sinus arrest. Not infrequently, a patient presents with episodes of atrial fibrillation that are followed by sinus arrest after termination because of overdrive suppression of the sinus node. Tachycardia-bradycardia syndrome also is known as bradycardia-tachycardia syndrome, sick sinus syndrome, and tachy-brady syndrome.

tachycardia cycle length (TCL). The period of time, or average period of time, from one complex to the next in a sensed tachycardia.

tachycardia-induced tachycardia. In certain clinical situations, the initial presence of one tachyarrhythmia may serve to induce a second tachyarrhythmia. Examples of this phenomenon include atrioventricular node reentry inducing right ventricular outflow tract tachycardia, a pulmonary vein tachycardia inducing either atrial fibrillation or atrial flutter, or atrioventricular reentrant tachycardia inducing atrial fibrillation.

tachycardia-recognition count. The number of tachycardia cycles that must be sensed by a pacemaker before the antitachycardia response is activated. The tachycardia-recognition count is a preset or programmable function of the tachycardia-terminating algorithm of antitachycardia devices. Various antitachycardia devices use different terms for this function.

tachycardia-recognition rate. The tachycardia rate that must be sensed by a pacemaker before the antitachycardia response is activated. The tachycardia-recognition rate is a preset or programmable function of the tachycardia-terminating algorithm of antitachycardia devices. Various antitachycardia devices use different terms for this function.

tachycardia redetection. In implanted defibrillators, once a tachycardia has been detected by fulfilling criteria programmed for the tachycardia detection zone, before delivery of a shock after charging, the device will check whether the tachycardia is still present and fulfills detection criteria if tachycardia redetection is programmed "on." Should the tachycardia have terminated during the charge, therapy will not be delivered. If tachycardia redetection is not programmed "on," the shock is delivered at the end of charge (committed shock).

tachycardia-terminating algorithm. The defined process and guidelines within the circuitry of an antitachycardia pacemaker which control the antitachycardia mechanism. The algorithm defines certain requirements that must be met, for example, determination of when activation of the antitachycardia mechanism is appropriate, what antitachycardia mechanism is to be used, what critically timed interval is to be delivered, and when the antitachycardia mechanism should stop. See also *tachycardia-recognition count, tachycardia-recognition rate*.

tachycardia-terminating pacing. See *anti-tachycardia pacing.*

tachycardia zone. Programmed detection zone in implanted cardioverter-defibrillators where sensed events are programmed to be detected as tachycardia, usually based on the cycle length.

tachy detection rates. In implanted defibrillators, continuous sensing of ventricular or atrial electrograms occurs. A programmable feature in most devices is a detection zone where the sensed events will be detected as a tachyarrhythmia. Once the tachyarrhythmia is detected in the tachy detect zone, programmed therapy may be delivered; if no therapy is programmed, the device in this zone works as a monitoring tool.

tachy zones. Detection zones programmed in atrial or ventricular defibrillators where various rates of either ventricular tachycardia or atrial tachycardia will be detected and appropriate programmed therapy delivered.

tamponade. A potential complication of temporary or permanent lead placement. If true tamponade occurs with hemodynamic compromise, immediate intervention is required. The incidence of tamponade as a complication of device implantation is uncertain but is uncommon.

target rate. A term used by some device manufacturers to refer to the optimal rate for typical patient activity.

target vein. 1. For left ventricular lead implantation, a particular portion, usually on the lateral wall of the right ventricle, is targeted for lead implantation. One or more veins may drain this target site and are referred to as the target veins. Common target veins are the lateral vein or lateral branches of a posterolateral or anterolateral vein. 2. In cardiac ablation, the site of origin of ectopy or tachycardia inducing atrial fibrillation may arise from a venous structure, such as a pulmonary vein or superior vena cava. This venous site of origin is sometimes termed a target vein for isolation.

TARP. Abbreviation for *total atrial refractory period.*

TCL. Abbreviation for *tachycardia cycle length.*

TDI. Abbreviation for *tissue Doppler imaging.*

TdP. Abbreviation for *torsades de pointes.*

TE. Abbreviation for *electrode temperature.*

telemetered information. Any stored or live-acquisition data that are retrieved from a pulse generator. Examples of telemetered information include the following tables or figures: *counters, long QT syndrome, mode switching,* and *pacemaker-mediated tachycardia.* See also *remote monitoring, telemetry.*

telemetry. The transmission of signals containing coded data from one electronic unit to another via radiofrequency or electromagnetic signals. In pacing, telemetry refers to the capability to interrogate a pacemaker with an external device to receive information about pacemaker function and intrinsic cardiac activity. Telemetered information may include the programmed pacemaker parameters, battery status, pacemaker model, or serial number, event records, and real-time telemetric measurements such as impedance and energy delivered. See also *remote monitoring, telemetered information.*

telemetry coil. A component of pacemaker circuitry that is an antenna for radiofrequency telemetry communication and enables the transmission of information between the pacemaker and the programmer.

telemetry link. An adequate radiofrequency signal that permits communication between devices, represented on some programmers by a display.

telescoping sheath technique. A technique used for lead extraction whereby a set of sheaths is placed with one sheath fitting over the other. This technique allows more effective disruption of fibrous (scar) tissue. The inner sheath may be a laser sheath, and, after forward manipulation during lasing, the outer nonlaser sheath is moved forward via the pathway created by the laser. This two-sheath system may be more successful than a single-sheath approach, and, once the lead is removed along with the inner sheath, the outer sheath can remain in place and a new lead may be passed through it.

temperature sensing. The determination of body temperature by the use of a thermistor, a resistor made of semiconductors that have resistance that varies rapidly and predictably with temperature. In pacing, temperature sensors have been used to measure changes in body temperature, incorporated into the pacing lead to measure the core body temperature. Temperature sensing has been used in rate-adaptive pacing systems to control pacing rate, but it is no longer used. See also *rate-adaptive pacing.*

temporary lead. An endocardial or epicardial pacing lead intended for short-term use, usually in conjunction with an external pacemaker. A temporary lead also is referred to as a temporary catheter. See also *lead*.

and cardiac events or to allow electrophysiologic studies in the absence of pacemaker output pulses.

temporary pacing. Pacing from an external, battery-powered pacemaker. An external pacemaker

Temporary Leads

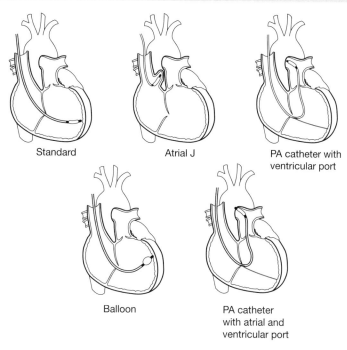

Standard Atrial J PA catheter with ventricular port

Balloon PA catheter with atrial and ventricular port

From Furman S, Hayes DL, Holmes DR Jr. A practice of cardiac pacing. 3rd ed. Mount Kisco (NY): Futura Publishing Company, Inc.; 1993. p. 231-60. Copyrighted and used with permission of Mayo Foundation for Medical Education and Research.

temporary pacemaker. An external, reusable, battery-powered pacemaker used to support the heart until a permanent pacemaker is implanted, or to control rhythm disturbances after cardiac surgery, myocardial infarction, or other transient conduction system disturbance. Temporary pacemakers usually have adjustable parameters, such as output and sensitivity. Temporary single- and dual-chamber pacemakers are available. Temporary pacemaker most commonly refers to an endocardial or epicardial temporary device, but external or transcutaneous pacing also is a type of temporary pacing. See also *external pacemaker, transcutaneous pacing.*

temporary pacemaker inhibition (TPI). A function of some programmers in which the pacemaker can be inhibited temporarily in order to permit assessment of intrinsic rhythm

emits controlled electrical impulses transcutaneously or via temporary pacing leads to the myocardium. Temporary pacing may be used as an emergency intervention in patients with symptomatic bradycardias. Temporary pacing also is referred to as external pacing. See also *temporary pacemaker, transcutaneous pacing.*

temporary parameter. Function on some device programmers that allows parameter values to be changed on a temporary basis and returned to original settings if needed.

tendon of Todaro. The superior boundary of the triangle of Koch. The tendon of Todaro is a right atrial ridge containing the commissure of the valves of the inferior vena cava and coronary sinus. See also *triangle of Koch.*

TENS. Abbreviation for *transcutaneous electrical nerve stimulation.*

terminal. See *lead connector.*

terminal cap. See *lead terminal cap.*

terminal crest. The terminal crest is formed during fetal development at the junction of the sinus venosus and the primordial right atrium. The superior portion of the terminal crest is the approximate site of the sinoatrial node. The atrial myocardium near the terminal crest is a relatively frequent site of origin of automatic atrial tachycardia. See also *crista terminalis.*

terminal pin. See *lead terminal pin.*

termination window. The segment of a reentry tachycardia circuit into which an impulse can be delivered to terminate a tachycardia. The delivered impulse causes the repolarized tissue in front of the impulse to depolarize but leaves the stimulation site refractory to the oncoming wave front of the reentrant circuit. This activity breaks the tachycardia. The window size, that is, the amount of time available to successfully interrupt the reentrant circuit, depends on the tachycardia rate, the size of the reentrant loop, and the refractory periods of tissue in the circuit. The termination window may be altered by body position, physiologic conditions, or drug therapy. The termination window is also referred to as the termination zone.

termination zone. See *termination window.*

tetrodotoxin. A poison that potently blocks the fast inward sodium channel during the resting state. Tetrodotoxin is used experimentally in vitro.

thebesian valve. A valve located at the ostium of the coronary sinus. The valve may be very small and rudimentary or may almost completely cover the orifice of the coronary sinus. A large thebesian valve may make entering the coronary sinus for electrophysiology and left ventricular pacing procedures difficult. A large thebesian valve often occurs in conjunction with a subeustachian ridge pouch.

theophylline. Classified as a methylxanthine, this drug is used primarily as a bronchodilator. However, theophylline has been advocated as a pharmacologic treatment for sinus node disease, specifically for bradycardia.

theoretical battery capacity. The calculated capacity of a battery to store charge. Theoretical battery capacity is based on the type and the amount of cathodal or anodal material available. See also *battery capacity, deliverable battery capacity, maximum available battery capacity.*

theoretical longevity. A calculated value of the time from the beginning of life to recommended replacement time for pulse generators. The calculation is based on battery capacity, programmed parameters, and accelerated battery test data.

therapeutic radiation. The treatment of disease by means of radiation. In pacing, exposure of a permanent pacemaker to therapeutic radiation may result in sudden lack of output of the pacemaker or in runaway pacemaker. Therapeutic radiation may damage the complementary metal-oxide semiconductor.

therapy initiation. In implantable cardioverter-defibrillators, this term designates delivery of the first antitachycardia pacing pulse or the initiation of capacitor charging for high-voltage therapy.

therapy summary. Telemetered information from an implantable cardioverter-defibrillator which summarizes all therapies delivered since the prior interrogation.

therapy zone. When a tachyarrhythmia has been detected, therapies may be programmed "on" or "off." When therapies that may include antitachycardia pacing or shock are programmed "on," the zone is referred to as a therapy zone. A detection zone with no therapies programmed "on" is referred to as a monitor zone.

thermal conduction. During ablative procedures, energy delivery at the catheter-myocardial interface results in heating. The heat may be conducted to neighboring structures, referred to as thermal conduction.

thermal injuries. Inadvertent injury to nontargeted structures during ablative procedures. Thermal injury may cause damage to, for example, coronary arterial vessels or neighboring lung tissue.

thermistor. Type of temperature sensor located in ablation electrodes to allow feedback titration of ablation energy delivery. Thermistors are resistors that are thermally sensitive. See also *thermocouples.*

Thermocool catheter. Trademark for a type of ablation catheter used in conjunction with an electroanatomic mapping system (CARTO) that utilizes internal irrigation to cool the catheter, allowing greater energy delivery and perhaps more complete transmural lesion formation.

thermocouples. Temperature sensors located in electrodes used for ablation. A thermocouple

Third-Degree AV Block

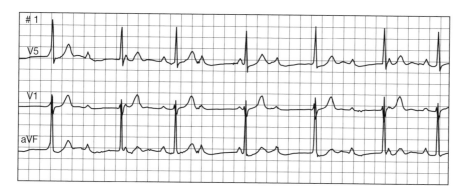

allows temperature monitoring during radio-frequency ablation, and this feedback is used to monitor appropriate power delivery. See also *thermistor*.

third-degree AV block. The inability of impulses to conduct from the atria to the ventricles. Third-degree AV block may be congenital or acquired. A junctional or ventricular ectopic focus usually compensates by generating a slow escape rhythm. Third-degree AV block may be an indication for temporary or permanent pacing. Third-degree AV block also is referred to as complete heart block. See also *first-degree AV block, second-degree AV block*.

third-degree (complete) heart block. See *third-degree AV Block*.

third-degree heart block. See *third-degree AV block*.

third-degree sinus node exit block. A complete disruption of sinus node conduction in which the sinus node discharges but none of its impulses are conducted to the atrial myocardium because of exit block. Third-degree sinus node exit block can be diagnosed only by recording the sinus node electrogram. See also *first-degree sinus node exit block, second-degree sinus node exit block, sinus node exit block*.

thoracic impedance monitoring. See *transthoracic impedance*.

three-dimensional mapping. Some methods used for mapping of tachyarrhythmias that allow three-dimensional reconstruction of the chamber or chambers that have been mapped. Three-dimensional mapping may be used to map the site of earliest activation of automatic tachycardias or the circuit and slow zones relevant in reentrant arrhythmia.

Three-dimensional mapping also may be used in sinus rhythm to identify sites of abnormal myocardial tissue (e.g., scars). See also *CARTO system, noncontact mapping*.

threshold. 1. In cellular electrophysiology, the minimum level of a stimulus that will evoke a response in excitable tissue, that is, the membrane potential at which a cell will generate an action potential. 2. In pacing, a measurement of the minimum electrical stimulation (pacemaker output pulse) required to consistently elicit a cardiac depolarization. The threshold also is the minimum spontaneous intrinsic signal required for consistent sensing by the pacemaker circuitry. Pacing and sensing thresholds may vary in response to physiologic changes resulting from factors such as maturation, myocardial infarction, drug therapy, and defibrillation. Thresholds can be measured invasively with a pacing systems analyzer. If the pacemaker is programmable, thresholds can be measured noninvasively by decreasing the voltage or pulse duration. Threshold is expressed in terms of amplitude (voltage or current), pulse duration, charge, or energy. See also *antiarrhythmic agent, defibrillation threshold, pacing threshold, sensing threshold*.

threshold evolution. See *threshold maturation*.

threshold margin test (TMT). See *safety margin test*.

threshold maturation. The change from acute threshold levels to chronic threshold levels. In pacing, maturation refers to the condition of the tissue around lead electrodes as scar tissue forms at the electrode-myocardial interface. Pacemaker function may be altered as a result of maturation because sensing or pacing thresholds may shift upward during the acute phase of maturation and subsequently decrease to lower levels during the chronic phase. Temporary loss of sensing or pacing that may occur during the maturation process may be corrected by noninvasive programming. See also *acute pacing threshold, chronic pacing threshold, pacing threshold, peak threshold, sensing threshold.*

threshold search. A term used as part of some autothreshold algorithms to describe the mechanism by which the threshold is determined.

tiered therapy. A description of the ability of newer implantable cardioverter-defibrillators to deliver different types of therapies in an attempt to terminate ventricular tachycardias of different rates.

tilt. A measurement of the percentage of voltage that dissipates from a capacitor after it discharges during delivery of a shock. Tilt = (Vi – Vf)/Vi, where Vi is the initial voltage and Vf is the final voltage. Delivery of a shock with a small value for tilt may not deliver enough voltage to successfully terminate an arrhythmia. Conversely, a shock with a very high tilt value may reinitiate the arrhythmia. For a given impedance, the duration (pulse width) of a shock varies as a function of the tilt. For a monophasic shock, some data suggest 50% to 80% as the most efficacious tilt. Tilt depends on the exponential decay time constant RC, that is, lower defibrillation capacitance or lower load resistance to higher tilt.

tilt-table testing (TTT). The technique used to provoke neurocardiogenic syncope in susceptible patients. While blood pressure and cardiac rate and rhythm are continuously monitored, patients are passively tilted upright to an angle of 60° to 85° for a period of time that varies in different protocols (15-60 minutes). If no abnormal response occurs during this time, the patient is returned to the supine position and a graded dose of isoproterenol may be infused, followed by repeat upright tilting for periods of 5 minutes at each dose. An abnormal response consists of a sudden drop in blood pressure (hypotension) during upright tilt. This hypotension often is accompanied by bradycardia. See also *neurocardiogenic syncope.*

time constant. A performance characteristic of electronic timing circuits or pulse generators. An exponential voltage decays to 63% of its initial value over a period of time equal to the time constant of the circuit. The time constant is equal to the product of the capacitance and the resistance of the circuit. For example, the period of an RC oscillator is longer for either larger values of resistance or capacitance. More importantly, the tilt of an exponential defibrillation waveform increases for smaller values of defibrillation capacitance or of patch impedance.

time-dependent refractoriness. The lack of excitability of tissue despite repolarization and return of membrane potential to the resting voltage. Time-dependent refractoriness may be a mechanism responsible for acceleration-dependent aberration.

time domain analysis. Assessment of the amplitude of a signal as a function of time, such as in signal-averaged electrocardiogram analysis. See also *frequency domain analysis.*

timing cycle. Timing periods that define device function. These intervals are predefined and specific and determine aspects of pacing or defibrillation (e.g., the ventriculoatrial interval, atrial escape interval). Timing cycles are measured and described in milliseconds.

timing diagram. A diagram provided or drawn schematically that defines specific elements of the behavior of a pacemaker, implantable cardioverter-defibrillator, or cardiac resynchronization device. These diagrams are often helpful for troubleshooting. Some programmers are capable of creating a timing diagram; timing diagrams also can be created manually.

timolol. A nonselective, β-adrenergic blocking agent without intrinsic sympathomimetic activity. Timolol is metabolized predominantly by the liver. For side effects, see *β-adrenergic blocking drugs.*

tine. A passive-fixation endocardial lead-tip configuration. Tines are made of silicone or polyurethane and are barblike appendages that protrude backward from the distal tip of the pacing lead. The tines are designed to be entrapped within the trabeculae of the heart in order to reduce the likelihood of lead dislodgement. See also *distal-tip electrode.*

tissue Doppler imaging (TDI). Echocardiographic imaging tool useful for assessing ventricular synchronization. Doppler imaging usually is used to image the velocity of blood flow (red blood cells); with tissue Doppler imaging, the myocardial tissue velocities are imaged typically with a color-coded system. Tissue

Doppler imaging is the basis for assessing synchronization of ventricular myocardial contraction, by comparing either two myocardial contraction velocity sites with each other or their timing with the QRS deflection on the electrocardiogram.

tissue Doppler strain echocardiography. Variant of tissue Doppler imaging in which the tissue velocities at two myocardial sites are compared with each other and related to the distance between these two sites (velocity 1 – velocity 2 ÷ distance). See also *tissue Doppler imaging.*

tissue tracking. A method based on tissue Doppler echocardiography for the assessment of longitudinal apical myocardial motion which assesses systolic displacement of myocardium.

titanium. A noncorrosive, hypoallergenic, biocompatible metallic element. Pacemaker cases usually are made of titanium.

titanium nitride. A material used to coat the electrode tip. This material has been shown to reduce polarization during stimulation with an electrode with a platinum-iridium surface.

TMT. Abbreviation for *threshold margin test.*

torque. A force that produces or tends to produce a rotating or twisting motion. In pacing, torque must be compensated for in the manipulation and insertion of catheters and endocardial pacing leads.

torque wrench. A tool designed to tighten pacemaker setscrews.

torsades de pointes (TdP). Polymorphic ventricular tachycardia associated with a long QT interval. Torsades de pointes is so named because it appears that the QRS complexes are twisting around a center axis. The rhythm often self-terminates but tends to recur. Disagreement exists as to whether the underlying mechanism is afterdepolarizations or dispersion of refractoriness.

total atrial refractory interval. See *total atrial refractory period.*

total atrial refractory period (TARP). The amount of time during which the pacemaker atrial sensing amplifier is unresponsive to input signals. In some pacemakers, however, the sensing circuitry is alert for extraneous signals during the latter portion of the total atrial refractory period, so that this portion of the total atrial refractory period is relatively refractory rather than absolutely refractory. In the dual-chamber pacing mode (DDD), the total atrial refractory period is composed of two intervals, the atrioventricular interval and the postventricular atrial refractory period. The total atrial refractory period also is referred to as the maximum rate interval. It is expressed in milliseconds.

totally porous electrode. An electrode in which a network of interstices are distributed uniformly throughout the electrode to facilitate tissue ingrowth. Totally porous electrodes are fabricated by sintering an inner core of platinum-iridium wire with a loose screen of fine platinum-iridium wire pads. See also *porous electrode, porous-surface electrode.*

total recovery time. The time required for the atria to return to basic cycle length after rapid atrial overdrive pacing. The total recovery time is used to assess sinus node function. Prolongation of the total recovery time indicates impaired sinus node automaticity or conduction. Normal recovery time usually has a duration of less than 5 seconds, occurs within four to six beats, and has a gradual shortening of cycle length. See also *sinus node recovery time.*

TPI. Abbreviation for *temporary pacemaker inhibition.*

tracking. The delivery of a pacemaker output stimulus at timed intervals after sensed intrinsic atrial activity. Tracking may occur in VDD, DDD, DDDR, and VAT pacing. It is used to maintain atrioventricular synchrony by synchronizing ventricular pacing with sensed atrial activity. Tracking also is referred to as atrial tracking. See also *maximum tracking rate, maximum tracking rate interval.*

tracking preference. A programmable parameter that is intended to maintain atrial-tracked ventricular pacing in DDD(R) and VDD(R) modes by temporarily reducing the postventricular atrial refractory period to reestablish atrial-tracked ventricular pacing inappropriately lost due to atrial events occurring in postventricular atrial refractory period.

traction. The act of pulling. In pacing, traction can be attempted in the removal of an implanted pacing lead.

trailing edge. The voltage downslope of a depolarization recording on an electrocardiogram or an intracardiac electrogram. In pacing and defibrillation, the trailing edge also refers to the voltage downslope of a recorded pacemaker output pulse or defibrillator shock. •

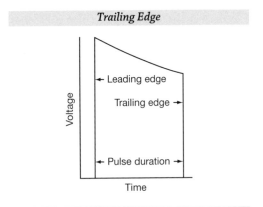

Trailing Edge

train stimulation. See *high-frequency stimulation*.

transceiver. The combination of a radio transmitter and receiver, usually in the same housing and sharing the same components. In pacing, a transceiver is used in the external programmer to generate the carrier signal for transmission to the implanted pacemaker and to receive the modulated carrier signal from the pacemaker.

transcutaneous electrical nerve stimulation (TENS). A technique to reduce pain by electrical stimulation through the skin. TENS application should be used cautiously in pacemaker-dependent patients and patients with an implantable cardioverter-defibrillator. Theoretically, TENS could cause clinically significant electromagnetic interference. Pacemaker-dependent patients and patients with an implantable cardioverter-defibrillator should initially be tested with the TENS unit while being monitored to be certain that no interference occurs.

transcutaneous pacing. External pacing in which adhesive pads are placed externally on the chest wall and current is delivered to cause ventricular depolarization. A transcutaneous pacemaker can be set to the desired pulses per minute. This is frequently uncomfortable for the patient, but often it is lifesaving until temporary transvenous pacing can be established.

transesophageal electrogram. See *esophageal electrogram*.

transesophageal pacing. See *esophageal pacing and recording*.

transient outward currents. Transient outward current I_{TO1} is a potassium current that is a brief repolarizing current occurring in phase 1 of the action potential. Transient outward currents shorten action potential duration by speeding up the cycling of channels that open later during the action potential. Another transient outward current is a chloride current called I_{TO2}. See also I_{TO}.

transient outward potassium current. See I_{TO}.

transistor. An electronic circuit component consisting of a semiconductor material to which three electrical contacts are made. Transistors can provide amplification, oscillation, or switching functions.

transitional cells. Transitional cells are cardiac cells that are intermediate in histologic appearance between Purkinje fibers and the working cardiac myocytes. Transitional cells are found between atrial myocardial cells and the atrioventricular node and also between atrioventricular nodal cells and the Purkinje fiber-like tissue of the His bundle.

transitional electrode impedance. The opposition to current occurring as a direct result of current flow through the electrode-myocardial interface. Transitional electrode impedance can be calculated by subtracting the lead conductor resistance from the total lead impedance.

transition zone. The region in the atrioventricular conduction axis between the atrium and the atrioventricular node.

transmembrane potential. The potential gradient, measured in millivolts, that exists across the membrane of cardiac cells. Transmembrane potentials determine the excitability level of cardiac cells and change during depolarization.

transmission rate. The number of information elements transmitted per unit time. Transmission rate is dependent on the type of carrier signal used in the communication process. In programming and telemetry, the transmission rate is maximized by the use of high-frequency radio signals or modulation to transmit large quantities of data in a short period of time. See also *baud*.

transmural dispersion of repolarization. See *tridimensional dispersion of repolarization*.

transmural reentry. The reentry circuit may involve the myocardium adjacent to the endocardial surface, mid myocardial cells, and the myocardial cells adjacent to the epicardial surface. Parts of the reentry circuit may be located more endocardially, and the slow zone may be located at either a mid myocardial or an epicardial site or vise versa. For ablation of transmural reentrant circuits, both endocardial and epicardial approaches may be required. See also *reentrant ventricular tachycardia*.

transseptal approach. One method for gaining access to the left heart chambers to perform catheter ablation of left free-wall accessory pathways. The ablation catheter is passed via a sheath that has been placed from the right atrium to the left atrium through the atrial septum.

transtelephonic monitoring (TTM). Transmission, via telephone lines, of electrocardiograms or telemetry information from an implanted pacemaker or cardioverter-defibrillator, or monitoring of documentation of symptomatic paroxysmal rhythm disturbances. The information sent is converted into transmission signals by a special transmitter and is then reconverted into a representation of the original signal by a special receiver so the information can be displayed graphically. Typically, transtelephonic monitoring is used to transmit information from the patient at home to a physician's office or follow-up clinic. Information that is frequently transmitted via transtelephonic monitoring includes electrocardiographic tracings, pacing rate, magnet rate, and pulse duration, although current technology allows transmission of much more data. See also *multiplex transmission*.

transthoracic impedance. The impedance presented to a system of two or more electrodes located within, or on, the chest. Transthoracic impedance is affected by the location of the electrodes and the composition of the body tissues. See also *impedance*.

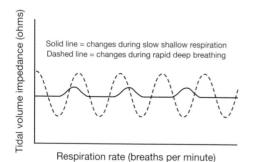

Transthoracic Impedance

Solid line = changes during slow shallow respiration
Dashed line = changes during rapid deep breathing

Tidal volume impedance (ohms)

Respiration rate (breaths per minute)

transthoracic lead. A temporary epicardial lead that is inserted through the chest wall. The

electrode is inserted into the myocardium or affixed to the epicardium with sutures. Transthoracic leads placed at the time of cardiac surgery are connected to an external temporary pacemaker. See also *temporary lead*.

transthoracic pacing. A term used to describe several types of temporary pacing. Transthoracic pacing most currently is used to describe a temporary pacing technique whereby a lead is passed through the thoracic wall. Transthoracic pacing refers either to the use of temporary epicardial leads or to an older method of emergency temporary pacing that was accomplished via an electrode passed through a large trocar that was blindly passed through the myocardium into an intracardiac space. The term sometimes is used inappropriately to describe transcutaneous or external pacing.

transthoracic shock. An external cardioversion or defibrillation shock applied across the chest wall.

transvenous. Inserted or performed through a vein. In pacing, the transvenous approach is used most commonly to insert and pass an endocardial pacing lead into and through a central venous structure into the right side of the heart. Some defibrillation leads may be placed transvenously.

transvenous defibrillation lead system. See *nonthoracotomy lead system*.

transvenous lead. See *endocardial lead*.

transvenous pacing. See *endocardial pacing*.

trend. In pacing, a telemetric feature of some rate-adaptive pacemakers that allows evaluation of the sensor-indicated rate by means of a graph that displays rate against time for a definable duration. This allows estimation of the appropriateness of rate adaptation for an individual patient's level of activity.

triangle of Koch. The region bounded by the tendon of Todaro, the septal leaflet of the tricuspid valve, and the coronary sinus ostium. The atrioventricular node is located at the apex of the triangle of Koch. See also *tendon of Todaro*. •

tridimensional dispersion of repolarization. Temporal differences in repolarization exist between ventricular myocardial cells in different locations. These differences may also occur in three dimensions, that is, between the endocardial, mid myocardial, and epicardial ventricular myocardial layers. See also *dispersion of repolarization, repolarization*.

Triangle of Koch

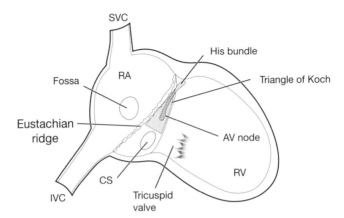

trifascicular block. The slowing or block of conduction in all three major divisions of the bundle branch system (right bundle branch, left anterior fascicle, and posterior fascicle). Trifascicular block presents most frequently as right bundle branch block with left anterior fascicular block and first-degree atrioventricular block. It must be determined whether the first-degree atrioventricular block is due to slowing of conduction in the left posterior fascicle or in the atrioventricular node.

trigeminy. An arrhythmia characterized by repeating patterns of three beats, with one premature ventricular contraction following two normal beats.

triggered activity. A mechanism of arrhythmias caused by afterdepolarizations that arise from the preceding action potential. Triggered rhythms may be initiated by programmed stimulation. Typically, the coupling interval of the first complex of the tachycardia demonstrates a direct relationship to the coupling interval of the initiating extrastimulus. Arrhythmias associated with digitalis toxicity may be due to triggered activity.

triggered automaticity. Triggered automaticity is a mechanism of arrhythmia generation that results from triggered depolarizations. Triggered depolarization may result from either early or late afterdepolarization and cause premature systoles or atrial, His-Purkinje, or ventricular tachycardias. Triggered automaticity results from calcium overload and is often made worse with rapid pacing (unlike abnormal automaticity, which is suppressed with rapid pacing). The worsening with rapid stimulation results from increased calcium flux, which increases the depolarizing currents generated during calcium efflux from the cytosol (sodium, calcium exchanger).

triggered pacing. Pacing in which an output pulse is delivered to the heart whenever intrinsic activity or noise is sensed. Triggered pacing may be atrial or ventricular. If the pacemaker output pulse is delivered into a P wave or a QRS complex, there is no electrical or hemodynamic effect on the heart because the tissue is refractory. Triggered pacing is used to test the sensing function of a pacemaker in relation to intrinsic conduction, to diagnose tracking of myopotentials or electromagnetic interference, to pace patients who are frequently exposed to electromagnetic interference or myopotential inhibition, to terminate tachycardias, and to perform noninvasive electrophysiologic studies. See also *atrial-triggered pacing mode (AAT), VVT.*

triple extrastimuli. Use of three extrastimuli, either atrial or ventricular, during electrophysiologic study, typically after an eight-beat drive train. Triple extrastimuli testing is a routine part of an electrophysiologic study when trying to induce a reentrant ventricular tachycardia.

tripolar sensing. See *differential bipolar sensing.*

truncated exponential waveform. The shape of the shock wave delivered by all implantable cardioverter-defibrillators available today. The capacitors are charged initially to a given voltage and then release this shock wave with

Twiddler's Syndrome

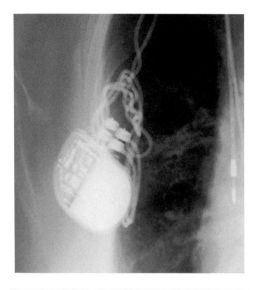

exponential decay. The capacitors are not allowed to discharge completely, and thus the waveform is cut off (truncated) while voltage still remains. The implantable cardioverter-defibrillators used today typically deliver biphasic waveform shocks. See also *tilt*.

Trypanosoma cruzi. The species of a sporozoan parasite responsible for Chagas' disease. Chagas' disease can result in conduction system disease that requires permanent pacing.

T shock. A method of inducing ventricular fibrillation during defibrillation threshold testing at implantation of a cardioverter-defibrillator. Energy, typically 0.62 to 1.5 J, is delivered at the approximate height peak of the T wave (venerable period) to induce ventricular fibrillation.

TTM. Abbreviation for *transtelephonic monitoring*.

TTT. Abbreviation for *tilt-table testing*.

T-type calcium channels. One type of calcium channel (see also *L-type calcium channels*). T-type calcium channels play a significant role in sinus node pacemaker activity where their small depolarizations generate an inward current that contributes to the oscillatory potentials typical of pacemaker cells. T-type calcium channels do not have an important role in depolarization of atrial, ventricular, or His-Purkinje cells. T-type calcium channels may be important also in cell proliferative signaling.

T wave. The low-frequency wave that follows the

ST segment on an electrocardiogram. The T wave represents repolarization (phase 3) of the ventricular myocardium. Generally, the normal T-wave vector is in the same direction as the QRS vector in any given lead.

T-wave alternans. Changes in the amplitude and polarity of the T wave, sometimes seen on electrocardiography or with specialized testing. Increased T-wave alternans is a marker for increased propensity for ventricular arrhythmias.

T-wave recycling. Resetting the pacemaker timing cycle when a T wave is sensed by the pacemaker and interpreted as an R wave. T-wave recycling represents oversensing by the pacemaker.

twiddler's syndrome. The conscious or unconscious rotation of an implanted pacemaker by a patient. Constant manipulation of the pacemaker through the overlying tissue causes coiling of the pacing lead(s), and this may result in lead fracture or gradual shortening and eventual dislodgement of the lead. Many cases of apparent twiddler's syndrome may not be due to manipulation of the pacemaker by the patient but rather to passive rotation of the pacemaker in a loose pocket.

two-dimensional reentry. The reentry circuit may involve both the endocardial and the mid myocardial layers or the mid myocardial and subepicardial layers of the ventricular myocardium. If the endocardium and mid myocardium are involved, ablation may require higher power delivery from an endocardial catheter. Alternatively, if both the subepicardium and the mid myocardium are involved, both endocardial and epicardial ablation may be required. See also *reentry, three-dimensional mapping*.

2:1 AV block. Atrioventricular block characterized by conduction to the ventricles with ventricular depolarization with every other P wave. It may represent Mobitz I or Mobitz II AV block.

2:1 block response. A variable block upper-rate response that occurs when the interval between consecutive P waves is shorter than the total atrial refractory period and only every other P wave is sensed. Ventricular output pulses occur only after the sensed P waves, which results in 2:1 block. See also *block response, pseudo-Wenckebach response, upper rate response, variable block response*.

2:1 retrograde conduction in ventricular tachycardia. During ventricular tachycardia, in some patients, retrograde conduction to the atrium via either the atrioventricular node or an accessory pathway may occur. Sometimes, particularly when retrograde conduction is through an accessory pathway, 2:1 retrograde ventriculoatrial block may be present during ventricular tachycardia. This results in one atrial depolarization for every two ventricular tachycardia beats.

u

UAR. Abbreviation for *upper activity rate*.

Uhl's anomaly. Congenital abnormality of the right ventricle, possibly an extreme form of right ventricular dysplasia. The right ventricular free wall is extremely thin and parchment-like. Problems associated with this abnormality may include reentrant right ventricular arrhythmia and perforation of the ventricle in attempting to place a sink lead or perform catheter-based procedures in the right ventricle.

UKPACE. See *United Kingdom Pacing and Cardiovascular Events*.

ultrarapid delayed rectifier potassium channel. Repolarizing currents that are carried by potassium channels that open after the initial depolarizing event were called delayed rectifier or delayed potassium currents (see also *delayed rectifier*). Ultrarapid delayed rectifier channels (I_{Kur}) are delayed potassium currents seen in the atrial myocardium where the action potential is short.

ULV. Abbreviation for *upper limit of vulnerability*.

uncommon AV nodal reentry. See *atypical AV nodal reentry*.

underdrive pacing. Competitive pacing with asynchronous stimulation at a rate below that of the tachycardia rate. Underdrive pacing can terminate a tachycardia circuit, provided that one of the randomly timed stimuli falls in the termination window of the tachycardia. Underdrive pacing usually is ineffective for termination of a tachycardia faster than 160 beats per minute.

undersensing. Failure of the pacemaker circuitry to sense intrinsic cardiac activity. Undersensing may cause the pacemaker to emit inappropriately timed, asynchronous, or competitive output pulses. In defibrillators, undersensing may cause lack of detection of an arrhythmia. See also *oversensing*.

unidirectional block. Cardiac conduction that occurs in only one direction. Unidirectional block may be caused by functional or permanent block. For example, unidirectional block is present in concealed accessory pathways that conduct only in the retrograde direction. Conduction pathways that have unidirectional block often are involved in reentrant arrhythmias. See also *reentry*.

unidirectional programming. One-way pacemaker programming. In unidirectional programming, commands are transmitted from the programmer to the pacemaker, but information is not transmitted from the pacemaker to the programmer. See also *bidirectional programming, telemetry*.

unifilar lead. A pacing lead whose conductor is composed of a single wire. Because there is no redundancy in a unifilar lead, fracture of the wire results in conduction failure. A unifilar lead also is more susceptible to stresses, such as flexion, that can result in lead failure.

Unipolar Electrode System

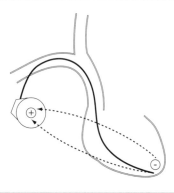

unipolar electrode system. An electrical system with one pole, or a system that requires only one pole for operation. In a conventional unipolar pacing system, one electrode (the cathode) is external to the pacemaker and is located on or within the heart. The other electrode (the anode) is the metal pacemaker case. Current flows from the cathode to the anode to complete the circuit. Unipolar pacemakers typically have better intrinsic signal strength but are more susceptible to electromagnetic interference and are associated with a higher incidence of extracardiac stimulation than bipolar systems. See also *bipolar electrode system, electrode configuration, unipolar lead.*

unipolar lead. A pacing lead with one electrical pole, which is external to the pacemaker and usually is located in the heart. The stimulating cathode typically is located at the distal tip of the endocardial lead, and the anode is the pacemaker case. The cathode must be placed in the heart chamber that is to be paced or sensed.

unipolar split cathodal configuration. See *split cathodal configuration.*

United Kingdom Pacing and Cardiovascular Events (UKPACE). This trial compared DDD with VVI pacing modes in patients 70 years or older requiring permanent pacing for second- or third-degree atrioventricular block. This trial showed no significant difference between pacing modes in the primary end point of all-cause mortality or in the composite secondary end point of cardiovascular deaths, atrial fibrillation, heart failure hospitalizations, cerebrovascular accidents or thromboembolic events, and reoperation (Toff WD, Camm AJ, Skehan JD, United Kingdom Pacing and Cardiovascular Events Trial Investigators. Single-chamber versus dual-chamber pacing for high-grade atrioventricular block. N Engl J Med. 2005;353:145-55).

universal pacing. See *dual-chamber pacing (DDD).*

universal programmer. A theoretical device that would allow external, noninvasive programming of a wide variety of pacemakers made by different manufacturers. Current pacemaker programming is accomplished by programmers that are manufacturer-specific.

upper activity rate (UAR). An upper rate that is programmed independently from the upper tracking rate or upper rate limit. It is the fastest rate that can be achieved in response to signals from a rate-responsive sensor.

upper limit of vulnerability (ULV). The phenomenon in which there is a maximum energy level, above which shocks delivered to the ventricle during repolarization will no longer induce ventricular fibrillation. This upper limit of vulnerability correlates closely with the defibrillation threshold. These observations, among others, led to the upper limit of vulnerability hypothesis of defibrillation, which states that shocks that fail to defibrillate the heart may actually stop and then reinitiate fibrillation.

upper rate behavior. Generic term that can be applied to pulse generator response when the programmed upper rate is achieved. The term is sometimes used more specifically to describe the behavior that occurs when the sensed atrial rate exceeds the maximum tracking rate or

Upper Rate Pseudo-Wenckebach and 2:1 Response

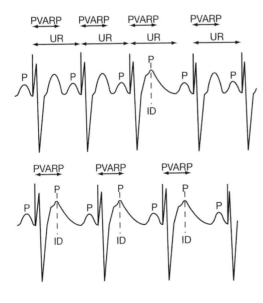

UR, upper rate. Modified from Hayes DL, Levine PA. Pacemaker timing cycles. In: Ellenbogen KA, editor. Cardiac pacing. Boston: Blackwell Scientific Publications; 1992. p. 263-308. Used with permission.

maximum sensor rate. See the figures *DDD: upper rate behavior* and *DDDR: upper rate behavior*.

upper rate interval (URI). See *maximum tracking rate interval*.

upper rate limit (URL). See *maximum tracking rate*.

upper rate response (URR). The preset or programmable response of a dual-chamber pacemaker that occurs when the atrial rate exceeds the limit at which ventricular output pulses can maintain 1:1 synchrony. The upper rate response is designed to limit the maximum pacing rate of the ventricle while maintaining, to some extent, the benefits of atrioventricular synchrony. Upper rate responses include fallback, 2:1 block, rate smoothing, variable block, and pseudo-Wenckebach response. See also *block response, fallback, pseudo-Wenckebach response, rate smoothing, sensor-driven rate-smoothing, 2:1 block response, variable block response*.

upper sensor rate. An upper activity rate that specifically reflects the maximum rate the sensor is allowed to achieve.

upright tilt testing. See *tilt-table testing*.

URI. Abbreviation for *upper rate interval*.

URL. Abbreviation for *upper rate limit*.

URR. Abbreviation for *upper rate response*.

use-dependent block. The increasing block of ion channels by a drug at faster rates. Use-dependent block is due to inadequate time, during electrical diastole, for the drug to dissociate from the channel. The rate at which a given drug exhibits use-dependent block depends on its time constant of recovery from block.

Use of Metoprolol CR/XL to Maintain Sinus Rhythm After Conversion From Persistent Atrial Fibrillation (METAFER). This study was designed to assess the safety and efficacy of metoprolol controlled release/extended release (CR/XL) for patients with a history of persistent atrial fibrillation that had been successfully cardioverted to determine whether the drug would reduce recurrent atrial fibrillation. Patients were randomized to either long-acting metoprolol (CR/XL) or placebo. Metoprolol CR/XL did reduce recurrent atrial fibrillation after cardioversion to normal sinus rhythm when compared with placebo (Kuhlkamp V, Schirdewan A, Stangl K, Homberg M, Ploch M, Beck OA. Use of metoprolol CR/XL to maintain sinus rhythm after conversion from persistent atrial fibrillation: a randomized, double-blind, placebo-controlled study. J Am Coll Cardiol. 2000;36:139-46).

U wave. The small positive deflection following the T wave as seen on an electrocardiogram. U waves are best seen on electrocardiographic leads V_3 to V_5. Prominent U waves may be caused by digitalis, hypokalemia, and various antiarrhythmic agents. U waves may represent repolarization of the ventricular Purkinje fibers.

V

V. Abbreviation for *volt*. Letter used in the NBG code for ventricle. See the table *NBG code*. Also, the chemical symbol for *vanadium*.

V_1. The ventricular response to S_1, the drive stimulus. See also *S_1*.

V_2. The ventricular response to S_2, the first extrastimulus. See also *S_2*.

V_1-V_2 interval in refractory. The V_1-V_2 interval is the shortest coupling interval between two consecutive ventricular stimuli, usually the last beat of the drive train and the first extrastimulus (V_2), where ventricular capture of the second extrastimulus occurs. V_1 refers to the ventricular response to S_1, which is the drive train stimulus, and V_2 refers to the ventricular response or captured electrogram in response to S_2, usually the first extrastimulus.

VA. Abbreviation for *ventriculoatrial*.

VA conduction. See *retrograde conduction*.

VA conduction system effective refractory period. During ventricular pacing, for a given drive cycle (V_1 to V_1), the longest V_1 to V_2 interval at which V_2 does not cause an atrial depolarization. See also *effective refractory period*.

VA conduction system functional refractory period. During ventricular pacing, for a given drive cycle (V_1 to V_1), the shortest A_1 to A_2 interval generated in response to a V_1 to V_2 interval. See also *functional refractory period*.

VA conduction system relative refractory period. During ventricular pacing, for a given drive cycle (V_1 to V_1), the longest V_1 to V_2 interval at which the V_2 to A_2 interval exceeds the V_1 to A_1 interval. See also *relative refractory period*.

VA conduction test. Some pulse generators have had the capability of conducting a test to determine the presence of VA conduction and VA conduction time. A VA conduction test may be accompanied by pacing the ventricle and recording the interval from the ventricular paced event to the next atrial sensed event.

VA conduction time. The amount of time required for a depolarizing impulse from the ventricular myocardium to be conducted to the atrial myocardium. VA conduction time also is referred to as the VA interval.

VA dissociation. Independent rhythms controlling the atria and ventricles. See also *AV dissociation*.

vagally induced tachycardia. See *postvagal tachycardia*.

vagal modulation. Input to the heart and vasculature occurring via the vagus nerve and modulating electrical properties in the heart. These effects primarily occur with reference to the sinoatrial node, atrioventricular node, and, to a lesser extent, the atrial and pulmonary venous myocardium.

vagotonia. Increased vagal tone, sometimes in athletes, during ablation near the pulmonary venous ostium or in certain disease states.

vagus nerve. The 10th cranial nerve, which carries parasympathetic fibers to most of the body.

VA interval. See *atrial escape interval, VA conduction time*.

Val-HeFT. See *Valsartan Heart Failure Trial*.

Valsalva maneuver. Voluntary forced exhalation against a closed glottis. The Valsalva maneuver creates an increase in aortic pulse pressure and an increase in heart rate during the maintained strain phase (phase 2). Reflex vagal output to the heart occurs during the overshoot phase (phase 4) and causes slowing of the heart rate. Because of this vagal effect, the Valsalva maneuver may be used to terminate a supraventricular tachycardia that has the atrioventricular node as part of its circuit.

Valsartan Heart Failure Trial (Val-HeFT). This trial assessed the effect of valsartan on patients with class II, III, and IV heart failure. Valsartan significantly reduced the combined end point of mortality and morbidity and improved clinical signs and symptoms in patients with heart failure when added to standard therapy (Cohn JN, Tognoni G, Valsartan Heart Failure Trial Investigators. A randomized trial of the angiotensin-receptor blocker valsartan in chronic heart failure. N Engl J Med. 2001;345:1667-75).

valve of Vieussens. Normally occurring valve-like structure found at the orifice of the posterior lateral ventricular vein. The valve of Vieussens may sometimes make it difficult to place a left ventricular pacing lead in the posterior lateral ventricular vein. The vein of Marshall, one of the primary atrial veins, often arises in the same location as the posterior ventricular valve and valve of Vieussens.

valves. The structures within the heart (tricuspid, mitral, pulmonary, and aortic) that open and close and thereby allow or stop the flow of blood. May also refer to smaller structures in the cardiac veins that prevent backflow of blood but also may obstruct the advancement of a guiding sheath during left ventricular lead placement. A venogram may be helpful for identifying the presence of a venous valve before placement of the lead.

vanadium (V). A metallic element used in silver-lithium-vanadium cells. See also *silver-vanadium cell chemistry*.

variable AV interval. A term used to describe two different AV interval behaviors of some dual-chamber pacemakers. Variable AV interval may refer to a rate-variable AV interval, in which the AV interval is shorter after a sensed atrial event than after a paced atrial event. The variable AV interval also may be referred to as the variable AV delay. See also *differential AV interval, rate-variable AV interval*.

variable block response. An upper rate response that has been incorporated in some pacemakers in which the interval between consecutive P waves is shorter than the total atrial refractory period. As a consequence, some of the P waves fall in the total atrial refractory period and are not sensed. Ventricular output pulses occur after sensed P waves, resulting in a variable block. The apparent degree of block, for example, 4:3, 3:2, 2:1, depends on the maximum tracking rate of the ventricular channel and the intrinsic atrial rate. See also *block response, pseudo-Wenckebach response, 2:1 block response, upper rate response*.

variable hysteresis. In pacing, lengthening of the pacing interval in response to sensed intrinsic activity in which the degree of lengthening is dependent on intrinsic heart rate. The escape interval is adapted automatically to the preceding cardiac cycle and can be programmed as a percentage of the intrinsic rate.

Vario test. A feature available in some pulse generators that automatically evaluates capture. Although variations exist, this feature generally involves stepping down the pulse amplitude to determine the point at which loss of capture occurs.

vasodepressor response. Parasympathetic response that results in a fall in systemic pressure as a result of vascular dilatation. This response occurs during an abnormal tilt-table study and may give rise to syncope.

vasodepressor syncope. See *neurocardiogenic syncope*.

vasovagal syncope (VVS). See *neurocardiogenic syncope*.

VAT. The NBG code for atrial-synchronized ventricular pacing, that is, P-wave synchronized pacing. In the VAT mode, pacing occurs in the ventricle, sensing occurs in the atrium, and the mode of response is triggered. VAT pacing is of historical interest only. It was abandoned because intrinsic ventricular activity was not sensed, and thus competition with the intrinsic rhythm could and did occasionally occur. In

VDD Pacing

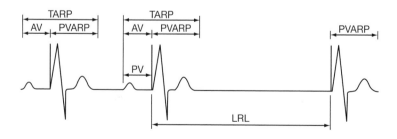

acute or unstable conditions, an asynchronous ventricular pacing stimulus during the vulnerable period could initiate malignant arrhythmias. See also *P-wave synchronous pacing*.

VDD. The NBG code for atrial-synchronized ventricular-inhibited pacing. In the VDD mode, pacing occurs in the ventricle, sensing occurs in both the atrium and the ventricle, and the mode of response is inhibited or triggered. See also *atrial-synchronized ventricular-inhibited pacing mode*.

VDDR. VDD pacing with rate-adaptive capability. The designation of VDDR is used by manufacturers to designate a device that operates in a P-synchronous mode except when it is sensor-driven, in which case the pacing mode may be VVIR or DDDR, depending on the specific device.

VDG. Abbreviation for *ventricular depolarization gradient*.

VDI mode. Ventricular pacing, dual-chamber sensing; responds only by inhibition by intrinsic chamber activity.

vector mapping. Method of using the electrocardiographic vector of depolarization to map the origin of the ventricular arrhythmia, atrial arrhythmia, or sites of cardiac pacing.

VEGM, ventricular EGM. Abbreviation for *ventricular electrogram*.

VEI. Abbreviation for *ventricular escape interval*.

vein of Marshall. Tributary of the coronary sinus that may allow an adequate site for stable atrial pacing and sensing.

vena cava. Large vein structure that returns deoxygenated blood from the body to the right side of the heart. As it pertains to device implantation, vessel through which endocardial leads pass before placement.

venoplasty. Angioplasty, often using low-pressure balloon, to dilate stenotic segments in the venous system. With reference to pacemaker-related and ablation-related procedures, venoplasty is sometimes required in the superior vena cava or subclavian venous system to gain access to the heart for placement of pacemaker leads. Coronary venous stenosis also may occur, requiring venoplasty to allow placement of left ventricular pacing leads or to allow catheter access to ablate epicardial ventricular arrhythmias or accessory pathways.

venous access. Process of gaining entry to the venous system for endocardial lead placement.

The most common sites for venous entry are the axillary, subclavian, and cephalic veins.

venous Corrigan waves. See *cannon waves*.

venous cutdown. A surgical procedure used to visually access a vein. In pacing, a venous cutdown may be used to visualize the cephalic vein for the insertion of an endocardial pacing lead.

VENTAK CHF. Study to determine whether biventricular pacing decreases the need for appropriate antitachycardia therapy. In a randomized crossover trial, patients received a cardiac resynchronization–implantable cardioverter-defibrillator device with a transvenous right ventricular lead and a left ventricular lead placed via thoracotomy. Of the 54 patients enrolled, 32 could be analyzed. In this relatively small trial, the investigators concluded that, in patients with standard indications for an implantable cardioverter-defibrillator who had congestive heart failure, left ventricular systolic dysfunction, and an intraventricular conduction delay, an implantable cardioverter-defibrillator is less frequently required with biventricular pacing. They also concluded that biventricular therapy did not obviate an implantable cardioverter-defibrillator but did diminish the need for appropriate tachyarrhythmia therapy in selected patients (Higgins SL, Yong P, Sheck D, McDaniel M, Bollinger F, Vadecha M, et al, Ventak CHF Investigators. Biventricular pacing diminishes the need for implantable cardioverter defibrillator therapy. J Am Coll Cardiol. 2000;36:824-7).

VENTAK CHF-CONTAK CD study. See *CONTAK-CD trial*.

ventricle. One of the lower two chambers of the heart. Blood from the right ventricle passes through the pulmonary outflow tract to the lungs, where it is oxygenated. Blood from the left ventricle passes through the aorta and is returned to the body. In ventricular pacing, the pacing lead is placed in contact with the right ventricular endocardium or myocardium, and successful stimulation causes depolarization of both ventricles, which together form one functional syncytium. See also *atrial myocardium, atrium, ventricular myocardium*.

ventricular activation. Normal electrical stimulation of the lower chambers, through the His bundle and the Purkinje system. Abnormal ventricular activation leads to intraventricular conduction disturbances and can affect optimization of atrioventricular synchrony.

ventricular alert period. The amount of time from the end of the ventricular refractory period to the next sensed or paced ventricular event. During the ventricular alert period, the pacemaker circuitry can respond to sensed activity. Intrinsic ventricular activity sensed during the ventricular alert period will terminate the ventricular alert period and will initiate either an inhibited or a triggered response from the pacemaker, depending on the programmed mode. If intrinsic ventricular activity is not sensed during the ventricular alert period, the pacemaker will produce a ventricular output pulse at the end of the alert period.

ventricular arrhythmia. Broad term used to describe abnormal ventricular rhythm. See also *ventricular fibrillation, ventricular tachycardia.*

ventricular asynchronous pacing mode (VOO). The pacing mode in which the ventricles are paced at a fixed rate independent of any intrinsic cardiac activity. In ventricular asynchronous pacing, intrinsic cardiac electrical activity is not sensed, and thus the competition with the intrinsic rhythm may occur. In acute or unstable cardiac conditions, an asynchronous ventricular pacing stimulus that occurs during the vulnerable period may initiate malignant arrhythmias. Ventricular asynchronous pacing may be used as backup pacing or as a magnet mode of response. It also may be used temporarily for reversion or control of ventricular rhythm disturbances. See also *asynchronous pacing, ventricular pacing.*

ventricular-based timing. Pacemaker timing that is based on a ventricular event and the subsequent atrial event (i.e., the VA interval). See also *ventricular-based timing system.*

ventricular-based timing system. A ventricular-based timing system in which the VA interval is fixed. A ventricular sensed event occurring during the VA interval resets the timer, causing it to begin again. A ventricular sensed event occurring during the AV interval terminates the AV interval and initiates the VA interval. If there is intact conduction through the AV node following an atrial pacing stimulus such that the AR interval (atrial stimulus to sensed R wave) is shorter than the programmed AV interval, the resulting paced rate will accelerate by a small amount. For example, assume a pacemaker is programmed to a lower rate of 60 beats per minute (i.e., a pacing interval of 1,000 milliseconds). With a programmed AV interval of 200 milliseconds, the VA interval would be 800 milliseconds (VA interval = lower rate interval – AV interval). If AV nodal function permitted conduction in 150 milliseconds (AR interval = 150 milliseconds), the conducted or sensed R wave would then inhibit the ventricular output and reset the VA interval, which would remain stable at 800 milliseconds. The resulting interval between consecutive atrial pacing stimuli would be 950 milliseconds (VA interval + AR interval), or a rate of 63 beats per minute, which is slightly greater than the programmed lower rate.

ventricular bigeminy. Single premature ventricular complexes that are coupled to each supraventricular beat. Thus, in ventricular bigeminy, every other complex is ventricular in origin.

ventricular blanking period. A short preset or programmable interval in dual-chamber pacemakers during which the ventricular sensing amplifiers are disabled. Ventricular blanking

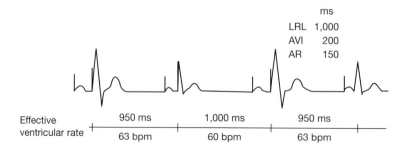

Ventricular-Based Timing System

	ms
LRL	1,000
AVI	200
AR	150

Effective ventricular rate

950 ms	1,000 ms	950 ms
63 bpm	60 bpm	63 bpm

is initiated by an atrial output pulse and is designed to eliminate ventricular sensing of the atrial stimulus (crosstalk). See also *blanking period, crosstalk*.

ventricular burst pacing. Pacing maneuver used during electrophysiologic studies to induce ventricular tachycardia or reentrant arrhythmias. Relatively short couple ventricular pacing is performed, usually at a cycle length of about 200 milliseconds, to induce the arrhythmia.

ventricular capture. Depolarization of the ventricles following the delivery of a pacemaker output pulse. Ventricular capture may be confirmed on an electrocardiogram by the appearance of a ventricular pacing stimulus followed by ventricular depolarization and subsequent repolarization waveforms.

ventricular capture management. An automatic function that determines pacing threshold by stimulating at various output settings. When the threshold is determined, the output is adjusted to maintain a safety margin to ensure consistent capture within a defined range of values.

ventricular cycle length (VV). See *VV interval*.

ventricular decremental pacing. Continuous ventricular pacing in which the cycle length is gradually decreased, causing an increase in the pacing rate. In normal VA conduction systems, the VA interval lengthens progressively as the cycle length decreases until Wenckebach-type block occurs. See also *atrial decremental pacing, incremental pacing*.

ventricular-demand pacing mode (VVI). See *ventricular-inhibited pacing mode*.

ventricular depolarization. The electrical process in which polarized ventricular myofibrils are discharged and produce a contraction. Ventricular depolarizations are represented by QRS complexes on an electrocardiographic recording.

ventricular depolarization gradient (VDG). See *paced depolarization integral*.

ventricular double counting. A complication associated with some cardiac resynchronization devices in which a single R wave may be sensed as two ventricular events if the conduction delay between ventricular leads is significant.

ventricular ectopy. An abnormal rhythm initiated by ectopic focus in the ventricles. See also *ectopic focus*.

ventricular effective refractory period (VERP). During ventricular pacing, the longest S_1 to S_2 interval at which S_2 does not cause a ventricular depolarization. See also *effective refractory period*.

ventricular electrogram (VEGM, ventricular EGM). An intracardiac electrogram recorded from the ventricular myocardium. See also *electrogram*.

ventricular escape interval (VEI). The maximum amount of time between a paced or sensed ventricular event and the next consecutive ventricular output pulse. The ventricular escape interval is determined by the programmed lower rate limit. In dual-chamber pacing, the ventricular evoked response often is recorded from the stimulating electrode or other intracardiac electrodes to control various aspects of pacemaker function, such as rate response and output intensity.

ventricular escape rhythm. A slow arrhythmia (typically less than 40 beats per minute) that originates from a ventricular ectopic focus.

ventricular evoked response (VER). When a pacemaker stimulus is applied or stimulation of the ventricular myocardium occurs during electrophysiologic procedures, a local electrogram is detected that indicates capture of the myocardium at the electrode-myocardial tissue contact site, referred to as the ventricular evoked response. Usually, once the local ventricular myocardium is activated, activation proceeds to the remaining myocardium and the QRS is inscribed on the surface 12-lead electrocardiogram. If an evoked response is seen but there is no manifest QRS complex on the surface electrocardiogram, exit block has likely occurred from the site of local activation. The ventricular evoked response is also used in capture management features in certain pacemakers. In these, automated algorithms use the presence or absence of the ventricular evoked response to determine whether ventricular capture has or has not occurred from the delivered stimulus, allowing a threshold test to be performed.

ventricular extrastimulus. In electrophysiology, the delivery of electrical impulses from an external source to the ventricle. Ventricular extrastimuli are delivered after every 8 beats of the basic paced ventricular cycle until ventricular refractoriness is reached.

ventricular fibrillation (VF). A malignant ventricular arrhythmia characterized by continuous uncoordinated contraction of the ventricles.

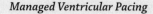

Managed Ventricular Pacing

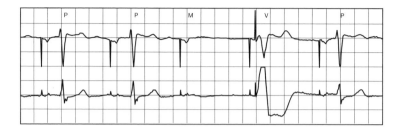

Ventricular fibrillation results in continuous quivering and twitching of the ventricles and in cessation of blood flow from the heart. Ventricular fibrillation is life-threatening.

ventricular flutter (VFl). A repetitive, regular, rapid ventricular arrhythmia at a rate of more than 250 beats per minute. Ventricular flutter is represented on an electrocardiogram by the merging of QRS complexes with T waves and often gives the appearance of sine waves.

ventricular functional refractory period. During ventricular pacing, the shortest V_1 to V_2 interval generated in response to an S_1 to S_2 interval. See also *functional refractory period*.

ventricular fusion beats. 1. In reference to the 12-lead electrocardiographic interpretation of wide QRS tachycardias, ventricular fusion beats occur when, during ventricular tachycardia, some supraventricular conducted beats also depolarize the myocardium. The resultant electrocardiographic morphology is a hybrid between that with ventricular tachycardia and normally conducted beats. 2. During a paced rhythm, premature ventricular complexes or conducted beats also may participate in ventricular depolarization, giving rise to ventricular fusion beats. 3. Rarely during ventricular tachycardia, the second focus of tachycardia or a second reentrant loop may alter the morphology of the QRS complex from ventricular fusion. 4. In the diagnosis for the critical zone requiring ablation for reentrant ventricular tachycardia, a pacing maneuver called entrainment (see *entrainment*) is performed. When the ventricle is paced during tachycardia, ventricular fusion beats may occur and are very useful for analyzing both the arrhythmogenic mechanisms and the characteristic of the ventricular tachycardia circuit.

ventricular high-rate diagnostic feature. A diagnostic feature of some pacemakers that

identify and store rhythms that meet predefined criteria for an inappropriately fast ventricular rhythm.

ventricular-inhibited pacing mode (VVI). The single-chamber pacing mode in which the pacemaker inhibits its ventricular output pulse in response to intrinsic ventricular activity sensed during the ventricular alert period. If an intrinsic ventricular complex is not sensed, the pacemaker will deliver a ventricular output pulse at the programmed or preset rate interval. Ventricular-inhibited pacing also is referred to as ventricular-demand pacing.

ventricular lead. An epicardial or endocardial, unipolar or bipolar, active or passive fixation lead designed for use in ventricular pacing. An endocardial ventricular lead is positioned most commonly in the right ventricular apex. Several different ventricular lead-tip configurations are available to ensure secure contact between the electrode and the endocardium or myocardium. See also *active fixation, endocardial lead, epicardial lead, fin, passive fixation, tine*.

ventricular myocardium. The muscular walls of the lower two chambers of the heart. The ventricular myocardium is relatively thick compared with the atrial myocardium. See also *ventricle*.

ventricular outflow tract tachycardias. See *outflow tract ventricular tachycardia*.

ventricular output pulse. A pacemaker stimulus delivered to the ventricle. The ventricular output pulse is recorded on the electrocardiogram and on the intracardiac electrogram as a vertical deflection.

ventricular pacing. Pacing in the ventricle, used therapeutically to prevent ventricular asystole or bradycardia. See also *VOO, VVI, VVT*.

ventricular pacing avoidance algorithm. An algorithm the purpose of which is to promote intrinsic ventricular conduction without compromising patient safety. It is generally an atrial-based pacing mode that decreases the percentage of ventricular pacing by operating primarily in an AAIR mode and provides ventricular back-up pacing based on preset criteria (e.g., when a certain AR interval is surpassed) after a certain number of atrial events are sensed without an intervening ventricular event.

ventricular parasystole. An independent rhythm arising from a protected focus within the ventricles. Ventricular parasystole is identified on a surface electrocardiogram by noncoupled premature ventricular complexes separated by a relatively constant interectopic interval or a multiple of that interval. Fusion complexes often are present. See also *modulated parasystole, parasystole.*

ventricular preexcitation. See *preexcitation.*

ventricular premature complex (VPC). See *premature ventricular complex.*

ventricular premature depolarization (VPD). See *premature ventricular complex.*

ventricular rate. The frequency of ventricular contractions, either intrinsic or paced, measured in beats per minute.

ventricular rate regularization. A feature designed to reduce V-V cycle length variability during conducted atrial arrhythmias by altering the ventricular pacing rate. Minimizing ventricular cycle length variability in patients with atrial arrhythmias has been shown to make such arrhythmias better tolerated.

ventricular rate stabilization algorithm. See *ventricular rate regularization.*

ventricular refractory interval (VRI). See *ventricular refractory period.*

ventricular refractory period (VRP). In pacing, an interval of the timing cycle following a sensed or paced ventricular event. The ventricular channel is totally unresponsive to incoming signals or waveforms during the majority of

Ventricular Rate Regularization

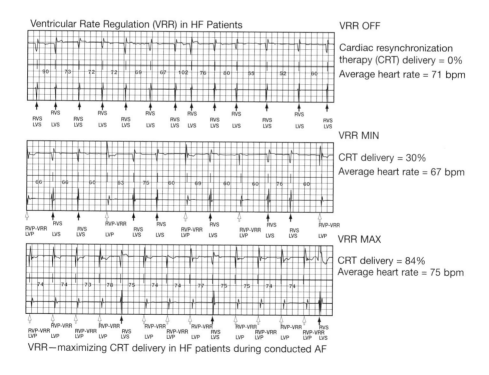

VRR—maximizing CRT delivery in HF patients during conducted AF

From Guidant Corporation [homepage on the Internet]. Natick (MA): Boston Scientific Corporation; c2007 [updated 2004 Jun; cited 2006 Nov 6]. CONTAK RENEWAL TR: Cardiac Resynchronization Therapy Pacemaker. Available from: http://www.guidant.com/products/ProductTemplates/CRM/Contak_Renewal_TR.shtml. Used with permission.

the ventricular refractory period. However, in some pacemakers, the sensing circuitry is alert for extraneous signals during a portion of the ventricular refractory period. The ventricular refractory period also may be referred to as the ventricular refractory interval.

ventricular relative refractory period. During ventricular pacing, the longest S_1 to S_2 interval at which the S_2 to V_2 interval exceeds the S_1 to V_1 interval. See also *relative refractory period*.

ventricular remodeling. A change in ventricular architecture. Patients with a dilated or ischemic cardiomyopathic state often have ventricular remodeling that results in left ventricular enlargement (e.g., increase in left ventricular end-diastolic and end-systolic volumes and dimensions).

ventricular resynchronization. See *biventricular pacing, cardiac resynchronization therapy*.

ventricular safety pacing (VSP). See *safety pacing*.

ventricular standstill. Failure of the ventricles to depolarize in response to atrial impulses, such as in complete heart block. If an escape focus does not take over impulse initiation, ventricular standstill is life-threatening and requires immediate intervention.

ventricular tachyarrhythmia. Term used to describe abnormally fast ventricular rhythms. See also *ventricular fibrillation, ventricular tachycardia*.

ventricular tachycardia (VT). A fast rhythm (more than 120 beats per minute) that has its entire circuit or focus within the ventricles. Ventricular tachycardia may be monomorphic or polymorphic. By definition, nonsustained ventricular tachycardia lasts longer than three complexes and less than 30 seconds before terminating spontaneously. Although most ventricular tachycardias probably are due to re-entry, the underlying mechanism also may be triggered activity or abnormal automaticity.

ventricular tachycardia induction. The initiation of ventricular tachycardia by artificial means such as programmed ventricular stimulation.

ventricular tracking limit (VTL). The maximum rate at which the ventricle can be paced in response to tracking of triggering by a sensed atrial event. See also *maximum tracking rate*.

ventricular triggered pacing (VVT). See *VVT*.

ventricular-triggered pacing mode (VVT). The single-chamber pacing mode in which a ventricular output pulse is delivered synchronously with each sensed QRS complex. Ventricular-triggered pacing is used to avoid inhibition of a ventricular output pulse in response to intrinsic activity that is erroneously recognized as QRS complexes, such as myopotentials and electromagnetic interference. See also *triggered pacing*.

ventriculoatrial conduction. Retrograde transmission of electrical signals from the ventricles to the atria. See also *retrograde conduction*.

ventriculoatrial conduction system effective refractory period. See *VA conduction system effective refractory period*.

ventriculoatrial conduction system functional refractory period. See *VA conduction system functional refractory period*.

Ventricular Tachycardia

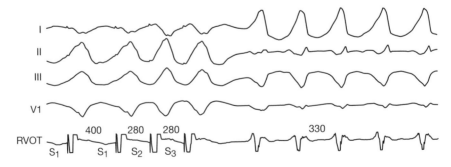

Induction of ventricular tachycardia by two extrastimuli (S_2, S_3) following an eight-beat ventricular pacing drive, the last two complexes of which are shown (S_1). Intervals are in milliseconds.

ventriculoatrial conduction system relative refractory period. See *VA conduction system relative refractory period.*

ventriculoatrial conduction time. See *VA conduction time.*

ventriculoatrial dissociation. Lack of conduction from the ventricles to the atria.

ventriculoatrial intervals. The time in milliseconds for retrograde transmission of electrical signals from the ventricles to the atria.

ventriculotomy. Opening the ventricle at the time of surgery, such as to perform subendocardial resection of a ventricular tachycardia focus.

VER. Abbreviation for *ventricular evoked response.*

verapamil. A class IV calcium-channel blocking antiarrhythmic agent that slows sinus node automaticity and atrioventricular nodal conduction time, prolongs atrioventricular nodal refractoriness, and blocks the slow pathway in atrioventricular nodal reentry. Verapamil has no effect on atrial or ventricular refractoriness. It has efficacy in the treatment of supraventricular tachycardias and some ventricular tachycardias, such as those that may be caused by delayed afterdepolarizations. Verapamil is metabolized by the liver. Its side effects include bradycardias, congestive heart failure, and constipation.

veratridine. A toxin that blocks the inward fast sodium current. Veratridine is used experimentally in vitro.

VERP. Abbreviation for *ventricular effective refractory period.*

vessel dilator. A device that is placed over a guidewire and used to enlarge the opening into a vessel and thus facilitate the insertion of a catheter or pacing lead. The vessel dilator should be removed before the catheter or lead is inserted. Vessel dilators are designed to minimize tissue damage and to minimize the occurrence of vessel dissection.

VF. Abbreviation for *ventricular fibrillation.*

VFl. Abbreviation for *ventricular flutter.*

VF zone. In implantable cardioverter-defibrillators, the detection zone for the most rapid ventricular arrhythmias, typically faster than 180 beats per minute. Intended to detect ventricular fibrillation, but very rapid ventricular tachycardias and ventricular flutter also may be detected in this zone.

V-H intervals. During invasive electrophysiologic study, the interval measured during ventricular pacing or wide QRS tachycardia between the ventricular electrogram and the beginning of the retrograde His bundle deflection.

vibration sensor. See *piezoelectric crystal.*

Vieussens valve. See *valve of Vieussens.*

viewing port. A small, clear-epoxy area in the pacemaker connector block that allows direct visualization of the lead terminal pin within the pacemaker aperture. If the lead terminal pin is visible through the viewing port, the pin is beyond the setscrew and it can be assumed that proper connection with the pacemaker circuitry at the connector block has been made.

VIGOR-CHF. See *VIGOR in Congestive Heart Failure.*

VIGOR in Congestive Heart Failure (VIGOR-CHF). An extension of the Pacing Therapies in Congestive Heart Failure (PATH-CHF) trial, in which a single DDD pulse generator with an epicardial left ventricular lead was implanted in patients with inclusion criteria similar to those of PATH-CHF. Patients were randomized (in a double-blinded design) to either VDD biventricular pacing or no pacing (ODO). After 6 weeks, patients in the ODO group had reprogramming to VDD biventricular pacing. At 10 weeks, the patients had programming to their optimal pacing settings and were followed up at 3-month intervals. The study was never completed as intended, in favor of the Comparison of Medical, Pacing, and Defibrillation Therapies in Heart Failure (COMPANION) study (oral communication, December 2001) (Saxon LA, Boehmer JP, Hummel J, Kacet S, De Marco T, Naccarelli G, et al, the VIGOR CHF and VENTAK CHF Investigators. Biventricular pacing in patients with congestive heart failure: two prospective randomized trials. Am J Cardiol. 1999;83:120D-3D).

virtual electrode. See *effective electrode.*

vitreous carbon. Carbon that has been treated to have a glass-like finish. Vitreous carbon is used in the manufacture of some pacing electrodes. It provides a roughened texture to the electrode surface yet maintains the corrosion-resistant characteristics of carbon. See also *carbon.*

volt (V). The international unit of potential difference. One volt is equal to the potential difference between two points. One volt produces a current of 1 ampere through a resistance of 1 ohm.

voltage. The electrical force or potential difference that makes current move through a conductor.

VOO Pacing

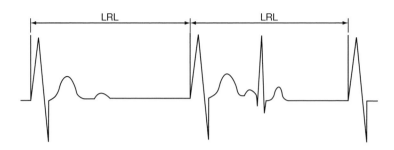

From Hayes DL, Levine PA. Pacemaker timing cycles. In: Ellenbogen KA, editor. Cardiac pacing. Boston: Blackwell Scientific Publications; 1992. p. 263-308. Used with permission.

Voltage is related to current (I) and resistance (R) by Ohm's law, V = IR. Voltage is expressed in volts.

voltage clamping. A technique used to analyze currents in whole cells or patches of membrane from cells by suddenly changing the membrane voltage and keeping it stable.

voltage deflection. See *stimulus artifact*.

voltage doubler. A type of voltage multiplier designed to allow greater output voltages, approximately twice as large as the voltage normally supplied by the circuit. In pacing, the output of a lithium power source usually ranges from 2 to 3.5 V per cell. A voltage doubler may be used to provide a twofold increase in pacemaker output. See also *voltage multiplier*.

voltage mapping. Method of electrophysiologic mapping for reentrant tachycardias in which tachycardia is not induced but a detailed map of the local amplitudes of the bipolar or unipolar electrograms is created. Areas of low voltage, particularly between scarred areas and anatomical structures that are electrically inert, such as the atrioventricular valves, are targeted for ablation.

voltage multiplier. A device designed to allow greater output voltages. When a voltage multiplier is used, the voltage supplied by the circuit is increased by a factor of 2, 3, 4, and so on. In pacing, a voltage multiplier provides an electrical circuit that allows, for example, the delivery of 5 V or 7.5 V from a cell whose voltage is less than 3 V.

voluntary standard (VS-1). See *VS-1*.

VOO. The NBG code for ventricular asynchronous pacing. The ventricle is paced at a fixed rate, and neither chamber is sensed. See also *ventricular asynchronous pacing mode*.

VOOR. The NBG code for ventricular asynchronous pacing with sensor-driven rate response.

VVI Pacing

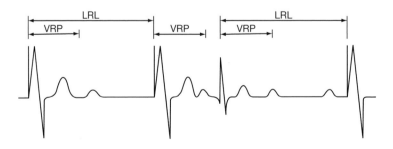

Modified from Hayes DL, Levine PA. Pacemaker timing cycles. In: Ellenbogen KA, editor. Cardiac pacing. Boston: Blackwell Scientific Publications; 1992. p. 263-308. Used with permission.

VPC. Abbreviation for *ventricular premature complex*. See *premature ventricular complex*.

VPD. Abbreviation for *ventricular premature depolarization*. See *premature ventricular complex*.

VPS-I. See *North American Vasovagal Pacemaker Study (VPS-I)*.

VPS-II. See *North American Vasovagal Pacemaker Study II*.

VRI. Abbreviation for *ventricular refractory interval*.

VRP. Abbreviation for *ventricular refractory period*.

VS-1 (voluntary standard #1). A designation for connectors of implantable cardiac rhythm management devices, such as pacemakers and pacemaker leads. It was used before the adoption of the formal IS-1 standard (see *IS-1*). Two versions existed: VS-1 A with O-ring seals located on the lead connector (and not in the pulse generator) and VS-1 B, with O-ring seals on the lead connector and in the pulse generator. VS-1 lead connectors are similar to IS-1 connectors, and some pulse generators are still manufactured to accept both IS-1 and VS-1 leads.

VSP. Abbreviation for *ventricular safety pacing*. See *safety pacing*.

VT. Abbreviation for *ventricular tachycardia*.

VTL. Abbreviation for *ventricular tracking limit*.

VT zone. Ventricular tachycardia zone. In programming implantable cardioverter-defibrillator therapies, a separate set of therapies can be programmed for ventricular tachycardia (sometimes differently for slow and fast ventricular tachycardias). The detection criteria for this zone (VT zone) are different from those usually programmed for ventricular fibrillation (VF zone) in that the rates of the tachycardia required for detection in this zone are lower and usually detection must occur for each consecutive beat (i.e., even if one beat does not meet the detection criteria, the counters will be restarted until consecutive beats, usually greater than 12, occur and therapies can be initiated). Therapies set for the VT zone typically involve antitachycardia pacing before delivery of shock.

vulnerability. The property of the heart that predisposes it to tachycardia or fibrillation if stimulated during a portion of recovery. Vulnerability may be caused by dispersion of refractoriness due to nonhomogeneous recovery of the myocardium at a given point in time following depolarization. See also *vulnerable period*.

VVIR Pacing

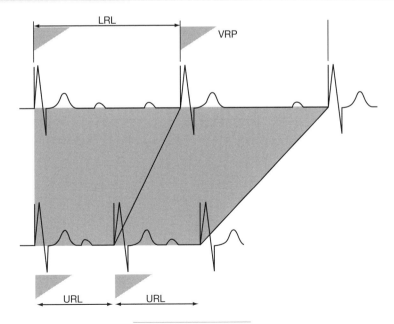

Modified from Hayes DL. Timing cycles of permanent pacemakers. Cardiol Clin. 1992;10:593-608. Used with permission.

vulnerable period. The time during repolarization of the myocardium when the occurrence of a premature impulse may produce a series of repetitive responses, such as tachycardia or fibrillation. The tachycardia or fibrillation may be sustained and may occur in either the atria or the ventricles. See also *vulnerability*.

VVI. The NBG code for ventricular-inhibited pacing. Pacing and sensing occur in the ventricle, and the mode of response is inhibited. See also *ventricular-inhibited pacing mode*. •

VV interval. In pacing, the amount of time elapsing between successive ventricular output pulses. The VV interval is measured from one pacemaker output stimulus to the next on an electrocardiogram or intracardiac electrogram. The VV interval is a measurement of programmed rate and is expressed in milliseconds. The VV interval also is referred to as the ventricular cycle length. See also *cycle length*.

VVIR. The NBG code for ventricular-inhibited rate-adaptive pacing. Pacing and sensing occur in the ventricle, the mode of response is inhibited, and the pacemaker is capable of rate adaptation via a sensor that monitors some physiologic or nonphysiologic parameter. •

VVS. Abbreviation for *vasovagal syncope*.

VVT. The NBG code for ventricular-triggered pacing. Pacing and sensing occur in the ventricle, and the mode of response is triggered. See also *ventricular-triggered pacing mode*.

VVTR. An uncommon mode designation that would represent ventricular-triggered pacing with a rate-adaptive sensor.

W

W. Abbreviation for *watt*.

wand. The telemetry coil of a telemetric programmer. A wand usually is disk-shaped or handle-shaped and is connected to the programmer by a flexible cable to facilitate positioning of the wand over an implanted device. In some newer devices, the wand may need to be briefly positioned over the pulse generator for recognition of the specific device but subsequent programming can be done remotely (i.e., without the wand over the pulse generator) via a radiofrequency link.

wandering atrial pacemaker. The shift of impulse formation from site-to-site within the sinus nodal, atrial, and atrioventricular junctional tissue. A wandering pacemaker causes variation in heart rate, in P-wave morphology, and in the PR interval. Wandering atrial pacemakers usually do not require therapy.

WARAD. Abbreviation for *window of atrial rate acceleration detection*.

warm-up. Progressive shortening in the cycle length of a tachycardia at its onset until the stable tachycardia rate is attained. Warm-up is more typical of automaticity, and sometimes of triggered activity, than of reentry. Warm-up also is used to describe the recovery of the basic cycle length following periods of rapid overdrive pacing.

watt (W). The international unit of electrical power. One watt is dissipated when 1 ampere of current flows through a resistance of 1 ohm. Watts are equivalent to joules per second.

watt-hour (W-h). The amount of energy converted or consumed at a rate of 1 watt during a period of 1 hour. One joule is equal to 1 watt delivered for 1 second, and thus 1 watt-hour is equal to 3,600 joules.

waveform. The shape, or morphology, of an electrical signal recorded as a function of time on, for example, an oscilloscope, electrocardiogram, or intracardiac electrogram.

wave front. During electrical excitation of myocardial tissue from a localized portion of myocardium excited by either an automatic focus or an exit from a reentrant circuit, the excitation spreads to the remainder of the viable myocardium. This spread of excitation occurs as a wave front.

wavelength. In a periodic wave, the distance between two points of corresponding phase in consecutive cycles. In pacing and defibrillation, wavelength may be calculated at the distance from the leading edge of a traveling impulse to the end of its refractory tail. In this case, wavelength is equal to the product of the conduction velocity and the refractory period.

wavelets. The small reentrant impulses created when the uniform wave action of atrial flutter breaks up. Wavelets are the mechanism by which atrial flutter degrades to atrial fibrillation. The small circulating wavelets encounter areas of tissue that are refractory, and the wavelets thus create multiple reentrant patterns distant to the initial site. The result is chaotic atrial activity, such as fibrillation.

Wedensky effect. The tendency of myocardial cells to have a lower stimulation threshold when threshold determination is completed from higher to lower outputs than if the determination is completed from lower to higher outputs. The Wedensky effect occurs as a result of the hyperpolarized state created across the myocardial cell membranes from the delivery of electrical stimulation of high output. See also *threshold*.

Wedensky facilitation. The capability of an impulse that is blocked to lower the threshold of tissue distal to the region of block and allow subsequent excitation or conduction of the next impulse. Wedensky facilitation may explain some instances of supernormal excitability. However, it remains unclear whether Wedensky facilitation occurs in the human heart.

wedge-tip lead. See *flange*.

Wenckebach block. See *Mobitz type I second-degree AV block, second-degree sinus node exit block*.

Wenckebach interval (WI). In a dual-chamber pacemaker capable of P-wave tracking, the amount of time that the atrioventricular interval is extended during the pseudo-Wenckebach response to an atrial rate that exceeds the preset or programmed upper rate limit of the pacemaker. The Wenckebach interval is expressed in milliseconds.

Wenckebach point. The lowest rate in incremental atrial pacing at which 1:1 atrioventricular conduction is no longer possible through the normal conduction pathway and, therefore, Mobitz type I second-degree atrioventricular block occurs. The Wenckebach point occurs between 130 and 190 beats per minute in a normal conduction system. See also *atrial decremental pacing*.

Wenckebach response. See *pseudo-Wenckebach response*.

W-h. Abbreviation for *watt-hour*.

WI. Abbreviation for *Wenckebach interval*.

wide-area circumferential ablation. One of the common ablation techniques used in attempting to treat atrial fibrillation. With wide-area circumferential ablation, radiofrequency energy is delivered to the atrial myocardium a few millimeters proximal to the pulmonary vein atrial junction. Circumferential ablative lesions are placed typically encompassing both left-sided pulmonary veins in one circle and both right-sided pulmonary veins in another circle. Often with wide-area circumferential ablation, these circular ablative lesions are connected to each other with a superior ablation line and the circumferential ablation around the left-sided pulmonary veins is connected with another linear ablation to the mitral anulus.

wide complex tachycardia. Any arrhythmia that demonstrates QRS duration more than 100 milliseconds. The three general mechanisms are 1) supraventricular tachycardia with aberration, 2) ventricular tachycardia, and 3) preexcited tachycardia, such as in antidromic tachycardia and atrial flutter with conduction over an accessory pathway. In consecutive patients presenting to an emergency department, the most common cause is ventricular tachycardia.

wide QRS complex tachycardia. Tachycardias with ventricular rates more than 100 beats a minute associated with a QRS duration of more than 120 milliseconds. Wide QRS tachycardias may arise from ventricular tachycardia, supraventricular tachycardia conducting to the ventricle with bundle branch block (either right or left bundle branch block), or supraventricular

arrhythmias associated with antegrade conduction to the ventricles via an accessory pathway (preexcited tachycardias).

Wiener-Rosenblueth theory. The seminal work of Norbert Wiener and Arturo Rosenblueth, who developed a mathematical formulation attempting to explain conduction of impulses in a network of connected excitable elements, such as in cardiac muscle. This laid the groundwork for the mathematical analysis of both cardiac arrhythmias and wave-front propagation in neural tissues.

Wilkoff locking stylet. See *locking stylet*.

window of atrial rate acceleration detection (WARAD). Interval used to detect changes in the atrial rates, specifically atrial rate acceleration. The interval is calculated when the present atrial interval is compared with preceding normal (sensed or paced) atrial intervals. Acceleration is detected if there is a 62.5% decrease in the cycle length when the cycle length itself is longer than 750 milliseconds or a 75% decrease in the cycle length if the cycle length itself measures 750 milliseconds or less.

wire. A single metal strand or group of strands, bare or insulated, that serves as a conductor of electricity. In pacing, a wire is the metal conductor of a pacing lead. Wire also is used to refer to temporary pacing leads or temporary catheters. See also *catheter, conductor, temporary lead*.

wire-cage electrode. An endocardial lead-tip electrode configuration. A wire-cage electrode is a small, metal, cylindrical mesh that protrudes from the distal end of some passive fixation leads. The electrode design provides a stimulation surface with a small surface area to create an intense current field and facilitates lead stability by tissue growth into the mesh framework. Wire-cage electrodes are not commonly used. See also *electrode*.

wire resistance. The portion of the pacing system impedance contributed by the wire conductors. The resistance of the conductors is determined by the material, the length, and the diameter of the wires.

Wolff-Parkinson-White (WPW) syndrome. The occurrence of an accessory atrioventricular connection that causes preexcitation of the ventricles. Wolff-Parkinson-White syndrome often causes paroxysmal supraventricular tachycardia and, in some individuals with a very rapid ventricular response, may lead to

Wolff-Parkinson-White Syndrome

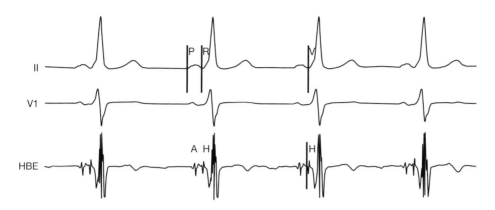

Surface and intracardiac leads demonstrating ventricular preexcitation by an atrioventricular accessory connection in a patient with Wolff-Parkinson-White syndrome. Note the short PR (112 ms) and HV (14 ms) intervals.

ventricular fibrillation. Wolff-Parkinson-White syndrome is defined by the presence of a short PR interval and a delta wave on the surface electrocardiogram along with evidence of supraventricular tachycardia. Technically, a concealed accessory pathway (one with retrograde conduction only) does not constitute Wolff-Parkinson-White syndrome. See also *delta wave*.

WPW syndrome. Abbreviation for *Wolff-Parkinson-White syndrome*.

X

x-ray identification. See *radiopaque identification letters*.

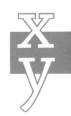

y

Y-adapter. A special device that connects two leads and allows them to be plugged into a single pacing or sensing port on the pulse generator.

Z

Z. Abbreviation for *impedance*.

zener diode. A semiconductor element of an electronic circuit that produces a large increase in current when a particular value of reverse voltage occurs. Zener diodes usually are made of silicone. In a pacemaker, a zener diode is used to prevent circuitry damage due to cardioversion, defibrillation, and other potentially damaging electrical currents by shunting these unusually large currents away from the pacemaker circuitry. See also *shunting circuit*.

zero-dimensional reentry. Reentrant circuits occur with a wave front typically propagating around an obstacle, such as a myocardial infarction scar, that has three dimensions. Such large obstacles constitute a common form of reentry called anatomic reentry. Sometimes the scar may be very small or planar, that is, less than three dimensions. If the size of this scar or obstacle is progressively decreased and eventually becomes a single point without dimensions, then functional reentry around a zero-dimensional object may be said to occur. As the radius of the obstacle decreases, the nature of the wave front that is propagating in a reentrant circuit also changes from periodic motion to a spiral wave.

zinc-mercuric oxide (HgOZn). A battery chemistry in which the anode is mercuric oxide and the cathode is zinc. Zinc-mercuric oxide batteries provide 1.35 V of energy per battery cell. Zinc-mercuric oxide battery chemistry has an internal electrochemical reaction that produces hydrogen gas, which subsequently creates internal pressure. The battery and pacemaker case cannot be sealed hermetically because the hydrogen gas must be vented. Zinc-mercuric oxide batteries commonly are referred to as mercury-zinc batteries.

zone of reset. During a reentrant arrhythmia, extrastimuli placed by pacing the myocardium may terminate the arrhythmia when coupled too early or be unable to penetrate into the circuit if very late coupled to the preceding beat. Appropriately placed extrastimuli can reset the tachycardia. The range of coupling intervals in which reset occurs is called the zone of reset. See also *entrainment, resetting*.

zone of slow conduction. A region of the myocardium in which an impulse travels at an abnormally slow rate and thus allows the more rapidly conducting tissue ahead of the impulse to repolarize. The zone of slow conduction is the critical link in many reentrant circuits. When ablation of a reentrant ventricular tachycardia is attempted, the zone of slow conduction is the area that is sought during mapping, because ablation of this site is most likely to yield success. See also *ablation*.

zonula occludens protein-1. The zonula occludens protein-1 is a membrane-associated component at cell junctions. This protein is found at both tight and adherens junctions at sites of cell-to-cell contact.

z ratio. The z ratio, also called the z score or z value, is a statistical value equal to the population being divided by the standard deviation. It is an example of a standard score typically associated with normal distribution.

Appendix A

Appendix B

A	Ampere
AC	Alternating current
ACC	American College of Cardiology
ACE	Angiotensin-converting enzyme
ADC	Analog-to-digital converter
ADL	Activities of daily living
AEGM	Atrial electrogram
AEI	Atrial escape interval
AF	Atrial fibrillation
AFl	Atrial flutter
AGC	Automatic gain control
AgLiVaO5	Silver-vanadium cell chemistry
A-h	Ampere-hour
AHA	American Heart Association
AICD	Automatic implantable cardioverter-defibrillator
AID	Automatic implantable defibrillator
AMS	Automatic mode switching
ANF	Atrial natriuretic factor
ANP	Atrial natriuretic peptide
ANS	Autonomic nervous system
ANSI	American National Standards Institute
AP	Atrial paced event
4-AP	4-aminopyridine
APC	Atrial premature complex
APD	Action potential duration, atrial premature depolarization
ARP	Absolute refractory period, atrial refractory period
ART	Antidromic reciprocating tachycardia
ARVD	Arrhythmogenic right ventricular dysplasia
AS	Atrial sensed event
ATP	Adenosine triphosphate, antitachycardia pacing
AV	Atrioventricular
AVD	AV delay
AVI	AV interval
AVN	AV node
AVNRT	AV nodal reentrant tachycardia
AVRT	AV reentrant tachycardia

BBB	Bundle branch block
BBR	Bundle branch reentry
BCL	Burst cycle length
bit	Binary digit
BNP	B-type natriuretic peptide
BOL	Beginning of life
BPEG	British Pacing and Electrophysiology Group
bpm	Beats per minute
C	Capacitor, carbon, coulomb
CAEP	Chronotropic assessment exercise protocol
cAMP	Cyclic adenosine monophosphate
CED	Coverage with Evidence Determination
cGMP	Cyclic guanine monophosphate
CHB	Complete heart block
CMOS	Complementary metal-oxide semiconductor
CMRR	Common-mode rejection ratio
CMS	Centers for Medicare and Medicaid Services
CO	Cardiac output
CPR	Cardiopulmonary resuscitation
CRT	Cardiac resynchronization therapy
CRT-D	Cardiac resynchronization therapy with defibrillation-cardioversion
Cs	Cesium
CSM	Carotid sinus massage
CSNRT	Corrected sinus node recovery time
CWS	Chest wall stimulation
DAC	Digital-to-analog converter
DAD	Delayed afterdepolarization
DAO	Dynamic atrial overdrive
DBS	Drawn-brazed strand
DBT	Device-based testing
DC	Direct current
DCM	Dilated cardiomyopathy
DF-1	Debrillation connector standard #1
DFT	Defibrillation threshold
DLC	Delayed longitudinal contraction
DSA	Defibrillator systems analyzer
DSP	Dexamethasone sodium phosphate
DTI	Doppler tissue imaging
E	Electrical field strength, energy
EAD	Early afterdepolarization
EAR	Electrogram amplitude reduction
ECG	Electrocardiogram

EDVI	End-diastolic volume index
EGM	Electrogram
EHR	Extended high rate
EKG	Electrocardiogram
ELT	Endless-loop tachycardia
EMF	Electromagnetic field
EMI	Electromagnetic interference
EOL	End of life
EOS	End of service
EP	Electrophysiology
EPROM	Erasable programmable read-only memory
EPS	Electrophysiologic study
ERI	Elective replacement indicator
ERP	Effective refractory period
ESC	Environmental stress cracking
ESWL	Extracorporeal shock-wave lithotripsy
ETO	Ethylene oxide
f	Frequency
FDA	Food and Drug Administration
FET	Field effect transistor
FFRW	Far-field R wave
FFT	Fast Fourier transform
FRP	Functional refractory period
GCV	great cardiac vein
HBE	His-bundle electrogram
HCM	Hypertrophic cardiomyopathy
HDE	Humanitarian device exemption
HEI	Hysteresis escape interval
HERG	Human ether-a-go-go
HgOZn	Zinc-mercuric oxide
HIFU	High-intensity focused ultrasonography
HRA	High right atrial electrogram, high right atrium
HRS	Heart Rhythm Society
HUD	Humanitarian use device
HUT	Head-up tilt
HV	High voltage
I	Current
IAB	Intra-atrial block
IART	Intra-atrial reentrant tachycardia
ICD	Implantable cardioverter-defibrillator
ICE	Intracardiac echocardiography
ICEG	Intracardiac electrogram
ICV	Inferior caval vein

ID	Intrinsic deflection
IDE	Investigational device exemption
IECG	Intracardiac electrogram
IEGM	Intracardiac electrogram
IHR	Intrinsic heart rate
ILR	Implantable loop recorder
ILVT	Idiopathic left ventricular tachycardia
IP$_3$	Inositol triphosphate
IPG	Implantable pulse generator
IS-1	International pacemaker cavity and lead connector standard #1
ISA	Intrinsic sympathomimetic activity
ISD	Implant support device
ISO	International Organization for Standardization
IST	Inappropriate sinus tachycardia
IVC	Inferior vena cava, isovolumic contraction
IVCD	Interventricular conduction delay
IVD	Interventricular delay
J	Current density, joule
JET	Junctional ectopic tachycardia
K	Potassium
LAS	Low-amplitude signal
laser	Light amplification by stimulated emission of radiation
LASF	Left anterior superior fascicle
LBB	Left bundle branch
LBBB	Left bundle branch block
LED	Light-emitting diode
LGL	Lown-Ganong-Levine (syndrome)
Li	Lithium
LiCuS	Lithium-cupric sulfide
LiI	Lithium iodide
LIPV	Left inferior pulmonary vein
LiVO$_5$	Lithium-vanadium-pentoxide
LMS	Left midseptal
LRI	Lower rate interval
LRL	Lower rate limit
LSPV	Left superior pulmonary vein
LVEF	Left ventricular ejection fraction
LVOT	Left ventricular outflow tract
LVPP	Left ventricular protection period
mA	Milliampere
MAP	Monophasic action potential
MAR	Mean atrial rate

MAS	Measured average sensor
MCV	Middle cardiac vein
MEA	Multielectrode array
MEAM	Magnetic electroanatomic map
MIBG	Meta-iodobenzylguanidine
μA	Microampere
μC	Microcoulomb
μJ	Microjoule
MIO	Metal-induced oxidation, metal ion oxidation
mm	Millimeter
MOSFET	Metal-oxide semiconductor field-effect transistor
MPI	Myocardial performance index
MRI	Magnetic resonance imaging, maximum rate interval
ms	Millisecond
MSR	Maximum sensor rate
MTI	Maximum tracking interval
MTR	Maximum tracking rate
MTRI	Maximum tracking rate interval
mV	Millivolt
MV	Minute ventilation
MVP	Managed ventricular pacing
MW	Microwave
Na	Sodium
NAPA	N-Acetylprocainamide
NASPE	North American Society of Pacing and Electrophysiology
NCAP	Noncompetitive atrial pacing
NiCd	Nickel-cadmium
NIEPS	Noninvasive electrophysiologic study
NIPS	Noninvasive programmed stimulation
NMR	Nuclear magnetic resonance (imaging)
N_2O	Nitrous oxide
NPJT	Nonparoxysmal junctional tachycardia
NSR	Normal sinus rhythm
NSVT	Nonsustained ventricular tachycardia
NYHA	New York Heart Association (classification)
Ω	Ohm
OPT	Optimized pharmacologic therapy
ORT	Orthodromic reciprocating tachycardia
PA	Pulmonary artery
PAC	Premature atrial complex
PAT	Paroxysmal atrial tachycardia
PAVB	Postatrial ventricular blanking
PCL	Paced cycle length

PCMT	Pacemaker circus-movement tachycardia
PC shock	Programmer-commanded shock
PCV	Percutaneous coronary venoplasty, posterior cardiac vein
PD	Potential difference
PDF	Probability density function
PDI	Paced depolarization integral
PEI	Preejection interval
PES	Programmed electrical stimulus
PI	Preexcitation index
PIA	Pacemaker-induced arrhythmia
PJRT	Permanent form of junctional reciprocating tachycardia
PM	pacemaker
PMA	Premarket approval
PMAA	Premarket approval application
PMT	Pacemaker-mediated tachycardia
POR	Power-on reset
POTS	Postural orthostatic tachycardia syndrome
PPI	Postpacing interval
ppm	Pulses per minute
PRR	Pulse repetition rate
PSA	Pacemaker systems analyzer
PSP	Postshock pacing
PSVT	Paroxysmal supraventricular tachycardia
PTER	Patient-triggered event record
Pt-Ir	Platinum-iridium
PV	Pulmonary vein
PVAB	Postventricular atrial blanking
PVARP	Postventricular atrial refractory period
PVC	Premature ventricular complex
PW	Pulse width
PWD	Pulsed-wave Doppler, pulse width duration
Q	Charge
QOL	Quality of life
R	Resistance
RAAVD	Rate-adaptive AV delay
RAM	Random-access memory
RBBB	Right bundle branch block
RCA	Radiofrequency catheter ablation
RDR	Rate drop response
rf	Radiofrequency
RF	Radiofrequency energy
RFA	Radiofrequency ablation
RFCA	Radiofrequency catheter ablation

ri	Internal longitudinal resistance
RMS	Root mean squared
RMVT	Repetitive monomorphic ventricular tachycardia
RNRVAS	Repetitive nonreentrant ventriculoatrial synchronous (rhythm)
ROM	Read-only memory
RPM	Real-time position management
RRF	Rate-response factor
RRP	Relative refractory period
RRT	Recommended replacement time
RSPV	Right superior pulmonary vein
RVA	Right ventricular apex (electrogram)
RVD	Right ventricular dysplasia
RVOT	Right ventricular outflow tract
RVS	Right ventricular septal (pacing)
SA	Sinoatrial
SACT	Sinoatrial conduction time
SAECG	Signal-averaged electrocardiography
SAV	Sensed AV interval
SCA	Sudden cardiac arrest
SCD	Sudden cardiac death
SCL	Sinus cycle length
SCV	Superior caval vein
SMDA	Safe Medical Device Act of 1990
SNE	Sinus node electrogram
SNR	Signal-to-noise ratio
SNRT	Sinus node recovery time
SOCA	Segmental ostial catheter ablation
SPWMD	Septal-posterior wall motion delay
SSS	Sick sinus syndrome
st	Application of an applied stimulus in electrophysiologic testing
SV	Stroke volume
SVC	Superior vena cava
SVT	Supraventricular tachycardia
TARP	Total atrial refractory period
TCL	Tachycardia cycle length
TDI	Tissue Doppler imaging
TdP	Torsades de pointes
T_E	Electrode temperature
TENS	Transcutaneous electrical nerve stimulation
TMT	Threshold margin test
TPI	Temporary pacemaker inhibition

TTM	Transtelephonic monitoring
TTT	Tilt-table testing
UAR	Upper activity rate
ULV	Upper limit of vulnerability
URI	Upper rate interval
URL	Upper rate limit
URR	Upper rate response
V	Vanadium, volt
VA	Ventriculoatrial
VDG	Ventricular depolarization gradient
VEGM	Ventricular electrogram
VEI	Ventricular escape interval
VER	Ventricular evoked response
VERP	Ventricular effective refractory period
VF	Ventricular fibrillation
VFl	Ventricular flutter
VPC	Ventricular premature complex
VPD	Ventricular premature depolarization
VRI	Ventricular refractory interval
VRP	Ventricular refractory period
VS-1	Voluntary standard #1
VSP	Ventricular safety pacing
VT	Ventricular tachycardia
VTL	Ventricular tracking limit
VVS	Vasovagal syncope
W	Watt
WARAD	Window of atrial rate acceleration detection
W-h	Watt-hour
WI	Wenckebach interval
WPW	Wolff-Parkinson-White (syndrome)
Z	Impedance

Appendix C

Absolute refractory period	ARP
Action potential duration	APD
Activities of daily living	ADL
Adenosine triphosphate	ATP
Alternating current	AC
American College of Cardiology	ACC
American Heart Association	AHA
American National Standards Institute	ANSI
4-Aminopyridine	4-AP
Ampere	A
Ampere-hour	A-h
Analog-to-digital converter	ADC
Angiotensin-converting enzyme	ACE
Antidromic reciprocating tachycardia	ART
Antitachycardia pacing	ATP
Application of an applied stimulus in EP testing	st
Arrhythmogenic right ventricular dysplasia	ARVD
Atrial electrogram	AEGM
Atrial escape interval	AEI
Atrial fibrillation	AF
Atrial flutter	AFl
Atrial natriuretic factor	ANF
Atrial natriuretic peptide	ANP
Atrial paced event	AP
Atrial premature complex	APC
Atrial premature depolarization	APD
Atrial refractory period	ARP
Atrial sensed event	AS
Atrioventricular	AV
Automatic gain control	AGC
Automatic implantable cardioverter-defibrillator	AICD
Automatic implantable defibrillator	AID
Automatic mode switching	AMS
Autonomic nervous system	ANS
AV delay	AVD
AV interval	AVI

AV nodal reentrant tachycardia	AVNRT
AV node	AVN
AV reentrant tachycardia	AVRT
Beats per minute	bpm
Beginning of life	BOL
Binary digit	bit
British Pacing and Electrophysiology Group	BPEG
B-type natriuretic peptide	BNP
Bundle branch block	BBB
Bundle branch reentry	BBR
Burst cycle length	BCL
Capacitor	C
Carbon	C
Cardiac output	CO
Cardiac resynchronization therapy	CRT
Cardiac resynchronization therapy with defibrillation-cardioversion	CRT-D
Cardiopulmonary resuscitation	CPR
Carotid sinus massage	CSM
Centers for Medicare and Medicaid Services	CMS
Cesium	Cs
Charge	Q
Chest wall stimulation	CWS
Chronotropic assessment exercise protocol	CAEP
Common-mode rejection ratio	CMRR
Complementary metal-oxide semiconductor	CMOS
Complete heart block	CHB
Corrected sinus node recovery time	CSNRT
Coulomb	C
Coverage with Evidence Determination	CED
Current	I
Current density	J
Cyclic adenosine monophosphate	cAMP
Cyclic guanine monophosphate	cGMP
Defibrillation connector standard #1	DF-1
Defibrillation threshold	DFT
Defibrillator systems analyzer	DSA
Delayed afterdepolarization	DAD
Delayed longitudinal contraction	DLC
Device-based testing	DBT
Dexamethasone sodium phosphate	DSP
Digital-to-analog converter	DAC
Dilated cardiomyopathy	DCM

Direct current	DC
Doppler tissue imaging	DTI
Drawn-brazed strand	DBS
Dynamic atrial overdrive	DAO
Early afterdepolarization	EAD
Effective refractory period	ERP
Elective replacement indicator	ERI
Electrical field strength	E
Electrocardiogram	ECG, EKG
Electrode temperature	T_E
Electrogram	EGM
Electrogram amplitude reduction	EAR
Electromagnetic field	EMF
Electromagnetic interference	EMI
Electrophysiologic study	EPS
Electrophysiology	EP
End-diastolic volume index	EDVI
Endless-loop tachycardia	ELT
End of life	EOL
End of service	EOS
Energy	E
Environmental stress cracking	ESC
Erasable programmable read-only memory	EPROM
Ethylene oxide	ETO
Extended high rate	EHR
Extracorporeal shock-wave lithotripsy	ESWL
Far-field R wave	FFRW
Fast Fourier transform	FFT
Field effect transistor	FET
Food and Drug Administration	FDA
Frequency	f
Functional refractory period	FRP
Great cardiac vein	GCV
Head-up tilt	HUT
Heart Rhythm Society	HRS
High-intensity focused ultrasonography	HIFU
High right atrial electrogram, high right atrium	HRA
High voltage	HV
His-bundle electrogram	HBE
Human ether-a-go-go	HERG
Humanitarian device exemption	HDE
Humanitarian use device	HUD
Hypertrophic cardiomyopathy	HCM

Hysteresis escape interval	HEI
Idiopathic left ventricular tachycardia	ILVT
Impedance	Z
Implantable cardioverter-defibrillator	ICD
Implantable loop recorder	ILR
Implantable pulse generator	IPG
Implant support device	ISD
Inappropriate sinus tachycardia	IST
Inferior caval vein	ICV
Inferior vena cava, isovolumic contraction	IVC
Inositol triphosphate	IP_3
Internal longitudinal resistance	ri
International Organization for Standardization	ISO
International pacemaker cavity and lead connector standard #1	IS-1
Interventricular conduction delay	IVCD
Interventricular delay	IVD
Intra-atrial block	IAB
Intra-atrial reentrant tachycardia	IART
Intracardiac echocardiography	ICE
Intracardiac electrogram	ICEG
Intracardiac electrogram	IECG
Intracardiac electrogram	IEGM
Intrinsic deflection	ID
Intrinsic heart rate	IHR
Intrinsic sympathomimetic activity	ISA
Investigational device exemption	IDE
Joule	J
Junctional ectopic tachycardia	JET
Left anterior superior fascicle	LASF
Left bundle branch	LBB
Left bundle branch block	LBBB
Left inferior pulmonary vein	LIPV
Left midseptal	LMS
Left superior pulmonary vein	LSPV
Left ventricular ejection fraction	LVEF
Left ventricular outflow tract	LVOT
Left ventricular protection period	LVPP
Light amplification by stimulated emission of radiation	laser
Light-emitting diode	LED
Lithium	Li
Lithium-cupric sulfide	LiCuS
Lithium iodide	LiI

Lithium-vanadium-pentoxide . . . . LiVO$_5$
Low-amplitude signal . . . . LAS
Lower rate interval . . . . LRI
Lower rate limit . . . . LRL
Lown-Ganong-Levine (syndrome) . . . . LGL
Magnetic electroanatomic map . . . . MEAM
Magnetic resonance imaging . . . . MRI
Managed ventricular pacing . . . . MVP
Maximum rate interval . . . . MRI
Maximum sensor rate . . . . MSR
Maximum tracking interval . . . . MTI
Maximum tracking rate . . . . MTR
Maximum tracking rate interval . . . . MTRI
Mean atrial rate . . . . MAR
Measured average sensor . . . . MAS
Meta-iodobenzylguanidine . . . . MIBG
Metal-induced oxidation . . . . MIO
Metal ion oxidation . . . . MIO
Metal-oxide semiconductor field-effect transistor . . . . . MOSFET
Microampere . . . . μA
Microcoulomb . . . . μC
Microjoule . . . . μJ
Microwave . . . . MW
Middle cardiac vein . . . . MCV
Milliampere . . . . mA
Millimeter . . . . mm
Millisecond . . . . ms
Millivolt . . . . mV
Minute ventilation . . . . MV
Monophasic action potential . . . . MAP
Multielectrode array . . . . MEA
Myocardial performance index . . . . MPI
N-Acetylprocainamide . . . . NAPA
New York Heart Association (classification) . . . . NYHA
Nickel-cadmium . . . . NiCd
Nitrous oxide . . . . N$_2$O
Noncompetitive atrial pacing . . . . NCAP
Noninvasive electrophysiologic study . . . . NIEPS
Noninvasive programmed stimulation . . . . NIPS
Nonparoxysmal junctional tachycardia . . . . NPJT
Nonsustained ventricular tachycardia . . . . NSVT
Normal sinus rhythm . . . . NSR
North American Society of Pacing and Electrophysiology . . NASPE

Nuclear magnetic resonance (imaging) . . . . NMR
Ohm . . . . Ω
Optimized pharmacologic therapy . . . . OPT
Orthodromic reciprocating tachycardia . . . . ORT
Paced cycle length . . . . PCL
Paced depolarization integral . . . . PDI
Pacemaker . . . . PM
Pacemaker circus-movement tachycardia . . . . PCMT
Pacemaker-induced arrhythmia . . . . PIA
Pacemaker-mediated tachycardia . . . . PMT
Pacemaker systems analyzer . . . . PSA
Paroxysmal atrial tachycardia . . . . PAT
Paroxysmal supraventricular tachycardia . . . . PSVT
Patient-triggered event record . . . . PTER
Percutaneous coronary venoplasty, posterior cardiac vein . . PCV
Permanent form of junctional reciprocating tachycardia . . PJRT
Platinum-iridium . . . . Pt-Ir
Postatrial ventricular blanking . . . . PAVB
Postpacing interval . . . . PPI
Postshock pacing . . . . PSP
Postural orthostatic tachycardia syndrome . . . . POTS
Postventricular atrial blanking . . . . PVAB
Postventricular atrial refractory period . . . . PVARP
Potassium . . . . K
Potential difference . . . . PD
Power-on reset . . . . POR
Preejection interval . . . . PEI
Preexcitation index . . . . PI
Premarket approval . . . . PMA
Premarket approval application . . . . PMAA
Premature atrial complex . . . . PAC
Premature ventricular complex . . . . PVC
Probability density function . . . . PDF
Programmed electrical stimulus . . . . PES
Programmer-commanded shock . . . . PC shock
Pulmonary artery . . . . PA
Pulmonary vein . . . . PV
Pulsed-wave Doppler . . . . PWD
Pulse repetition rate . . . . PRR
Pulses per minute . . . . ppm
Pulse width . . . . PW
Pulse width duration . . . . PWD
Quality of life . . . . QOL

Radiofrequency ablation . . . . RFA
Radiofrequency catheter ablation . . . . RFCA, RCA
Radiofrequency energy . . . . rf, RF
Random-access memory. . . . . RAM
Rate-adaptive AV delay . . . . RAAVD
Rate drop response . . . . RDR
Rate-response factor . . . . RRF
Read-only memory . . . . ROM
Real-time position management . . . . RPM
Recommended replacement time. . . . . RRT
Relative refractory period . . . . RRP
Repetitive monomorphic ventricular tachycardia. . . . . . RMVT
Repetitive nonreentrant ventriculoatrial
    synchronous (rhythm) . . . . RNRVAS
Resistance. . . . . R
Right bundle branch block. . . . . RBBB
Right superior pulmonary vein. . . . . RSPV
Right ventricular apex (electrogram) . . . . RVA
Right ventricular dysplasia . . . . RVD
Right ventricular outflow tract. . . . . RVOT
Right ventricular septal (pacing) . . . . RVS
Root mean squared . . . . RMS
Safe Medical Device Act of 1990 . . . . SMDA
Segmental ostial cather ablation . . . . SOCA
Sensed AV interval . . . . SAV
Septal-posterior wall motion delay . . . . SPWMD
Sick sinus syndrome . . . . SSS
Signal-averaged electrocardiography . . . . SAECG
Signal-to-noise ratio . . . . SNR
Silver-vanadium cell chemistry. AgLiVaO5
Sinoatrial . . . . SA
Sinoatrial conduction time . . . . SACT
Sinus cycle length . . . . SCL
Sinus node electrogram . . . . SNE
Sinus node recovery time . . . . SNRT
Sodium . . . . Na
Stroke volume . . . . SV
Sudden cardiac arrest . . . . SCA
Sudden cardiac death . . . . SCD
Superior caval vein . . . . SCV
Superior vena cava . . . . SVC
Supraventricular tachycardia. . . . . SVT
Tachycardia cycle length. . . . . TCL

Temporary pacemaker inhibition . . . . TPI
Threshold margin test . . . . TMT
Tilt-table testing . . . . TTT
Tissue Doppler imaging . . . . TDI
Torsades de pointes . . . . TdP
Total atrial refractory period . . . . TARP
Transcutaneous electrical nerve stimulation . . . . TENS
Transtelephonic monitoring . . . . TTM
Upper activity rate . . . . UAR
Upper limit of vulnerability . . . . ULV
Upper rate interval . . . . URI
Upper rate limit . . . . URL
Upper rate response . . . . URR
Vanadium V
Vasovagal syncope . . . . VVS
Ventricular depolarization gradient . . . . VDG
Ventricular effective refractory period . . . . VERP
Ventricular electrogram . . . . VEGM
Ventricular escape interval . . . . VEI
Ventricular evoked response . . . . VER
Ventricular fibrillation . . . . VF
Ventricular flutter . . . . VFl
Ventricular premature complex . . . . VPC
Ventricular premature depolarization . . . . VPD
Ventricular refractory interval . . . . VRI
Ventricular refractory period . . . . VRP
Ventricular safety pacing . . . . VSP
Ventricular tachycardia . . . . VT
Ventricular tracking limit . . . . VTL
Ventriculoatrial . . . . VA
Volt V
Voluntary standard #1 . . . . VS-1
Watt . . . . W
Watt-hour . . . . W-h
Wenckebach interval . . . . WI
Window of atrial rate acceleration detection . . . . WARAD
Wolff-Parkinson-White (syndrome) . . . . WPW
Zinc-mercuric oxide . . . . HgOZn